12th
EDITION

Fitness & Wellness

Werner W. K. Hoeger
Boise State University

Sharon A. Hoeger
Amber L. Fawson
Cherie I. Hoeger
Fitness & Wellness, Inc.

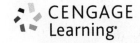
CENGAGE
Learning·

Australia • Brazil • Mexico • Singapore • United Kingdom • United States

CENGAGE Learning®

Fitness & Wellness, 12th Edition
Werner W. K. Hoeger, Sharon A. Hoeger,
Amber L. Fawson, Cherie I. Hoeger

Product Manager: Krista Mastroianni

Content Developer: Alex Brady

Product Assistant: Victor Luu

Content Project Manager: Tanya Nigh

Art Director: Andrei Pasternak

Manufacturing Planner: Karen Hunt

Production Service and Compositor:
    MPS Limited

Photo and Text Researcher:
    Lumina Datamatics, Ltd.

Text Designer: Dare Porter

Cover Image: istock/Vasko

> For product information and technology assistance, contact us at
> **Cengage Learning Customer & Sales Support, 1-800-354-9706**
>
> For permission to use material from this text or product,
> submit all requests online at **www.cengage.com/permissions**
> Further permissions questions can be e-mailed to
> **permissionrequest@cengage.com**

Library of Congress Control Number: 2015949717

Student Edition:
ISBN: 978-1-305-63801-3

Loose-leaf Edition:
ISBN: 978-1-305-88130-3

Cengage Learning
20 Channel Center Street
Boston, MA 02210
USA

Cengage Learning is a leading provider of customized learning solutions with employees residing in nearly 40 different countries and sales in more than 125 countries around the world. Find your local representative at **www.cengage.com**.

Cengage Learning products are represented in Canada by Nelson Education, Ltd.

To learn more about Cengage Learning Solutions, visit **www.cengage.com**

Purchase any of our products at your local college store or at our preferred online store **www.cengagebrain.com**

Printed in Canada
Printed Number: 01   Print Year: 2016

Contents

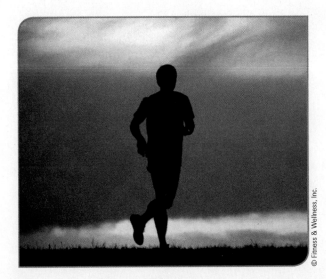

© Fitness & Wellness, Inc.

Chapter 4
Evaluating Fitness Activities 102

Chapter 5
Nutrition for Wellness 124

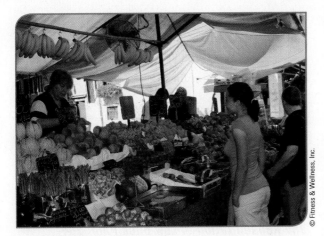

© Fitness & Wellness, Inc.

Chapter 6
Weight Management 153

Chapter 7
Stress Management 181

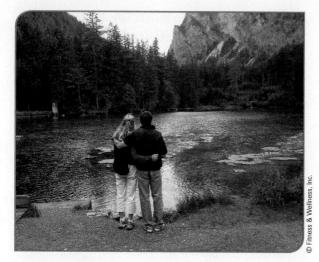

© Fitness & Wellness, Inc.

Chapter 8
A Healthy Lifestyle Approach 205

Chapter 9
Relevant Fitness and Wellness Issues 239

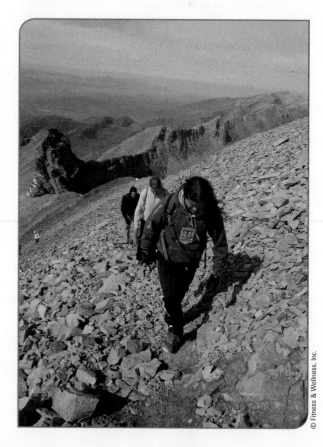

© Fitness & Wellness, Inc.

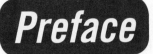

Preface

Most people go to college to learn how to make a living. Making a good living, however, won't help them unless they live a wellness lifestyle that will allow them to enjoy what they have. Unfortunately, the current American lifestyle does not provide the human body with sufficient physical activity to enhance or maintain adequate health. As a result, the importance of a sound fitness and wellness program is of utmost importance to lead a long and healthy life and reach one's potential and quality of life without physical limitations.

Science has clearly determined that a lack of physical activity is detrimental to health. In fact, the office of the Surgeon General has identified physical fitness as a top health priority by stating that the nation's top health goals include exercise, increased consumption of fruits and vegetables, smoking cessation, and the practice of safe sex. All four of these fundamental healthy lifestyle factors are addressed in this book.

Many of the behaviors we adopt in life are a product of our environment. Currently, we live in a "toxic" health/fitness environment. We are so habituated to our modern-day environment that we miss the subtle ways it influences our behaviors, personal lifestyles, and health each day. The epidemic of physical inactivity and obesity that is sweeping across America is so harmful to health that it actually increases the deterioration rate of the human body and leads to premature aging, illness, and death.

Only about one-half of the adults in the United States meet the recommended amount of weekly aerobic physical activity, whereas less than a fourth meet the guidelines for muscular (strength) fitness. Among those who meet the guidelines, many do not reap the full benefits because they simply do not know how to implement and stay with a program that will yield the desired results.

The good news is that lifetime wellness is within the grasp of most people. We know that most chronic and debilitating conditions are largely preventable. Scientific evidence has shown that improving the quality and length of our lives is a matter of personal choice.

A regular exercise program is as close as we get to the miracle pill that people look for to enjoy good health and quality of life over a now longer lifespan. Myriad benefits of exercise include enhanced functional capacity; increased energy; weight loss; improved mood, self-esteem, and physical appearance; and decreased risk for many chronic ailments, including obesity, cardiovascular disease, cancer, and diabetes. As stated as far back as 1982 in the prestigious *Journal of the American Medical Association,* "There is no drug in current or prospective use that holds as much promise for sustained health as a lifetime program of physical exercise."

This book offers you the necessary information to start on your path to fitness and wellness by adhering to a healthy lifestyle. The information in the following chapters and the subsequent activities at the end of each chapter will enable you to develop a personal program that promotes lifetime fitness, preventive health care, and personal wellness. The emphasis throughout the book is teaching you how to take control of your lifestyle habits so that you can do what is necessary to stay healthy and realize your optimal well-being.

What the Book Covers

As you study this book and complete the respective activities, you will learn to:

- understand the importance of good physical fitness and a wellness lifestyle in the achievement of good health and quality of life and a more productive and longer life.

- determine whether medical clearance is needed for your safe participation in exercise.

- learn behavior modification techniques to help you adhere to a lifetime fitness and wellness program.

- assess the health-related components of fitness (cardiorespiratory endurance, muscular strength and endurance, muscular flexibility, and body composition).

- write exercise prescriptions for cardiorespiratory endurance, muscular strength and endurance, and muscular flexibility.

- analyze your diet and learn the principles that govern sound nutrition.

- develop sound diet and weight-management programs.

- understand stress, lessen your vulnerability to stress, and implement a stress management program if necessary.

- implement a cardiovascular disease risk-reduction program.
- follow guidelines to reduce your personal risk of developing cancer.
- implement a smoking cessation program, if applicable.
- understand the health consequences of chemical dependency and irresponsible sexual behaviors and learn guidelines for preventing sexually transmitted infections.
- discern between myths and facts of exercise and health-related concepts.

New in the Twelfth Edition

All nine chapters in the 12th edition of *Fitness & Wellness* have been revised and updated according to recent advances published in the scientific literature and information reported at professional health, fitness, wellness, and sports medicine conferences. In addition to the chapter updates listed below, selected new figures and photographs are included in this edition. The following are the most significant chapter updates:

Chapter 1, Physical Fitness and Wellness

- Reorganization of chapter material to better highlight the importance of daily physical activity and non-exercise activity thermogenesis (NEAT)
- Updates to all statistics regarding disease risk, mortality, and healthcare costs in the United States and worldwide
- Updated information about exercise as a preventative health measure and its effectiveness as a treatment modality in comparison to drug treatments
- Exploration of the causes behind the United States' lagging life expectancy
- A new section on *Values and Behavior* that explains the way core values are formed with new information on the role of the prefrontal cortex of the brain in carrying out value-centered behavior
- Updated and expanded information about the brain and habit formation
- An introduction to mindfulness and willpower and their role in goal achievement

Chapter 2, Assessment of Physical Fitness

- An update on the benefits of cardiorespiratory endurance and muscular fitness

Chapter 3, Exercise Prescription

- New information on activity trackers under the heading *Monitoring Daily Physical Activity*
- New information on the importance of a proper cool-down following exercise
- An update on the importance of being physically active throughout the day, including the relevance of non-exercise activity thermogenesis
- The concepts of myofibrillar hypertrophy and sarcoplasmic hypertrophy are now included in this chapter
- New information on the timing, dose, and type of protein to be under the Dietary Recommendations for Strength Development
- Up-to-date information on modes of stretching and when to stretch under flexibility development

Chapter 4, Physical Fitness and Wellness

- Expanded information on high intensity interval training (HIIT) and its wide range of applications for peak performance, new exercisers, and patients with chronic illness
- Discussions of new fitness trends in areas including functional fitness, HIIT, outdoor training, cross training, and dance fitness

Chapter 5, Nutrition for Wellness

- Expanded information on the importance of a healthy diet to include less sugar, processed foods, refined carbohydrates, and unhealthy fats
- Thorough coverage of the concept of chronic low-grade inflammation
- Expanded information on the important role of adequate protein intake throughout each day for proper weight management and lean tissue development and preservation
- Additional information on the role of nutrient supplements
- Introduction to emotional eating and eating disorders not otherwise specified (EDNOS)
- Upgrades on current dietary guidelines for healthy people based on the most recent recommendations given in the literature

Chapter 6, Weight Management

- Updates to all statistics on the overweight and obesity problem in the United States based on the latest data from the Centers for Disease Control and Prevention

- Presentation of the theory on the role of light exposure and BMI
- Addition of two recent research studies on the role of strength training for proper visceral fat management in the Exercise and Weight Management section

Chapter 7, Stress Management

- New section on the damaging role of "technostress" in today's technology dependent age, including tips on managing tech-related stress at home, school, and in the work place
- New information on the importance of proper breathing as a natural mechanism to reduce stress
- Expanded information on the benefits of mindfulness meditation for stress management

Chapter 8, Physical Fitness and Wellness

- Expanded information about the critical role of physical inactivity and excessive sitting throughout the day as a disease-promoting unhealthy behavior
- Presentation of the 2013 American Heart Association and American College of Cardiology recommendations for heart disease and stroke prevention in the *Abnormal Cholesterol Profile* section and the recommendations for saturated fat replacement in the diet
- New information detailing the way cancer develops at the cellular level has been added to help students better understand the cause and effect of cancer risk and prevention
- Updates to all statistics regarding cancer and additional important preventative recommendations, including information on spices and teas and recommendations for limiting alcohol consumption
- New information outlining the latest research on distracted driving accidents and the cognitive processes behind a variety of driving scenarios
- Enhanced section on synthetic cannabinoids (known as synthetic marijuana or Spice) which are currently the most prevalent synthetic drugs in the United States
- Expanded introductory information detailing the types and causes of common STIs and whether they are curable or treatable

Chapter 9, Relevant Fitness and Wellness Issues

- Updates and new questions that address some of the most frequently discussed issues related to physical fitness and wellness, including changing behavior, sequence of aerobic and strength training, exercise

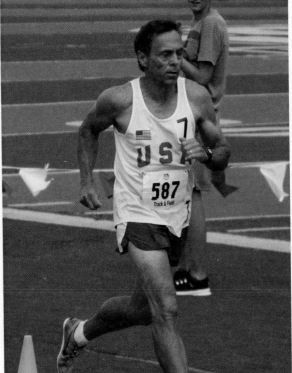

© Fitness & Wellness, Inc.

clothing, energy drinks, following a diet 24/7, excessive sugar in the diet, and exercise and aging

Additional Course Resources

- **Health MindTap for Fitness & Wellness.** Instant Access Code, ISBN-13: 978-1-305-86978-3.

  MindTap is well beyond an eBook, a homework solution or digital supplement, a resource center website, a course delivery platform, or a Learning Management System. More than 70% of students surveyed said it was unlike anything they have seen before. MindTap is a new personal learning experience that combines all your digital assets—readings, multimedia, activities, and assessments—into a singular learning path to improve student outcomes.

- **Diet & Wellness Plus.** The Diet & Wellness Plus App in MindTap helps you gain a better understanding of how nutrition relates to your personal health goals. It enables you to track your diet and activity, generate reports, and analyze the nutritional value of the food you eat! It includes over 55,000 foods in the database, custom food and recipe features, and the latest dietary references, as well as your goal and actual percentages of essential nutrients, vitamins, and minerals. It also helps you to identify a problem behavior and make a positive change. After completing the Wellness Profile Questionnaire, Diet & Wellness Plus will rate the level of concern for eight different areas of wellness, helping you determine the areas where you are most at risk. It then helps you put together a plan for positive change by helping you select a goal to work toward—complete with a reward for all your hard work.

The Diet & Wellness Plus App is accessed from the App dock in MindTap and can be used throughout the course for students to track their diet and activity and behavior change. There are activities and labs in the course that have students access the App to further extend learning and integrate course content.

- **Instructor Companion Site.** Everything you need for your course in one place! This collection of book-specific lecture and class tools is available online via **http://www.cengage.com/login**. Access and download PowerPoint presentations, images, instructor's manual, videos, and more.

- **Cengage Learning Testing Powered by Cognero.** Cengage Learning Testing Powered by Cognero is a flexible, online system that allows you to:
  - author, edit, and manage test bank content from multiple Cengage Learning solutions.
  - create multiple test versions in an instant.
  - deliver tests from your LMS, your classroom, or wherever you want.

- **Global Health Watch.** Instant Access Code, ISBN-13: 978-1-111-37733-5. Printed Access Card, ISBN-13: 978-1-111-37731-1.

Updated with today's current headlines, Global Health Watch is your one-stop resource for classroom discussion and research projects. This resource center provides access to thousands of trusted health sources, including academic journals, magazines, newspapers, videos, podcasts, and more. It is updated daily to offer the most current news about topics related to your health course.

- **Careers in Health, Physical Education, and Sports, 2e.** ISBN-13: 978-0-495-38839-5.

This unique booklet takes students through the complicated process of picking the type of career they want to pursue; explains how to prepare for the transition into the working world; and provides insight into different career paths, education requirements, and reasonable salary expectations. A designated chapter discusses some of the legal issues that surround the workplace, including discrimination and harassment. This supplement is complete with personal development activities designed to encourage students to focus on and develop better insight into their futures.

Acknowledgments

This book is dedicated to Dr. Herta Kipper for the unconditional support and love provided to the authors and her lifelong commitment to health and physical activity programs for older adults in the southern region of Austria.

This 12th edition of *Fitness & Wellness* was made possible through the contributions of many individuals. In particular, we would like to express our gratitude to the reviewers of the 12th edition. Their valuable comments and suggestions are most sincerely appreciated.

Reviewers for the 12th edition:

Craig Newton, Community College of Baltimore County

Kristin Bartholomew, Valencia College

Sharon Brunner, Carroll Community College

Carl Bryan, Central Carolina Community College

Rosanne Caputo, College of Staten Island

William Chandler, Brunswick Community College

Keith Fritz, Colorado Mesa University

Lurelia A. Hardy, Georgia Regents University

Cynthia Karlsson, Virginia Tech, Virginia Western Community College

Gloria Lambertz, Carroll College

Vince Maiorino, John Jay College

Craig Newton, Community College of Baltimore County

Nancy A. Winberg, Western Technical College

Bruce Zarosky, Lone Star College, Tomball

Kym Atwood, University of West Florida

Laura Baylor, Blue Ridge Community College

Laura Brieser-Smith, Front Range Community College

Cynthia Burwell, Norfolk State University

Lisa Chaisson, Houston Community College

Kelli Clay, Georgia Perimeter College

Karen Dennis, Illinois State University

Ali El-Kerdi, Philadelphia University

Leslie Hedelund, St. Clair County Community College

Scott Kinnaman, Northwest Nazarene University

Jerome Kotecki, Ball State University

Justin Kraft, Missouri Western State University

Wayne Lee, Jr., Delta State University

Julia Leischner, Benedictine University

Becky Louber, Northwest Nazarene University

Paul McDonald, Vermillion Community College

Kason O'Neill, East Tennessee State University

Kathryn Perry, Olivet College

William Pertet, Young Harris College

Deonna Shake, Abilene Christian University

Vicki Shoemaker, Lake Michigan College

Christine Sholtey, Waubonsee Community College

Carole Sloan, Henry Ford College

John Stroffolino, Germanna Community College

Linda Villarreal, Texas A&M International University

Reviewers for the 11th edition:

Chip Darracott, Georgia Regents University

Kathy Gieg, Missouri Baptist University

Laurelia Hardy, Georgia Regents University

Candace Hendershot, University of Findlay

Kevin B. Kinser, Tarrant County College

Linda J. Romaine, Raritan Valley Community College

William Russell, Missouri Western State University

Staci Jo Smith, Tarrant County College

Reviewers for the 10th edition:

Lisa Augustine, Lorain Community College

Vicki Boye, Concordia University

Michael Dupper, University of Mississippi

Nicholas Farkouh, College of Staten Island

Megan Franks, Lone Star College–North Harris

Misti Knight, Tarrant County College Northwest

Colleen Maloney-Hinds, California State University–San Bernadino

Reviewers for the ninth edition:

John Acquavivia, Northern Virginia Community College

Leslie K. Hickcox, Portland Community College

Rebecca Kujawa, Mother McAuley High School

Robin Kurotori, Ohlone College

Cathy McMillan, Western Illinois University

Jeff Meeker, Cornell College

Holly J. Molella, Dutchess Community College

Charles Pelitera, Canisius College

Marc Postiglione, Union County College

Andrea Pate Willis, Abraham Baldwin College

Sharon Woodard, Wake Forest University

Brief Author Biographies

Werner W. K. Hoeger is a Professor Emeritus of the Department of Kinesiology at Boise State University. He remains active in research and continues to lecture in the areas of exercise physiology, physical fitness, health, and wellness.

Dr. Hoeger completed his undergraduate and Master's degrees in physical education at the age of 20 and received his Doctorate degree with an emphasis in exercise physiology at the age of 24. He is a *Fellow* of the

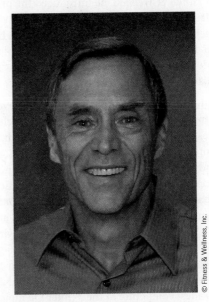

© Fitness & Wellness, Inc.

American College of Sports Medicine and also of the *Research Consortium* of *SHAPE America* (Society of Health and Physical Educators). In 2002, he was recognized as the *Outstanding Alumnus* from the *College of Health and Human Performance* at *Brigham Young University.* He was the recipient of the first *Presidential Award for Research and Scholarship* in the *College of Education* at *Boise State University* in 2004.

In 2008, he was asked to be the *keynote speaker* at the *VII Iberoamerican Congress of Sports Medicine and Applied Sciences* in Mérida, Venezuela, and was presented with the *Distinguished Guest of the City* recognition. In 2010, he was also honored as the *keynote speaker* at the *Western Society for Kinesiology and Wellness* in Reno, Nevada.

Dr. Hoeger uses his knowledge and personal experiences to write engaging, informative books that thoroughly address today's fitness and wellness issues in a format accessible to students. Since 1990, he has been the most widely read fitness and wellness college textbook author in the United States. He has published a total of 62 editions of his 9 fitness and wellness-related titles. Among the textbooks written for Cengage Learning are *Principles and Labs for Fitness and Wellness,* thirteenth edition; *Lifetime Physical Fitness & Wellness,* fourteenth edition; *Fitness and Wellness,* twelfth edition; *Principles and Labs for Physical Fitness,* tenth edition; *Wellness: Guidelines for a Healthy Lifestyle,* fourth edition; and *Water Aerobics for Fitness and Wellness,* fourth edition (with Terry-Ann Spitzer Gibson).

Dr. Hoeger was the first author to write a college fitness textbook that incorporated the "wellness" concept. In 1986, with the release of the first edition of *Lifetime Physical Fitness & Wellness,* he introduced the principle that to truly improve fitness, health, and quality of life, and to achieve wellness, a person needed to go beyond the basic health-related components of physical fitness. His work was so well received that every fitness author immediately followed his lead.

As an innovator in the field, Dr. Hoeger has developed many fitness and wellness assessment tools, including fitness tests such as the Modified Sit-and-Reach, Total Body Rotation, Shoulder Rotation, Muscular Endurance, and Muscular Strength and Endurance and Soda Pop Coordination Tests. Proving that he "practices what he preaches," he was the oldest male competitor in the 2002 Winter Olympics in Salt Lake City, Utah, at the age of 48. He raced in the sport of luge along with his then 17-year-old son Christopher. It was the first time in Winter Olympics history that father and son competed in the same event. In 2006, at the age of 52, he was the oldest competitor at the Winter Olympics in

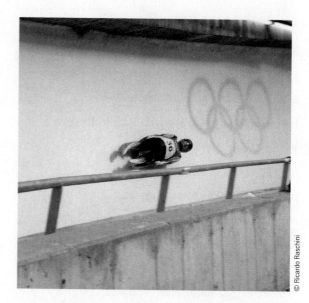

© Ricardo Raschini

Turin, Italy. In 2011, Dr. Hoeger raced in the 800-, 1,500-, and 5,000-meter events in track and field at the World Masters Track and Field (Athletic) Championships held in Sacramento, California. At different times and in different distances in 2012, 2013, 2014, and 2015, he reached All-American standards for his age group by USA Track and Field (USATF). In 2015, he finished third in the one mile run at the USATF Masters Indoor Track and Field National Championships, and third and fourth respectively in the 800- and 1,500-meters at the Outdoor National Senior Games.

Sharon A. Hoeger is Vice-President of Fitness & Wellness, Inc. of Boise, Idaho. Sharon received her degree in computer science from Brigham Young University. She is extensively involved in the research process used in

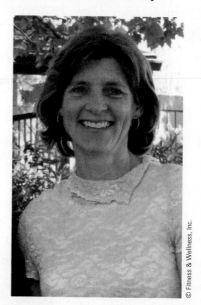

© Fitness & Wellness, Inc.

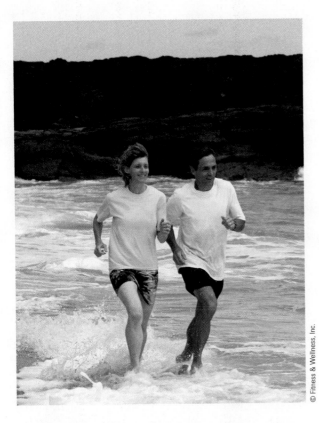

© Fitness & Wellness, Inc.

writing research and marketing copy for client magazines, newsletters, and websites; and contracting as a textbook copy editor for Cengage Learning (previously under Thomson Learning and the Brooks/Cole brand).

Amber and Cherie have been working for Fitness & Wellness, Inc. for several years and have now taken on a more significant role with the research, updates, and writing of the new editions. There is now a four-person team to sort through and summarize the extensive literature available in the health, fitness, wellness, and sports medicine fields. Their work has greatly enhanced the excellent quality of these textbooks. They are firm believers in living a healthy lifestyle, they regularly attend professional meetings in the field, and they are active members of the American College of Sports Medicine.

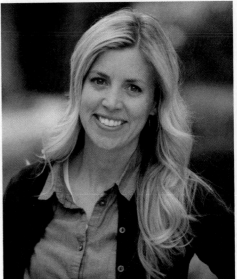

© Fitness & Wellness, Inc.

retrieving the most current scientific information that goes into the revision of each textbook. She is also the author of the software written specifically for the fitness and wellness textbooks. Her innovations in this area since the publication of the first edition of *Lifetime Physical Fitness & Wellness* set the standard for fitness and wellness computer software used in this market today.

Sharon is a co-author in five of the seven fitness and wellness titles. She also served as Chef de Mission (Chief of Delegation) for the Venezuelan Olympic Team at the 2006 Olympic Winter Games in Turin, Italy. Husband and wife have been jogging and strength training together for more than 39 years. They are the proud parents of five children, all of whom are involved in sports and lifetime fitness activities. Their motto: "Families that exercise together, stay together."

Amber L. Fawson and Cherie I. Hoeger received their degrees in English with an emphasis in editing for publication. For the past 15 years Amber has enjoyed working in the publication industry and has held positions as an Editorial Coordinator for *BYU Studies*, Assistant Editor for Cengage Learning, and freelance writer and editor for tertiary education textbooks and workbooks. During the last decade, Cherie has been working as a freelance writer and editor;

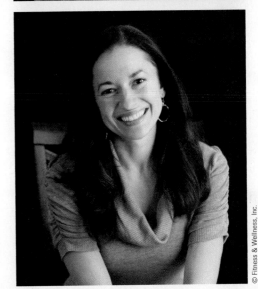

© Fitness & Wellness, Inc.

1

Introduction to Physical Fitness and Wellness

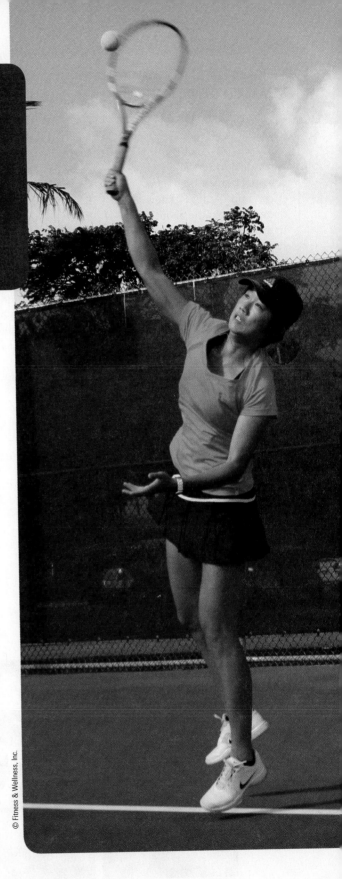

Daily physical activity is the miracle medication that people are looking for. It makes you look and feel younger, boosts energy, provides lifetime weight management, improves self-confidence and self-esteem, and enhances independent living, health, and quality of life. It further allows you to enjoy a longer life by decreasing the risk of many chronic conditions, including heart disease, high blood pressure, stroke, diabetes, some cancers, and osteoporosis.

Objectives

> Understand the importance of lifetime fitness and wellness.

> Learn the recommended guidelines for weekly physical activity.

> Define physical fitness and list components of health-related and skill-related fitness.

> Understand the benefits of a comprehensive fitness and wellness program.

> Learn motivational and behavior modification techniques to enhance compliance with a healthy lifestyle program.

> Learn to write SMART goals to aid with the process of change.

> Determine whether medical clearance is required for safe participation in exercise.

© Fitness & Wellness, Inc.

REAL LIFE STORY | Jordan's Experience

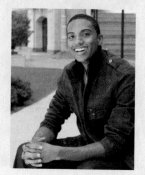

Last year as a freshman in college I was advised to enroll in a general ed fitness and wellness course. I played high school sports and thought I knew all there was to know about being fit and in shape. As the course started, I realized I didn't really know how important it was to exercise regularly and take good care of myself. It quickly became my favorite class, and I couldn't wait to try what I was learning.

I started cardio and strength workouts according to an exercise prescription I wrote myself. I didn't even know there was such a thing as an "exercise prescription." I even stretched once in a while and started to eat better. As I became more fit, I started to feel better about myself, I lost weight, I toned up, I had so much more energy, and I actually started to enjoy exercise. It is fun to work out! I now know that how well I will live the rest of my life has a lot to do with wellness choices I make. My goal is to never stop exercising and take good care of myself.

Most people believe school will teach them how to make a better living. A fitness and wellness course will teach you how to live better—how to truly live your life to its fullest potential. Real success is about more than money: Making a good living will not help you unless you live a wellness lifestyle that will allow you to enjoy what you have. Your lifestyle is the most important factor affecting your personal well-being, but most people don't know how to make the right choices to live their best life.

The benefits of an active and healthy lifestyle have been clearly substantiated by scientific evidence linking increased physical activity and positive habits to better fitness, health, and improved quality of life. Even though a few individuals live long because of favorable genetic factors, for most people, the quality of life during middle age and the "golden years" is more often related to wise choices initiated during youth and continued throughout life.

Unfortunately, the current way of life in most developed nations does not provide the human body with sufficient physical activity to maintain adequate health. Furthermore, many lifestyle patterns are such a serious threat to health that they actually speed up deterioration of the human body. In a few short years, lack of wellness leads to loss of vitality and gusto for life, as well as premature morbidity and mortality.

Even though most people in the United States believe a positive lifestyle has a great impact on health and longevity, most do not know how to implement a fitness and wellness program that will yield the desired results. Patty Neavill is an example of someone who frequently tried to change her life but was unable to do so because she did not know how to implement a sound exercise and weight

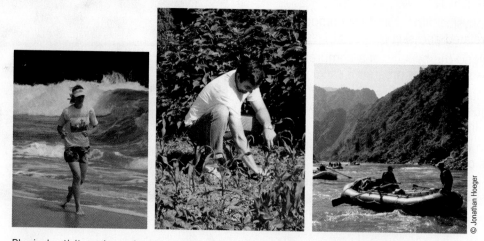

Physical activity and exercise lead to less disease, a longer life, and enhanced quality of life.

control program. At age 24, Patty, a college sophomore, was discouraged with her weight, level of fitness, self-image, and quality of life in general.

She had struggled with weight most of her life. Like thousands of other people, she had made many unsuccessful attempts to lose weight. Patty put aside her fears and decided to enroll in a fitness course. As part of the course requirement, she took a battery of fitness tests at the beginning of the semester. Patty's cardiorespiratory fitness and strength ratings were poor, her flexibility classification was average, she weighed more than 200 pounds, and she was 41 percent body fat.

Following the initial fitness assessment, Patty met with her course instructor, who prescribed an exercise and nutrition program such as the one presented in this book. Patty fully committed to carry out the prescription. She walked or jogged five times a week, worked out with weights twice a week, and played volleyball or basketball two to four times each week. Her daily caloric intake was set in the range of 1,500 to 1,700 calories. She took care to meet the minimum required amounts from the basic food groups each day, which contributed about 1,200 calories to her diet. The remainder of the calories came primarily from complex carbohydrates. By the end of the 16-week semester, Patty's cardiorespiratory fitness, strength, and flexibility ratings all had improved to the "good" category, she had lost 50 pounds, and her percent body fat had dropped to 22.5!

A thank-you note from Patty to the course instructor at the end of the semester read:

> *Thank you for making me a new person. I truly appreciate the time you spent with me. Without your kindness and motivation, I would have never made it. It's great to be fit and trim. I've never had this feeling before and I wish everyone could feel like this once in their life.*
>
> *Thank you, your trim Patty!*

Patty never had been taught the principles governing a sound weight loss program. She needed this knowledge, and, like most Americans who have never experienced the process of becoming physically fit, she needed to be in a structured exercise setting to truly feel the joy of fitness.

Of even greater significance, Patty maintained her aerobic and strength-training programs. A year after ending her calorie-restricted diet, her weight actually increased by 10 pounds—but her body fat decreased from 22.5 percent to 21.2 percent. As discussed in Chapter 6, the weight increase was related mostly to changes in lean tissue lost during the weight-reduction phase. Despite only a slight drop in weight during the second year following the calorie-restricted diet, Patty's

2-year follow-up revealed a further decrease in body fat, to 19.5 percent. Patty understands the new quality of life reaped through a sound fitness program.

1.1 *Lifestyle, Health, and Quality of Life*

Research findings have shown that physical inactivity and negative lifestyle habits pose a serious threat to health. Movement and physical activity are basic functions for which the human organism was created. Advances in modern technology, however, have all but eliminated the need for physical activity in daily life. Physical activity no longer is a natural part of our existence. This epidemic of physical inactivity is the second greatest threat to U.S. public health and is often referenced in new concerns about "Sitting Disease" and **"Sedentary Death Syndrome,"** or SeDS. (The number-one threat is tobacco use—the largest cause of preventable deaths.)

Today we live in an automated society. Most of the activities that used to require strenuous physical exertion can be accomplished by machines with the simple pull of a handle or push of a button. If people go to a store that is only a couple of blocks away, most drive their automobiles and then spend a couple of minutes driving around the parking lot to find a spot 10 yards closer to the store's entrance. During a visit to a multilevel shopping mall, nearly everyone chooses to ride the escalators instead of taking the stairs.

Automobiles, elevators, escalators, cell phones, remote controls, electric garage door openers—all are modern-day commodities that minimize the amount of movement and effort required of the human body.

With the developments in technology, three additional factors have changed our lives significantly and have had a negative effect on human health: nutrition, stress, and environment. Fatty foods, sweets, alcohol, tobacco, excessive stress, and environmental hazards (such as wastes, noise, and air pollution) have detrimental effects on people's health.

One of the most significant detrimental effects of modern-day technology has been an increase in **chronic diseases** related to a lack of physical activity. These include hypertension (high blood pressure), heart disease, diabetes, chronic low back pain, and obesity, among

---

GLOSSARY

Sedentary Death Syndrome (SeDS) Deaths that are attributed to a lack of regular physical activity.

Chronic diseases Illnesses that develop and last over a long time.

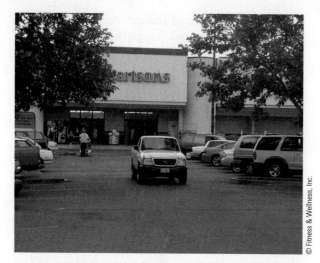

The epitome of physical inactivity is to drive around a parking lot for several minutes in search of a parking spot 10 to 20 yards closer to the store's entrance.

Figure 1.1 **Leading causes of death in the United States: 2013.**

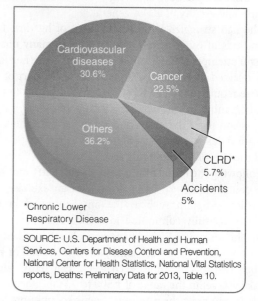

SOURCE: U.S. Department of Health and Human Services, Centers for Disease Control and Prevention, National Center for Health Statistics, National Vital Statistics reports, Deaths: Preliminary Data for 2013, Table 10.

others. They sometimes are referred to as **hypokinetic diseases**. ("Hypo" means low or little, and "kinetic" implies motion.) Lack of adequate physical activity is a fact of modern life that most people can avoid no longer. Worldwide, obesity now claims triple the number of victims as malnutrition. Over the last two decades the world has transitioned from a concern about how populations did not have enough to eat (though many still don't) to one about how an abundance of unhealthy food and physical inactivity are causing obesity, chronic diseases, and premature death. According to the World Health Organization (WHO), chronic diseases account for 60 percent of all deaths worldwide.[1] If we want to enjoy contemporary commodities and still expect to live life to its fullest, a personalized lifetime exercise program must become a part of our daily lives.

The leading causes of death in the United States today (see Figure 1.1) are lifestyle-related. About 53 percent of all deaths in the United States are caused by cardiovascular disease and cancer.[2] Almost 80 percent of these deaths could be prevented by adhering to a healthy lifestyle. The third leading cause of death—chronic lower respiratory (lung) disease—is related largely to tobacco use. Accidents are the fourth leading cause of death. Even though not all accidents are preventable, many are. Fatal accidents often are related to abusing drugs and not wearing seat belts.

Estimates indicate that more than half of disease is lifestyle-related, a fifth is attributed to environmental factors, and a tenth is influenced by the health care the individual receives. Only 16 percent is related to genetic factors. Thus, the individual controls as much as 84 percent of disease and quality of life. The data also indicate that most of the deaths that occur before age 65

are preventable. In essence, most people in the United States are threatened by the very lives they lead today.

1.2 *Life Expectancy*

Currently, the average **life expectancy** in the United States is 79.6 years (77.1 years for men and 81.9 years for women). In the past decade alone, life expectancy has increased by one year—the news, however, is not all good. The data show that people now spend an extra 1.2 years with a serious illness and an extra two years of disability.

Based on the WHO data, the United States ranks 33rd in the world for life expectancy (see Figure 1.2). Japan ranks first in the world with an overall life expectancy of 84.46 years. While the United States was once a world leader in life expectancy, over recent years, the increase in life expectancy in the United States has not kept pace with that of other developed countries.

Several factors may account for the current U.S. life expectancy ranking, including the extremely poor health of some groups (such as Native Americans, rural African Americans, and the inner-city poor) and fairly high levels of violence (notably homicides). The current trend is a widening disparity between those in the United States with the highest and lowest life expectancy. For example, males in Fairfax County, Virginia can expect to live as long as males in Japan, while those in Bolivar County, Mississippi have the same life expectancy as males in countries with much lower life expectancies, like Pakistan. Physical activity trends by United States county, in most cases, are aligned with life expectancy trends.[3]

Figure 1.2 Life expectancy at birth for selected countries as of December 2012.

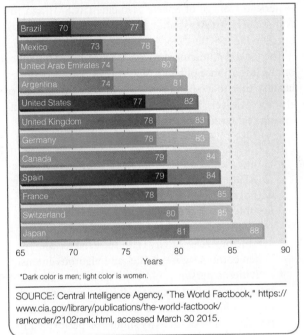

*Dark color is men; light color is women.

SOURCE: Central Intelligence Agency, "The World Factbook," https://www.cia.gov/library/publications/the-world-factbook/rankorder/2102rank.html, accessed March 30 2015.

While not a single country has managed to lower its obesity rate in more than 30 years, some countries have seen slower rises in obesity than the United States. A report by the Organisation for Economic Cooperation and Development (OECD) found that while the United States far outspent every other country in health care cost per capita, it also easily had the highest rates of obesity of all 36 OECD countries.[4]

Although life expectancy in the United States gradually increased by 30 years over the past century, scientists from the National Institute of Aging believe that in the coming decades the average life-span may decrease by as much as 5 years. This decrease in life expectancy will be related primarily to the growing epidemic of obesity. About 35 percent of the adult population in the United States is obese. The latest statistical update from the American Heart Association reported that the incidence of diabetes has been climbing dramatically each year in parallel step with the increased incidence of obesity.[5] Currently, one of ten adults has type 2 diabetes. If we are unable to change the current trend, by 2050 the number of adults suffering from diabetes could be one in three. This will be one in three of our current elementary to college-age youth. Diabetes is the third most expensive chronic disease to treat, preceded only by angina (heart disease) and hypertension, respectively. All three of these chronic conditions are linked with obesity.[6] Additional information on the obesity epidemic and its detrimental health consequences is given in Chapter 5.

1.3 *Importance of Increased Physical Activity*

The U.S. Surgeon General along with various other national and global health organizations has announced that poor health as a result of lack of physical activity is a serious public health problem that must be met head-on at once. Regular moderate physical activity provides substantial benefits in health and well-being for the vast majority of people who are not physically active. For those who are already moderately active, even greater health benefits can be achieved by increasing the level of physical activity.

Among the benefits of regular physical activity and exercise are a significant reduction in premature mortality and decreased risks for developing heart disease, stroke, metabolic syndrome, type 2 diabetes, obesity, osteoporosis, colon and breast cancers, high blood pressure, depression, and even dementia and Alzheimer's.[7] Regular physical activity also is important for the health of muscles, bones, and joints, and has been shown in clinical studies to improve mood, cognitive function, creativity, and short-term memory and enhance one's ability to perform daily tasks throughout life. It also can have a major impact on health care costs and helps maintain a high quality of life into old age.

Based on the abundance of scientific research on physical activity and exercise, a distinction has been established between physical activity and exercise. **Exercise** is considered a type of physical activity that requires planned, structured, and repetitive bodily movement to improve or maintain one or more components of physical fitness. A regular weekly program of walking, jogging, cycling, aerobics, swimming, strength training, and stretching exercises is an example of various types of exercise.

Physical activity is defined as bodily movement produced by skeletal muscles that requires the expenditure of energy and produces progressive health benefits. Examples of simple daily physical activity are walking to and from work and the store, taking the stairs instead of elevators and escalators, gardening, doing household chores, dancing, and washing

---

GLOSSARY

Hypokinetic diseases Diseases related to a lack of physical activity.

Life expectancy Number of years a person is expected to live based on the person's birth year.

Exercise A type of physical activity that requires planned, structured, and repetitive bodily movement done to improve or maintain one or more components of physical fitness.

Physical activity Bodily movement produced by skeletal muscles that requires energy expenditure and produces progressive health benefits.

the car by hand. Physical inactivity, by contrast, implies a predominantly sedentary lifestyle, characterized by excessive sitting throughout most days and a level of activity that is lower than that required to maintain good health.

Physical activity can be of light intensity or moderate to vigorous intensity. Extremely light expenditures of energy throughout the day needed to pick up children, set and clear the table, stand at a counter, take the stairs, or carry the groceries are of far greater significance in our overall health than we once realized. To better understand the impact of all intensities of physical activity, scientists created a new category of movement called **nonexercise activity thermogenesis (NEAT)**. Any energy expenditure that does not come from basic ongoing body functions (such as digesting food) or planned exercise is categorized as NEAT.[8] A person on an average day may expend 1300 calories simply maintaining vital body functions (the basal metabolic rate) and 200 calories digesting food (thermic effect of food). Any additional energy expended during the day is expended either through exercise or NEAT. Though it may not increase cardiorespiratory fitness as moderate or vigorous exercise will, NEAT can easily use more calories in a day than the planned exercise session itself. As a result, NEAT is extremely critical to keep daily energy balance in check. For example, people who spend most of the day working on their feet, such as a medical assistant or a stay-at-home parent, will expend an average of 700 daily calories more than a person who has a desk job that does not offer the option to stand, take walking breaks, or move about.

Moderate physical activity has been defined as any activity that requires an energy expenditure of 150 calories per day, or 1,000 calories per week. The general health recommendation is that people strive to accumulate at least 30 minutes of physical activity a minimum of 5 days per week. Whereas 30 minutes of continuous activity is preferred, on days when time is limited, 3 activity sessions of at least 10 minutes each provide about half the aerobic benefits. Examples of moderate physical activity are walking, cycling, playing basketball or volleyball, recreational swimming, dancing fast, pushing a stroller, raking leaves, shoveling snow, washing or waxing a car, washing windows or floors, and gardening.

1.4 *Federal Guidelines for Physical Activity*

Because of the importance of physical activity to our health, in October 2008 the U.S. Department of Health and Human Services issued Federal Physical Activity Guidelines for Americans for the first time. These guidelines complement international recommendations issued by the World Health Organization (WHO) and further substantiate previous recommendations issued by the American College of Sports Medicine (ACSM) and the American Heart Association (AHA) in 2007[9] and the U.S. Surgeon General in 1996.[10]

The federal guidelines provide science-based guidance on the importance of being physically active and eating a healthy diet to promote health and reduce the risk of chronic diseases. The federal guidelines include the following recommendations:[11]

Adults Between 18 and 64 Years of Age

- Adults should do 150 minutes a week of **moderate-intensity aerobic (cardio-respiratory) physical activity**, 75 minutes a week of **vigorous-intensity aerobic physical activity**, or an equivalent combination of moderate- and vigorous-intensity aerobic physical activity (also see Chapter 3). When combining moderate- and vigorous-intensity activities, a person could participate in moderate-intensity activity twice a week for 30 minutes and high-intensity activity for 20 minutes on another two days. Aerobic activity should be performed in episodes of at least 10 minutes long each, preferably spread throughout the week.
- *Additional health benefits* are provided by increasing to 5 hours (300 minutes) a week of moderate-intensity aerobic physical activity, 2 hours and 30 minutes a week of vigorous-intensity physical activity, or an equivalent combination of both.
- Adults should also do muscle-strengthening activities that involve all major muscle groups, performed on two or more days per week.

Older Adults (Ages 65 and Older)

- Older adults should follow the adult guidelines. If this is not possible due to limiting chronic conditions, older adults should be as physically active as their abilities allow. They should avoid inactivity. Older adults should do exercises that maintain or improve balance if they are at risk of falling.

Children 6 Years of Age and Older and Adolescents

- Children and adolescents should do 1 hour (60 minutes) or more of physical activity every day.
- Most of the 1 hour or more a day should be either moderate- or vigorous-intensity aerobic physical activity.
- As part of their daily physical activity, children and adolescents should do vigorous-intensity activity on at least three days per week. They also should do muscle-strengthening and bone-strengthening activities on at least three days per week.

Pregnant and Postpartum Women

- Healthy women who are not already doing vigorous-intensity physical activity should get at least 2 hours and 30 minutes (150 minutes) of moderate-intensity aerobic activity a week. Preferably, this activity should be spread throughout the week. Women who regularly engage in vigorous-intensity aerobic activity or high amounts of activity can continue their activity provided that their condition remains unchanged and they talk to their health care provider about their activity level throughout their pregnancy.

The guidelines state that some adults should be able to achieve calorie balance with 150 minutes of moderate physical activity in a week, while others will find they need more than 300 minutes per week.[12] This recommendation is based on evidence indicating that people who maintain healthy weight typically accumulate 1 hour of daily physical activity.[13] Between 60 and 90 minutes of moderate-intensity physical activity daily is recommended to sustain weight loss for previously overweight people.[14] And 60 to 90 minutes of activity per day provides additional health benefits.

The most recent data released in 2012 by the Centers for Disease Control and Prevention (CDC) indicate that only 19.8 percent of U.S. adults ages 18 and older meet the federal physical activity guidelines for both aerobic and muscular fitness (strength and endurance) activities, whereas 28.6 percent meet the guidelines for aerobic fitness. Another 46 percent of Americans are completely inactive during their leisure time (Figure 1.3).

Figure 1.3 Percentage of adults who did not meet and who met the 2008 federal guidelines for physical activity by gender.

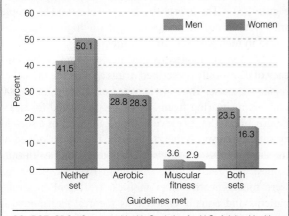

SOURCE: CDC, "Summary Health Statistics for U.S. Adults: Health Interview Survey, 2012," (February 2014) Table 26: Frequency distributions of participants in leisure-time aerobic and muscle-strengthening activities.

> **!**
> ### Critical Thinking
> Do you consciously incorporate physical activity into your daily lifestyle? • Can you provide examples? • Do you think you get sufficient daily physical activity to maintain good health?

1.5 *Benefits of Physical Fitness*

The benefits to be enjoyed from participating in a regular fitness program are many. In addition to a longer life (see Figure 1.4 and Figure 1.5), the greatest benefit of all is that physically fit people who lead a positive lifestyle have a healthier and better quality of life. These people live life to its fullest and have fewer health problems than inactive individuals who also indulge in negative lifestyle habits. Compiling an all-inclusive list of the benefits to be reaped through participation in a fitness program is a challenge, but the list provided in Table 1.1 summarizes many of these benefits.

In addition to the benefits listed in Table 1.1, **epidemiological** research studies linking physical activity habits and mortality rates have shown lower premature mortality rates in physically active people. Pioneer work in this area demonstrated that, as the amount of weekly physical activity increased, the risk of cardiovascular deaths decreased.[15] In this study, conducted among 16,936 Harvard alumni, the greatest decrease in cardiovascular deaths was observed in alumni who burned more than 2,000 calories per week through physical activity.

A landmark study subsequently upheld the findings of the Harvard alumni study.[16] Based on data from 13,344 individuals who were followed over an average of 8 years, the results confirmed that the level of cardiorespiratory fitness is related to mortality from all causes. These findings showed a graded and consistent inverse relationship between physical fitness and mortality, regardless of age and other risk factors.

---GLOSSARY---

Nonexercise activity thermogenesis (NEAT) Energy expended doing everyday activities other than exercise.

Moderate physical activity Any activity that requires an energy expenditure of 150 calories per day, or 1,000 calories per week.

Moderate-intensity aerobic physical activity Defined as the equivalent of

a brisk walk that noticeably increases the heart rate.

Vigorous-intensity aerobic physical activity Defined as an activity similar to jogging that causes rapid breathing and a substantial increase in heart rate.

Epidemiological Of the study of epidemic diseases.

Figure 1.4 Death rates by physical fitness levels.

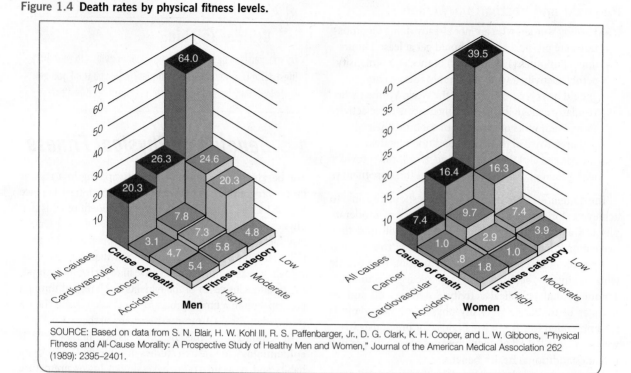

SOURCE: Based on data from S. N. Blair, H. W. Kohl III, R. S. Paffenbarger, Jr., D. G. Clark, K. H. Cooper, and L. W. Gibbons, "Physical Fitness and All-Cause Morality: A Prospective Study of Healthy Men and Women," Journal of the American Medical Association 262 (1989): 2395–2401.

Figure 1.5 Effects of fitness changes on mortality rates.

Death rate from all causes*

Initial assessment	Unfit	Unfit	Fit
5-year follow-up	Unfit	Unfit	Fit

Values shown: 122.0, 67.7, 39.6

*Death rates per 10,000 man-years observation.

SOURCE: S. N. Blair et al., "Changes in Physical Fitness and All-Cause Morality: A Prospective Study of Healthy Men and Women," Journal of the American Medical Association 273 (1995): 1193–1198.

In essence, the higher the level of cardiorespiratory fitness, the longer the life (see Figure 1.4). The death rate from all causes for the low-fit men was 3.4 times higher than for the high-fit men. For the low-fit women, the death rate was 4.6 times higher than for the high-fit women. The study also reported a greatly reduced rate of premature deaths, even at moderate fitness levels, which most adults can achieve easily. People gain further protection when they combine higher fitness levels with reduction in other risk factors such as hypertension, elevated cholesterol, cigarette smoking, and excessive body fat.

Additional research that looked at changes in fitness and mortality found a substantial (44 percent) reduction in mortality risk when the study participants abandoned a sedentary lifestyle and became moderately fit (see Figure 1.5).[17] The lowest death rate was found in people who were fit and remained fit, and the highest rate was found in men who remained unfit.

A 2013 study looked to specifically compare the efficacy of commonly prescribed drugs against the impact of regular exercise. The data is based on more than 14,000 patients recovering from stroke, being treated for heart failure, or looking to prevent Type 2 diabetes or a second episode of coronary heart disease. The study looked at the effectiveness of exercise versus drugs on health outcomes. The results were revealing: Exercise programs were more effective than medical treatment in stroke patients and equally effective as medical treatments in patients of diabetes and coronary heart disease. Only in the prevention of heart failure were diuretic drugs more effective in preventing mortality than exercise.[18]

Table 1.1 **Long-Term (Chronic) Benefits of Exercise**

Regular participation in exercise

- improves and strengthens the cardiorespiratory system.
- maintains better muscle tone, muscular strength, and endurance.
- improves muscular flexibility.
- enhances athletic performance.
- helps maintain recommended body weight.
- helps preserve lean body tissue.
- increases resting metabolic rate.
- improves the body's ability to use fat during physical activity.
- improves posture and physical appearance.
- improves functioning of the immune system.
- lowers the risk for chronic diseases and illness (including heart disease, stroke, and certain cancers).
- decreases the mortality rate from chronic diseases.
- thins the blood so it doesn't clot as readily (thereby decreasing the risk for coronary heart disease and strokes).
- helps the body manage cholesterol levels more effectively.
- prevents or delays the development of high blood pressure and lowers blood pressure in people with hypertension.
- helps prevent and control type 2 diabetes.
- helps achieve peak bone mass in young adults and maintain bone mass later in life, thereby decreasing the risk for osteoporosis.
- helps people sleep better.
- helps prevent chronic back pain.
- relieves tension and helps in coping with life stresses.
- raises levels of energy and job productivity.
- extends longevity and slows the aging process.
- improves and helps maintain cognitive function, decreasing the risk for dementia and Alzheimer's disease.
- promotes psychological well-being, including higher morale, self-image, and self-esteem.
- reduces feelings of depression and anxiety.
- encourages positive lifestyle changes (improving nutrition, quitting smoking, controlling alcohol and drug use).
- speeds recovery time following physical exertion.
- speeds recovery following injury or disease.
- regulates and improves overall body functions.
- improves physical stamina and counteracts chronic fatigue.
- reduces disability and helps to maintain independent living, especially in older adults.
- enhances quality of life: People feel better and live a healthier and happier life.

© Cengage Learning

Additional studies in this area have substantiated early findings and also indicated that primarily vigorous activities are associated with greater longevity.[19] Vigorous activity was defined as activity that requires a **MET** level equal to or greater than 6 METs (see Chapter 4, Table 4.1, page 116). This level represents exercising at an energy level of 6 times the resting energy requirement. Examples of vigorous activities used in the previous study include brisk walking, jogging, swimming laps, squash, racquetball, tennis, and shoveling snow. Results also indicated that vigorous exercise is as important as maintaining recommended weight and not smoking.

While it is clear that moderate-intensity exercise does provide substantial health benefits, the research data shows a dose-response relationship between physical activity and health. That is, greater health and fitness benefits occur at higher duration and/or intensity of physical activity.

Vigorous activities are preferable, to the extent of one's capabilities, because they are most clearly associated with better health and longer life. Compared to prolonged moderate-intensity activity, vigorous-intensity activity has been shown to provide the best improvements in

GLOSSARY

MET Short for metabolic equivalent; represents the rate of energy expenditure while sitting quietly at rest. This energy expenditure is approximately 3.5 milliliters of oxygen per kilogram of body weight per minute (mL/kg/min) or 1.2 calories per minute for a 70-kilogram person. A 3-MET activity requires three times the energy expenditure of sitting quietly at rest.

aerobic capacity, coronary heart disease risk reduction, blood pressure, blood glucose control, and overall cardiovascular health.[20]

A word of caution, however, is in order. Vigorous exercise should be reserved for healthy individuals who have been cleared to do so (see Activity 1.2) and who have been participating regularly in at least moderate-intensity activities.

While most of the chronic (long-term) benefits of exercise are well-established, what many people fail to realize is that there are *immediate benefits* derived by participating in just one single bout of exercise. Most of these benefits dissipate within 48 to 72 hours following exercise. The acute (immediate) benefits, summarized in Table 1.2, are so striking that they prompted Dr. William L. Haskell of Stanford University to state: "*Most of the health benefits of exercise are relatively short term, so people should think of exercise as a medication and take it on a daily basis.*" Of course, as you regularly exercise a minimum of 30 minutes 5 times per week, you will realize the impressive long-term benefits listed in Table 1.2.

In order to help the public better see exercise for its true benefits, the ACSM and the American Medical Association (AMA) have launched a nationwide "Exercise Is Medicine" program.[21] The initiative is in conjunction with the *Physical Activity Guidelines for Americans*, with the goal of improving the health and wellness of the nation through exercise prescriptions from physicians and health care providers. It calls on all physicians to assess and review every patient's physical activity program at every visit. "Exercise is medicine and it's free." All physicians should be prescribing exercise to all patients and participating in exercise themselves. Exercise is considered to be the much-needed vaccine in our era of widespread chronic diseases. As our understanding of human physiology deepens we are continually uncovering new reasons physical activity and exercise are powerful tools that the human body uses for both the treatment and the prevention of chronic diseases and premature death. Additional information on this program can be obtained by consulting the following Web site: http://www.exerciseis medicine.org/.

Table 1.2 Immediate (Acute) Benefits of Exercise

You can expect a number of benefits as a result of a single exercise session. Some of these benefits last up to 72 hours following your workout. Exercise

- increases heart rate, stroke volume, cardiac output, pulmonary ventilation, and oxygen uptake.
- begins to strengthen the heart, lungs, and muscles.
- enhances metabolic rate or energy production (burning calories for fuel) during exercise and recovery. For every 100 calories you burn during exercise you can expect to burn another 15 during recovery.
- uses blood glucose and muscle glycogen.
- improves insulin sensitivity (decreasing type 2 diabetes risk).
- immediately enhances the body's ability to burn fat.
- lowers blood lipids.
- improves joint flexibility.
- reduces low-grade (hidden) inflammation (see page 215 in Chapter 8).
- increases endorphins (hormones), naturally occurring opioids that are responsible for exercise-induced euphoria.
- increases fat storage *in muscle,* which can then be burned for energy.
- improves endothelial function (Endothelial cells line the entire vascular system, providing a barrier between the vessel lumen and surrounding tissue. Endothelial dysfunction contributes to several disease processes, including tissue inflammation and subsequent atherosclerosis.
- enhances mood and self-worth.
- provides a sense of achievement and satisfaction.
- decreases blood pressure the first few hours following exercise.
- decreases arthritic pain.
- leads to muscle relaxation.
- decreases stress.
- improves brain function.
- promotes better sleep (unless exercise is performed too close to bedtime).
- improves digestion.
- boosts energy levels.
- improves resistance to infections.

1.6 *Physical Fitness*

Individuals are physically fit when they can meet both the ordinary and the unusual demands of daily life safely and effectively without being overly fatigued and still have energy left for leisure and recreational activities. **Physical fitness** can be classified into health-related and skill-related fitness.

Health-Related Fitness

Health-related fitness has four components: cardiorespiratory endurance, muscular fitness, muscular flexibility, and body composition (see Figure 1.6).

1. *Cardiorespiratory endurance:* the ability of the heart, lungs, and blood vessels to supply oxygen to the cells to meet the demands of prolonged physical activity (also referred to as aerobic exercise).
2. *Muscular fitness (muscular strength and muscular endurance):* the ability of the muscles to generate force.
3. *Muscular flexibility:* the achievable range of motion at a joint or group of joints without causing injury.
4. *Body composition:* the amount of lean body mass and adipose tissue (fat mass) in the human body.

Skill-Related Fitness

Fitness in motor skills is essential in activities such as basketball, racquetball, golf, hiking, soccer, and water skiing. Good skill-related fitness also enhances overall quality of life by helping people cope more effectively in emergency situations (see Chapter 4). The components of **skill-related fitness** are agility, balance, coordination, power, reaction time, and speed (see Figure 1.7).

1. *Agility:* the ability to change body position and direction quickly and efficiently. Agility is important in sports such as basketball, soccer, and racquetball,

Figure 1.6 Health-related components of physical fitness.

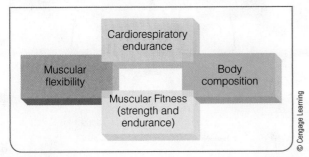

© Cengage Learning

Figure 1.7 Motor skill–related components of physical fitness.

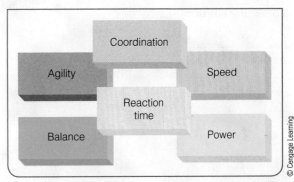

© Cengage Learning

in which the participant must change direction rapidly and at the same time maintain proper body control.
2. *Balance:* the ability to maintain the body in equilibrium. Balance is vital in activities such as gymnastics, diving, ice skating, skiing, and even football and wrestling, in which the athlete attempts to upset the opponent's equilibrium.
3. *Coordination:* integration of the nervous system and the muscular system to produce correct, graceful, and harmonious body movements. This component is important in a wide variety of motor activities such as golf, baseball, karate, soccer, and racquetball, in which hand-eye or foot-eye movements, or both, must be integrated.
4. *Power:* the ability to produce maximum force in the shortest time. The two components of power are speed and force (strength). An effective combination of these two components allows a person to produce explosive movements such as those required in jumping; putting the shot; and spiking, throwing, and hitting a ball.
5. *Reaction time:* the time required to initiate a response to a given stimulus. Good reaction time is important for starts in track and swimming; for

---GLOSSARY---

Physical fitness The general capacity to adapt and respond favorably to physical effort.

Health-related fitness A physical state encompassing cardiorespiratory endurance, muscular strength and endurance, muscular flexibility, and body composition.

Skill-related fitness Components of fitness important for successful motor performance in athletic events and in lifetime sports and activities.

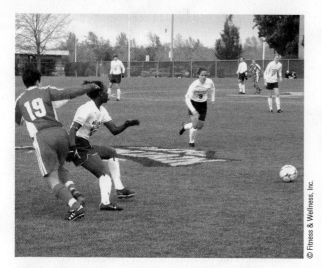

Good skill-related fitness enhances success in sports performance.

quick reactions when playing tennis at the net; and in sports such as table tennis, boxing, and karate.

6. *Speed:* the ability to propel the body or a part of the body rapidly from one point to another. Examples of activities that require good speed for success are soccer, basketball, stealing a base in baseball, and sprints in track.

In terms of preventive medicine, the main emphasis of fitness programs should be on the health-related components. Skill-related fitness is crucial for success in sports and athletics, and it also contributes to wellness. Improving skill-related fitness affords an individual more enjoyment and success in lifetime sports, and regular participation in skill-related fitness activities also helps develop health-related fitness. Further, total fitness is achieved by taking part in specific programs to improve health-related and skill-related components alike.

1.7 *Wellness*

After the initial fitness boom swept across the United States in the 1970s, it became clear that improving physical fitness alone was not always enough to lower the risk for disease and ensure better health. For example, individuals who run three miles a day, lift weights regularly, participate in stretching exercises, and watch their body weight can be classified as having good or excellent fitness. If these same people, however, have high blood pressure, smoke, are under constant stress, consume too much alcohol, and eat too many fatty and processed foods, they are exposing themselves to **risk factors** for disease of which they may not be aware.

Good health no longer is viewed as simply the absence of disease. The notion of good health has evolved notably in the past few years and continues to change as scientists learn more about lifestyle factors that bring on illness and affect wellness. Once the idea took hold that fitness by itself would not necessarily decrease the risk for disease and ensure better health, the wellness concept developed in the 1980s.

Wellness is an all-inclusive umbrella covering a variety of health-related factors. A wellness lifestyle requires the implementation of positive programs to change behavior and thereby improve health and quality of life, prolong life, and achieve total well-being. To enjoy a wellness lifestyle, a person has to practice behaviors that will lead to positive outcomes in seven dimensions of wellness: physical, emotional, intellectual, social, environmental, spiritual, and occupational (Figure 1.8). These dimensions are interrelated; one frequently affects the others. For example, a person who is "emotionally down" often has no desire to exercise, study, go to work, socialize with friends, or attend church.

The concept behind the seven dimensions of wellness shows that high-level wellness clearly goes beyond optimum fitness and the absence of disease. Wellness incorporates fitness, proper nutrition, stress management, disease prevention, social support, self-worth, nurturance (a sense of being needed), spirituality, personal safety, substance control and not smoking, regular physical examinations, health education, and environmental support.

For a wellness way of life, individuals must be physically fit and manifest no signs of disease, and they also

Figure 1.8 Dimensions of wellness.

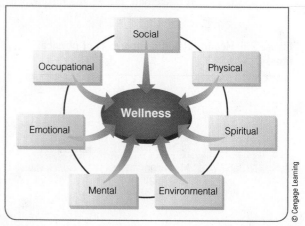

must avoid all risk factors for disease (such as physical inactivity, hypertension, abnormal cholesterol levels, cigarette smoking, excessive stress, faulty nutrition, or careless sex). Even though an individual tested in a fitness center might demonstrate adequate or even excellent fitness, indulgence in unhealthy lifestyle behaviors will increase the risk for chronic diseases and decrease the person's well-being. Additional information on wellness and how to implement a wellness program is given in Chapter 8.

Unhealthy behaviors contribute to the staggering U.S. health care costs. Risk factors for disease carry a heavy price tag. U.S. health care costs per capita are above $8,745 per year, and represent about 17.4 percent of the gross domestic product (GDP). In 1980, health care costs in the United States represented 8.8 percent of the GDP, and if the current trend continues, they are projected to reach almost 20 percent by 2019. This ratio far outpaces the spending of all other countries in the Organisation for Economic Co-operation and Development (OECD). The next closest country is the Netherlands, at 11.8 percent, and Canada ranks eighth, at 10.9 percent of GDP. According to the Institute of Medicine, up to a third of health care costs is wasteful or inefficient.

One of the reasons for the low overall ranking is the overemphasis on state-of-the-art cures instead of prevention programs. The United States is the best place in the world to treat people once they are sick, but the system does a poor job of keeping people healthy in the first place.

Risk factors for disease such as obesity and smoking carry a heavy price tag. The yearly medical costs for a person who is obese are $1,429 higher than for a person of normal weight. Looking at the country as a whole, the annual cost of obesity is $147 billion, the cost of smoking $289 billion. Regarding diseases, the annual cost of diabetes is $245 billion and costs for cardiovascular disease and stroke exceed $320 billion.[22] These figures include direct medical costs as well as lost productivity because of time away from work. As a comparison, the federal education budget is a dwarfed $80.9 billion. In a very tangible way, living a wellness way of life with a focus on disease prevention boosts both our quality of life and our economic progress.

1.8 *The Path to Fitness and Wellness*

Current scientific data and the fitness movement that began more than three decades ago in the United States have led many people to see the advantages of participating in fitness programs that will improve and maintain health. Because fitness and wellness needs vary from one person to another, exercise and wellness prescriptions must be personalized for best results. This book provides the necessary guidelines for developing a lifetime program to improve fitness and promote preventive health care and personal wellness. As you study the book and complete the assignments in each chapter, you will learn to

- Determine whether medical clearance is required for you to participate safely in exercise.
- Assess your overall level of physical fitness, including cardiorespiratory endurance, muscular fitness (strength and endurance), muscular flexibility, and body composition.
- Prescribe personal programs for total fitness development.
- Use behavior modification techniques that will allow you to change unhealthy lifestyle patterns.
- Develop sound diet and weight-control programs.
- Implement a healthy lifestyle program that includes prevention of cardiovascular diseases and cancer, stress management, and smoking cessation, if applicable.
- Discern myths from facts pertaining to exercise and health-related concepts.

1.9 *Behavior Modification*

Despite scientific evidence of the benefits derived from living a healthy lifestyle, many people still don't make healthy daily choices. To understand why this is so, one has to examine what motivates people and what actions are required to make permanent changes in behavior, which is called **behavior modification**.

GLOSSARY

Risk factors Characteristics that predict the chances for developing a certain disease.

Wellness The constant and deliberate effort to stay healthy and achieve the highest potential for well-being.

Behavior modification The process used to permanently change negative behaviors in favor of positive behaviors that will lead to better health and well-being.

Behavior Modification Planning

Healthy Lifestyle Habits

Research indicates that adherence to the following 12 lifestyle habits will significantly improve health and extend life:

1. Participate in a lifetime physical activity program.
2. Do not smoke cigarettes.
3. Eat right.
4. Avoid snacking.
5. Maintain recommended body weight through adequate nutrition and exercise.
6. Sleep seven to eight hours each night.
7. Lower your stress levels.
8. Drink alcohol moderately or not at all.
9. Surround yourself with healthy friendships.
10. Seek to live and work in a healthy environment.
11. Use the mind: Keep your brain engaged throughout life to maintain cognitive function.
12. Take personal safety measures to lessen the risk for avoidable accidents.

Try It

Look at the list above and indicate which habits are already a part of your lifestyle. What changes could you make to incorporate additional healthy habits into your daily life?

© Cengage Learning

Let's look at an all-too-common occurrence on college campuses. Most students understand that they should be exercising. They contemplate enrolling in a fitness course. The motivating factor might be enhanced physical appearance, health benefits, or simply fulfillment of a college requirement. They sign up for the course, participate for a few months, finish the course—and stop exercising! Various excuses are offered: too busy, no one to exercise with, already have the grade, inconvenient open-gym hours, or job conflicts. A few months later, they realize once again that exercise is vital and repeat the cycle (see Figure 1.9).

The information in this book will be of little value to you if you are unable to abandon negative habits and adopt and maintain new, healthy behaviors. Before looking at the physical fitness and wellness guidelines, you need to take a critical look at your behaviors and lifestyle—and most likely make some permanent changes to promote your overall health and wellness.

Change is incredibly difficult for most people. Our behaviors are based on our core values and actions that are rewarded. Whether we are trying to increase physical activity, quit smoking, change unhealthy eating habits, or reverse heart disease, it is human nature to resist change even when we know that change will provide substantial benefits in the near future.

People pursue change when it's rewarded (for example, lower health care premiums if you quit smoking) or they start contemplating change when there is a change in core values that will make them feel uncomfortable with the present behavior (for example, a long and healthy life is more important than smoking). Core values change when feelings are addressed. The challenge is to find ways that will help people understand the problems and solutions in a manner that will influence emotions and not just the thought process. Once the problem behavior is understood and "felt," the person may become uncomfortable with the situation and will be more inclined to address the problem behavior or adopt a healthy behavior.

Values and Behavior

Values are defined as the core beliefs and ideals that people have. Values govern behavior as people look to conduct themselves in a manner that is conducive to living and attaining goals consistent with their beliefs and what's important to them. People's values reflect who they are.

Figure 1.9 Exercise/exercise dropout cycle.

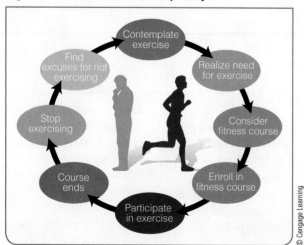

© Cengage Learning

Values are established through experience and learning, and their development is a lifelong process that influences all aspects of life. Personal values are first developed within family circles, schools, the media, and the culture where people grow up and live, according to what is acceptable or unacceptable, desirable or undesirable, good or bad, and rewarded or ignored/punished. Educational experiences play a key role in the establishment of values. Education is power: It provides people with knowledge to form opinions, allows them to better grasp future outcomes from today's choices, and forces them to question issues and take stands.

Values are also learned through examples and role models. People tend to emulate and adopt behaviors from people they admire, look up to, or view as heroes. Role models are most often parents, life heroes, siblings, classmates, sports figures, or people one sees on television or in movies, or reads and hears about through books or other media sources. As people look to develop values, they typically search for and emulate people of high ethical values and accomplishments that make them feel positive both about the people whose behaviors they are trying to emulate and themselves. Subsequently, the constant and habitual repetition of similar actions, behaviors, and expectations has a powerful conditioning effect on the mind and the role of the value for success in life.

Core values change throughout life based on education and the environment in which people live. Learning and gaining a belief about a particular issue is most critical in the establishment of values. For example, individuals who lead a sedentary lifestyle and never exercise lack an understanding of and don't experience the myriad benefits and vibrant quality of life obtained through fitness participation. Through a book, class, sports participation, or a friend, the person may first be exposed to exercise and an active lifestyle. The individual may then seek an environment wherein he/she can learn and actively participate in a physical activity or exercise program. The feelings of well-being and increased health, functional capacity, quality of life, and the education gained about the benefits of fitness in turn become the reward for program participation and lead to the development of the value that daily activity is vital for health and wellness.

The person, often subconsciously, learns to analyze the feelings experienced through participation that lead to the development of a new value. The value now sways the person's actions to live according to what is important to achieve wellness. This feeling of "fitness" often snowballs into the adoption of other healthy behaviors that further improve the individual's state of well-being. Of utmost importance in the maintenance of core values is to live the principles involved to reap the benefits. Thus, a constant and deliberate effort is required to be in an environment that rewards the behavior(s) the individual is trying to live.

Your Brain and Your Habits

Habits are a necessary tool for everyday brain function. Our minds learn to use familiar cues to carry out automatic behavior that has worked successfully in the past. While we carry out these automatic behaviors, we allow our minds to spend energy working on other tasks and puzzling through other problems. If you've ever found yourself driving a familiar route when you had intended to turn off and drive elsewhere, you are performing a habit.

Habits happen in familiar environments and not in new environments. Habits, however, can be changed by deliberate choice. During times of stress or when our minds are preoccupied with other problems, we are much more prone to return to and rely on habits, good or bad, and we are less likely to consider deliberate choice, core values, and long-term goals.

The striatum is a part of the brain that is activated by events that are rewarding, exciting, unexpected, and intense, as well as by cues from the environment that are associated with those events. The striatum memorizes events that are pleasurable and rewarding. Following repeated pairings with a reward, a behavior becomes a conditioned response that is now hard-wired in the brain. All it needs is a familiar environmental cue to set off the automatic behavior.

There are steps you can take to change unwanted habits or create helpful habits. First, take note of the situational cues or stressful experiences that trigger a habit. Next, as you are adopting a new habit, remember that repetition is critical. The more you repeat a new behavior under similar circumstances, the more likely you will develop the required circuitry in the striatum to make it a habit. Finally, realize that excessive stress (distress—see Chapter 7) often triggers old habits. You must prepare for an adequate response in these situations. If you made a mistake and did not adequately respond to that specific situation, chalk it up to experience and next time come back with the proper response.

Fortunately, there are greater forces at work in behavioral change than just pathways of automatic behavior. Change in core values often overrules instant rewards as we seek long-term gratification. An entirely separate portion of the brain, the prefrontal cortex, is responsible for reminding us of who we are and of the long-term goals we've created. As you work to change behavior you will notice competing desires, especially as you begin change. Find ways to guide yourself towards new behaviors by first recognizing that you have two desires, a short-term urge and a long-term desire. Take a few extra minutes to understand and visualize the reward you are seeking and to educate yourself about the best way to obtain it. Remind yourself often of your core values and look for opportunities throughout the day to align your behaviors with those core values.

Willpower

Understanding the concept of willpower, or self-control, is helpful in the process of behavioral change. Scientists have found that self-restraint against impulses can be built, like a muscle, if built slowly and gradually. Start with small choices and then build to acts of greater self-control. Studies have also found that willpower is a limited daily resource. It is highest in the morning and is depleted as we use it throughout the day, primarily when confronted with difficult challenges and stress. When you are planning to take on a significant task, help yourself be successful by choosing a time when you can put aside as many other demands and stressors as possible.

Studies indicate that willpower reserve can be increased through exercise, balanced nutrition, a good night's sleep, and quality time spent with important people in your life. On the other hand, willpower decreases in times of depression, anxiety, anger, and loneliness.

Motivation and Locus of Control

Motivation often explains why some people succeed and others do not. Although motivation comes from within, external factors are what trigger the inner desire to accomplish a given task. These external factors, then, control behavior.

Understanding **locus of control** is helpful to the study of motivation. People who believe they have control over events in their lives are said to have an internal locus of control. People with an external locus of control, by contrast, believe that what happens to them is a result of chance or environmental factors and is unrelated to their behavior. The latter group often has difficulty getting out of the precontemplation or contemplation stages.

People with an internal locus of control are apt to be healthier and have an easier time initiating and adhering to a wellness program than those who perceive that they have little control and think of themselves as powerless and vulnerable. People with an external locus of control also are at greater risk for illness. When illness does strike, restoring a sense of control is vital to regaining health.

Few people have either a completely external or a completely internal locus of control. They fall somewhere along a continuum. The more external, the greater is the challenge in changing and adhering to exercise and other healthy lifestyle behaviors. Fortunately, a person can develop a more internal locus of control. Understanding that most events in life are not determined genetically or environmentally helps people pursue goals and gain control over their lives. Three impediments, however, can keep people from entering the preparation or action stages: problems of competence, confidence, and motivation.

1. *Problems of competence.* Lacking the skills to get a given task done leads to less competence. If your friends play basketball regularly but you don't know how to play, you might not be inclined to participate. The solution to this problem of competence is to master the skills you need for participation. Most people are not born with all-inclusive natural abilities, including playing sports.

   A college professor continuously watched a group of students play an entertaining game of basketball every Friday at noon. Having no basketball skills, he was reluctant to play (contemplation stage). Eventually, however, the desire to join in the fun was strong enough that he enrolled in a beginning course at the college so he would learn to play the game (preparation stage). To his surprise, most of the students were impressed that he was willing to do this. Now, with greater competence, he is able to join in on Friday's "pick-up games" (action phase).

   Another alternative is to select an activity in which you are skilled. It may not be basketball, but

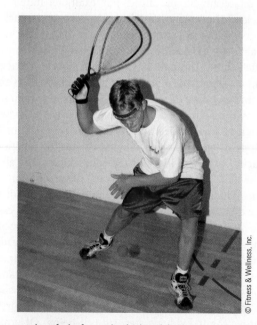

Many people refrain from physical activity because they lack the necessary skills to enjoy and reap the benefits of regular participation.

it could be aerobics. And don't be afraid to try new activities. Similarly, if your body weight is a problem, you could learn to cook low-calorie meals. Try different recipes until you find foods you like.

Patty's story at the beginning of this chapter exemplifies a lack of competence. Patty was motivated and knew she could do it, but she lacked the skills to reach her goal. All along, Patty was fluctuating between the contemplation and action stages. Once she mastered the skills, she was able to achieve and maintain her goal.

2. *Problems of confidence.* Problems with confidence arise when you have the skills but you don't believe you can get it done. Fear and feelings of inadequacy often interfere with the ability to perform the task.

Don't talk yourself out of something until you have given it a fair try. If the skills are there, the sky is the limit. Initially, try to visualize yourself doing the task and getting it done. Repeat this several times, then actually give it a try. You will surprise yourself.

Sometimes, lack of confidence sets in when the task seems to be insurmountable. In these situations, dividing a goal into smaller, realistic objectives helps to accomplish the task. You may know how to swim, but the goal of swimming a continuous mile could take you several weeks to accomplish. Set up your training program so you swim a little farther each day until you are able to swim the entire mile. If you don't meet your objective on a given day, try it again, reevaluate, cut back a little, and, most important, don't give up.

3. *Problems of motivation.* With problems of motivation, both the competence and the confidence are there, but individuals are unwilling to change because the reasons for change are not important to them. For example, a person begins contemplating a smoking cessation program when the reasons for quitting outweigh the reasons for smoking.

The lack of knowledge and lack of goals are the primary causes of unwillingness to change. Knowledge often determines goals, and goals determine motivation. How badly you want something dictates how hard you'll work at it. Many people are unaware of the magnitude of the benefits of a wellness program. When it comes to a healthy lifestyle, however, there may not be a second chance. A stroke, a heart attack, or cancer can have irreparable or fatal consequences. Greater understanding of what leads to disease may be all that is needed to initiate change.

Also, feeling physically fit is difficult to explain unless you have experienced it yourself. What Patty expressed to her instructor—fitness, self-esteem, confidence, health,

and quality of life—cannot be conveyed to someone who is constrained by sedentary living. In a way, wellness is like reaching the top of a mountain. The quiet, the clean air, the lush vegetation, the flowing water in the river, the wildlife, and the majestic valley below are difficult to explain to someone who has spent a lifetime within city limits.

Changing Behavior

The first step in addressing behavioral change is to recognize that indeed a problem exists. Five general categories of behaviors are addressed in the process of willful change:

1. Stopping a negative behavior
2. Preventing relapse of a negative behavior
3. Developing a positive behavior
4. Strengthening a positive behavior
5. Maintaining a positive behavior

Changing chronic, unhealthy behaviors to stable, healthy behaviors is often challenging. Change usually does not happen all at once but, rather, is a lengthy process with several stages.

The simplest model of change is the two-stage model of unhealthy behavior and healthy behavior. This model states that either you do it or you don't. Most people who use this model attempt self-change but end up asking themselves why they're unsuccessful: They just can't do it (start and adhere to exercise or quit smoking, for example). Their intention to change may be good, but to accomplish it, they need knowledge about how to achieve change. The following discussion may help.

The Transtheoretical Model for Changing Behavior

To aid in this process, psychologists James Prochaska, John Norcross, and Carlo DiClemente developed a behavioral change model.[23] The model's five stages are important to understanding the process of willful change. The stages of change describe underlying processes that people go through to change most problem behaviors and adopt healthy behaviors. Most frequently, the model is used to change health-related behaviors such as

---

GLOSSARY

Motivation The desire and will to do something.

Locus of control The extent to which a person

believes he or she can influence the external environment.

physical inactivity, smoking, nutrition, weight control, stress, and alcohol abuse.

The five stages of change are precontemplation, contemplation, preparation, action, and maintenance. A sixth stage of change, termination/adoption, was subsequently added to this model.

After years of study, researchers found that applying specific behavior-change techniques during each stage of the model increases the rate of success for change. Understanding each stage of this model will help you determine where you are in relation to your personal healthy-lifestyle behaviors. It also will help you identify techniques to make successful changes.

Precontemplation

People in the **precontemplation stage** are not considering or do not want to change a specific behavior. They typically deny having a problem and presently do not intend to change. These people are usually unaware or underaware of the problem. Other people around them, including family, friends, health care practitioners, and coworkers, however, identify the problem quite clearly.

Precontemplators do not care about the problem behavior and might even avoid information and materials that address the issue. They avoid free screenings and workshops that could help identify and change the problem, even if they receive financial incentives for attending. Frequently, these people actively resist change and seem resigned to accept the unhealthy behavior as their "fate."

Precontemplators are the most difficult people to reach for behavioral change. They often think that change isn't even a possibility. Educating them about the problem behavior is critical to helping them start contemplating the process of change. It is said that knowledge is power, and the challenge is to find ways to help them realize that they will be ultimately responsible for the consequences of their behavior. Sometimes they initiate change only when under pressure from others.

Contemplation

In the **contemplation stage**, people acknowledge that they have a problem and begin to think seriously about overcoming it. Although they are not quite ready for change yet, they are weighing the pros and cons. People may remain in this stage for years, but in their mind they are planning to take some action within the next six months or so. Education and peer support are valuable during this stage.

Preparation

In the **preparation stage**, people are seriously considering and planning to change a behavior within the next month. They are taking initial steps for change and may even try it for a short while, such as stopping smoking for a day or exercising a few times during this month. In this stage, people define a general goal for behavior change (say, to quit smoking by the last day of the month) and write specific actions to accomplish this goal (see the discussion on SMART goals, pages 21–22). Continued peer and environmental support are recommended during the preparation phase.

Action

The **action stage** requires the most commitment of time and energy by the individual. Here people are actively doing things to change or modify the problem behavior or to adopt a new healthy behavior. The action stage requires that the person follow the specific guidelines set forth for that specific behavior. For example, a person has actually stopped smoking completely, is exercising aerobically three times per week according to exercise prescription guidelines (see Chapter 3), or is maintaining a healthy diet.

Relapse, in which the individual regresses to a previous stage, is common during this stage. Once people maintain the action stage for six consecutive months, they move into the maintenance stage.

Maintenance

During the **maintenance stage**, the person continues to adhere to the behavior change for up to five years. The maintenance phase requires continuously adhering to the specific guidelines that govern the target behavior (for example, complete smoking cessation, aerobic exercise three times per week, or proper stress management techniques). At this time, a person works to reinforce the gains made through the various stages of change and strives to prevent lapses and relapses.

Termination/Adoption

Once a person has maintained a behavior more than five years, he or she enters the **termination/adoption stage** without fear of relapse. In the case of negative behaviors that have been terminated, this stage of change is referred to as termination. If the person has adopted a positive behavior for more than five years, this stage is designated the adoption stage. Many experts believe that after this period of time, any former addictions, problems, or lack of compliance with healthy behaviors no longer present an obstacle in the quest for wellness. The change has become a part of one's lifestyle. This phase is the ultimate goal for everyone who seeks a healthier lifestyle.

Use the form provided in Figure 1.10 to determine where you stand in respect to behaviors that you want to

Figure 1.10 Identifying your current stage of change.

Please indicate which response most accurately describes your current _____
behavior (in the blank space identify the behavior: smoking, physical activity, stress, nutrition, weight control, etc.).
Next, select the statement below (select only one) that best represents your current behavior pattern. To select the most
appropriate statement, fill in the blank for one of the first three statements if your current behavior is a problem behavior. (For example, you might say, "I currently smoke, and I do *not* intend to change in the foreseeable future," or "I currently *do not* exercise, but I am contemplating changing in the next 6 months.") If you have already started to make changes, fill in the blank in one of the last three statements. (In this case, you might say: "I currently *eat a low-fat diet*, but I have done so only within the last 6 months," or "I currently *practice adequate stress management techniques*, and I have done so for more than 6 months.") As you can see, you may use this form to identify your stage of change for any type of health-related behavior.

1. I currently _____, and I do not intend to change in the foreseeable future.

2. I currently _____, but I am contemplating changing in the next 6 months.

3. I currently _____ regularly but intend to change in the next month.

4. I currently _____, but I have done so only within the last 6 months.

5. I currently _____, and I have done so for more than 6 months.

6. I currently _____, and I have done so for more than 5 years.

STAGES OF CHANGE

1 = Precontemplation   4 = Action
2 = Contemplation   5 = Maintenance
3 = Preparation   6 = Termination/Adoption

© Cengage Learning

change or new ones that you wish to adopt. As you fill out this form, you will realize that you are at different stages for different behaviors. For instance, you may be in the termination stage for aerobic exercise and smoking, in the action stage for strength training, but only in the contemplation stage for a healthy diet. Realizing where you are at with respect to different behaviors will help you design a better action plan for a healthy lifestyle.

Using the form provided in Activity 1.1, pages 24–25, select two or three behaviors that you have targeted for the next three months. Developing new behavioral patterns takes time, and trying to work on too many components at once most likely will lower your chances for success. Start with components in which you think you will have a high chance for success.

Critical Thinking

What factors do you think keep you from participating in a regular exercise program? • How about factors that keep you from managing your daily caloric intake?

1.10 *The Process of Change*

When wellness is concerned, the sooner we implement a healthy lifestyle program, the greater are the health benefits and quality of life that lie ahead. Adopting the

GLOSSARY

Precontemplation stage Stage of change in which people are unwilling to change their behavior.

Contemplation stage Stage of change in which people are considering changing behavior in the next six months.

Preparation stage Stage of change in which people are getting ready to make a change within the coming month.

Action stage Stage of change in which people are actively changing a negative behavior or adopting a new, healthy behavior.

Relapse Slipping or falling back into unhealthy behavior(s) or failing to maintain healthy behaviors.

Maintenance stage Stage of change in which people maintain behavioral change for up to five years.

Termination/adoption stage Stage of change in which people have eliminated an undesirable behavior or maintained a positive behavior for more than five years.

following behavior modification principles can help change behavior.

Self-Analysis

If you have no interest in changing a behavior, you won't do it (precontemplator). A person who has no intention of quitting smoking will not quit, regardless of what anyone says or how strong the evidence is against it. As part of your self-analysis, you may want to prepare a list of reasons for continuing or discontinuing the behavior. When the reasons for changing outweigh the reasons for not changing, you are ready for the next step (contemplation stage).

Positive Outlook

Having a positive outlook means taking an optimistic approach from the beginning and believing in yourself. Studies of individuals who are trying to quit an addictive behavior have found that asking that person to reconnect with positive and meaningful goals in their life greatly improves chances for success.

Commitment

Write down your goals and, preferably, share them with others. In essence, you are signing a behavioral contract for change. You will be more likely to adhere to your program if others know you are committed to change.

Environment Control

In environment control, the person restructures the physical surroundings to avoid problem behaviors and decrease temptations. If you don't buy alcohol, you can't drink any. If you shop on a full stomach, you can reduce impulse buying of junk food.

Mindfulness

The simple act of being aware of thoughts and choices is a powerful tool. A person should not feel that having an urge means that they have to act on it. During an urge our mind may be experiencing some of the pleasure response it remembers from a specific past experience, like consuming a particular food. Our mind then notices that the act that caused the reward is missing. We are then driven by a desire to eat that food. A common technique of mindfulness is referred to as "urge surfing," which directs the person to notice the urge, pay attention to the way the urge feels as it builds, and then simply continue noticing it as the urge subsides. Professional behavioral therapists have found that having some kind of preemptive strategy for coping with urges, no matter how

simple, greatly improves an individual's chance of success for overcoming and choosing the desired behavior.

Behavior Analysis

Now you have to determine the frequency, circumstances, and consequences of the behavior to be altered or implemented. If the desired outcome is to consume less unhealthy fats, you first must find out what foods in your diet are high in those fats, when you eat them, and when you don't eat them (preparation stage). Knowing when you don't eat fatty foods points to circumstances under which you exert control of your diet and will help as you set goals.

Goal Setting

A **goal** motivates change in behavior. The stronger the goal, or desire, the more motivated you will be either to change unwanted behaviors or to implement new healthy behaviors. The final topic of this chapter, SMART goals, will help you write goals and prepare an action plan to achieve those goals. This will aid with behavior modification.

Helping Relationships

Surrounding yourself with people who will work toward a common goal with you or will encourage you along the way will be helpful. Attempting to quit smoking, for instance, is easier when the person is around others who are trying to quit as well. The person also may get help from friends who have quit already. Peer support is a strong incentive for behavior change. During this process, people who will not be supportive should be avoided. Friends who have no desire to quit smoking may tempt the person to smoke and encourage relapse. People who achieved the same goal earlier might not be supportive either. For instance, someone might say, "I can do six consecutive miles." The response should be, "I'm proud that I can jog three consecutive miles."

Countering

The process whereby you substitute healthy behaviors for a problem behavior, known as countering, is a critical part of the action and maintenance stages of changing behaviors.

Monitoring

During the action and maintenance stages, continuous behavior monitoring increases awareness of the desired outcome. Sometimes this principle in itself is sufficient to cause change. For example, keeping track of daily food intake reveals sources of unhealthy fats in the diet. This can help a person cut down gradually or completely eliminate some unhealthy-fat foods before consuming them.

Rewards

People tend to repeat behaviors that are rewarded and disregard those that are not rewarded or are punished. If you have successfully cut down your fat intake during the week, reward yourself by going to a show or buying a new pair of shoes. Do not reinforce yourself with destructive behaviors such as eating a high-fat dinner. If you fail to change a desired behavior (or to implement a new one), you may want to put off buying those new shoes. When a positive behavior becomes habitual, give yourself an even better reward. Treat yourself to a weekend away from home, buy a new bike, or get that tennis racket you always wanted.

1.11 *SMART Goals*

Only a well-conceived action plan will help you attain goals. Determining what you want to accomplish is the starting point, but to reach your goal you need to write **SMART** goals. The SMART acronym means that goals are *Specific, Measurable, Acceptable, Realistic,* and *Time-specific.*

1. *Specific.* When writing goals, state in a positive manner exactly what you would like to accomplish. For example, if you are overweight at 150 pounds and at 27 percent body fat, simply stating "I will lose weight" is not a specific goal. Instead, rewrite your goal to state, "I will reduce my body fat to 20 percent (137 pounds) in 12 weeks."

   Be sure to write down your goals. An unwritten goal is simply a wish. A written goal, in essence, becomes a contract with yourself. Show this goal to a friend or an instructor and have him or her witness the contract you made with yourself by signing alongside your signature.

   Once you have identified and written down a specific goal, write the specific **actions** that will help you reach that goal. These actions are the necessary steps required to reach your goal. For example, a goal might be to achieve recommended body weight. Several specific actions could be to

   (a) lose an average of one pound (or one fat percentage point) per week.

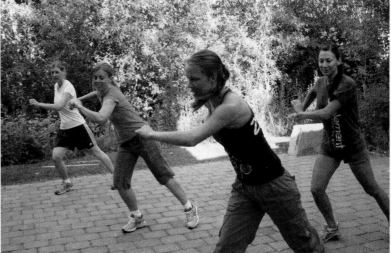
Social support enhances regular participation and the process of behavior modification.

   (b) monitor body weight before breakfast every morning.
   (c) assess body composition every three weeks.
   (d) limit fat intake to less than 25 percent of total daily caloric intake.
   (e) eliminate all pastries from the diet during this time.
   (f) walk/jog in the proper target zone for 60 minutes, 6 times per week.

2. *Measurable.* Whenever possible, goals and actions should be measurable. For example, "I will lose weight" is not measurable, but "I will reduce body fat to 20 percent" is measurable. Also note that all of the sample specific actions (a) through (f) in item 1 above are measurable. For instance, you can figure out easily whether you are losing a pound or a percentage point per week; you can conduct a nutrient analysis to assess your average fat intake; or you can monitor your weekly exercise sessions to make sure you are meeting this specific objective.

3. *Acceptable.* Goals that you set for yourself are more motivational than goals that someone else sets for you. These goals will motivate and

---

GLOSSARY

Goal The ultimate aim toward which effort is directed.

SMART An acronym for Specific, Measurable,

Acceptable, Realistic, and Time-specific goals.

Actions Steps required to reach a goal.

challenge you and should be consistent with other goals that you have. As you set an acceptable goal, ask yourself: Do I have the time, commitment, and necessary skills to accomplish this goal? If not, you need to restate your goal so that it is acceptable to you.

In instances where successful completion of a goal involves others, such as an athletic team or an organization, an acceptable goal must be compatible with those of the other people involved. If a team's practice schedule is set Monday through Friday from 4:00 p.m. to 6:00 p.m., it is unacceptable for you to train only three times per week or at a different time of the day.

Acceptable goals are also embraced with positive thoughts. Visualize and believe in your success. As difficult as some tasks may seem, where there's a will, there's a way. A plan of action, prepared according to the guidelines in this chapter, will help you achieve your goals.

4. *Realistic.* Goals should be within reach. If you currently weigh 190 pounds and your target weight (at 20 percent body fat) is 140 pounds, setting a goal to lose 50 pounds in a month would be unsound, if not impossible. Such a goal does not allow for the implementation of adequate behavior modification techniques or ensure weight maintenance at the target weight. Unattainable goals only set you up for failure, discouragement, and loss of interest.

On the other hand, do not write goals that are too easy to achieve and that do not challenge you. If a goal is too easy, you may lose interest and stop working toward it.

At times, problems arise even with realistic goals. Try to anticipate potential difficulties as much as possible and plan for ways to deal with them. If your goal is to jog for 30 minutes on 6 consecutive days, what are the alternatives if the weather turns bad? Possible solutions are to jog in the rain, find an indoor track, jog at a different time of day when the weather is better, or participate in a different aerobic activity such as stationary cycling, swimming, or step aerobics.

Monitoring your progress as you move toward a goal also reinforces behavior. Keeping an exercise log or doing a body composition assessment periodically enables you to determine your progress at any given time.

5. *Time-specific.* A goal always should have a specific date set for completion. The above example to reach 20 percent body fat in 12 weeks is time-specific.

The chosen date should be realistic but not too distant in the future. Allow yourself enough time to achieve the goal, but not too much time, as this could affect your performance. With a deadline, a task is much easier to work toward.

Goal Evaluation

In addition to the SMART guidelines provided above, you should conduct periodic evaluations of your goals. Reevaluations are vital for success. You may find that after you have fully committed and put all your effort into a goal, that goal may be unreachable. If so, reassess the goal.

Recognize that you will face obstacles and that you will not always meet your goals. Use your setbacks and learn from them. Rewrite your goal and create a plan that will help you get around self-defeating behaviors in the future. Once you achieve a goal, set a new one to improve upon or maintain what you have achieved. Goals keep you motivated.

In addition to previously discussed guidelines, throughout this book you will find information on behavioral change. For example, Chapter 3 includes the Exercise Readiness Questionnaire, tips to start and adhere to an exercise program, and how to set your fitness goals; Chapter 4 offers tips to enhance your aerobic workout; Chapter 6 gives suggestions on how to adhere to a lifetime weight management program; Chapter 7 sets forth stress management techniques; and Chapter 8 outlines a six-step smoking cessation plan.

1.12 *A Word of Caution Before You Start Exercise*

Even though exercise testing and participation is relatively safe for most apparently healthy individuals, a small but real risk exists for exercise-induced abnormalities in people with a history of cardiovascular problems and those who are at higher risk for disease. These people should be screened before initiating or increasing the intensity of an exercise program.

Before you engage in an exercise program or participate in any exercise testing, at a minimum you should fill out the Physical Activity Readiness Questionnaire (PAR-Q) found in Activity 1.2. A "yes" answer to any of these questions may signal the need for a physician's approval before you participate. If you don't have any "yes" responses, you may proceed to Chapter 2 to assess your current level of fitness.

Assess Your Behavior

. . . .

1. Are you aware of lifestyle factors that may negatively impact your health?

2. Do you accumulate at least 30 minutes of moderate-intensity physical activity five days per week?

3. Do you participate in vigorous-intensity physical activity a minimum of two times per week?

4. Do you make a constant and deliberate effort to stay healthy and achieve the highest potential for well-being?

Assess Your Knowledge

. . . .

1. Bodily movement produced by skeletal muscles is called
   a. physical activity.
   b. kinesiology.
   c. exercise.
   d. aerobic exercise.
   e. muscle strength.

2. The 2008 Federal Guidelines for Physical Activity state that adults between 18 and 64 years of age should
   a. do 2 hours and 30 minutes a week of moderate-intensity aerobic physical activity.
   b. do 1 hour and 15 minutes (75 minutes) a week of vigorous-intensity aerobic physical activity.
   c. do an equivalent combination of moderate- and vigorous-intensity aerobic physical activity listed under choices a and b above.
   d. do muscle-strengthening activities that involve all major muscle groups on two or more days per week.
   e. All of the above choices are correct.

3. The leading cause of death in the United States is
   a. cancer.
   b. accidents.
   c. chronic lower respiratory disease.
   d. diseases of the cardiovascular system.
   e. drug-related illness.

4. The constant and deliberate effort to stay healthy and achieve the highest potential for well-being is defined as
   a. health.
   b. physical fitness.
   c. wellness.
   d. health-related fitness.
   e. metabolic fitness.

5. Which of the following is not a component of health-related fitness?
   a. cardiorespiratory endurance
   b. body composition
   c. agility
   d. muscular strength and endurance
   e. muscular flexibility

6. Research on the effects of fitness on mortality indicates that the largest drop in premature mortality is seen between
   a. the average and excellent fitness groups.
   b. the least fit and moderately fit groups.
   c. the good and high fitness groups.
   d. the moderately fit and good fitness groups.
   e. The drop is similar among all fitness groups.

7. What is the greatest benefit of being physically fit?
   a. absence of disease
   b. a higher quality of life
   c. improved sports performance
   d. better personal appearance
   e. maintenance of ideal body weight

8. Which of the following is a stage in the behavioral modification model?
   a. recognition
   b. motivation
   c. relapse
   d. preparation
   e. goal setting

9. A precontemplator is a person who
   a. has no desire to change a behavior.
   b. is looking to make a change in the next six months.
   c. is preparing for change in the next 30 days.
   d. willingly adopts healthy behaviors.
   e. is talking to a therapist to overcome a problem behavior.

10. A SMART goal is effective when it is
    a. realistic.
    b. measurable.
    c. specific.
    d. acceptable.
    e. All are correct choices.

Correct answers can be found on page 307.

Activity 1.1 Behavior Modification: Stages of Change

Name _____ Date _____

Course _____ Section _____

Instructions

Please indicate which response most accurately describes your stage of change for three different behaviors (in the blank space identify the behavior: smoking, physical activity, stress, nutrition, weight control, etc.). Next, select the statement (select only one) that best represents your current behavior pattern. To select the most appropriate statement, fill in the blank for one of the first three statements if your current behavior is a problem behavior. (For example, you might say, "I currrently smoke and I do *not* intend to change in the foreseeable future," or "I currently *do not* exercise, but I am contemplating changing in the next 6 months.")

If you have already started to make changes, fill in the blank in one of the last three statements. (In this case, you might say: "I currently eat a *low-fat* diet but I have done so only within the last 6 months," or "I currently *practice adequate stress management techniques* and I have done so for more than 6 months.") You may use this technique to identify your stage of change for any type of health-related behavior.

Now write SMART goals (see pages 21–22) and identify three behavior modification principles (pages 20–21) that will aid you with the process of change.

Behavior 1: _____

1. I currently _____ , and I do not intend to change in the foreseeable future.

2. I currently _____ , but I am contemplating changing in the next 6 months.

3. I currently _____ regularly but intend to change in the next month.

4. I currently _____ , but I have done so only within the last 6 months.

5. I currently _____ , and I have done so for more than 6 months.

6. I currently _____ , and I have done so for more than 5 years.

Stage of change: (see Stages of Change list below) _____

Specific goal and date to be accomplished: _____

Principles of behavior modification to be used: _____

Behavior 2: _____

1. I currently _____ , and I do not intend to change in the foreseeable future.

2. I currently _____ , but I am contemplating changing in the next 6 months.

3. I currently _____ regularly but intend to change in the next month.

4. I currently _____ , but I have done so only within the last 6 months.

5. I currently _____ , and I have done so for more than 6 months.

6. I currently _____ , and I have done so for more than 5 years.

Stage of change: (see Stages of Change list below) _____

Specific goal and date to be accomplished: _____

Principles of behavior modification to be used: _____

Activity 1.1 **Behavior Modification: Stages of Change** *(continued)*

Behavior 3: _____

1. I currently _____, and I do not intend to change in the foreseeable future.

2. I currently _____, but I am contemplating changing in the next 6 months.

3. I currently _____ regularly but intend to change in the next month.

4. I currently _____, but I have done so only within the last 6 months.

5. I currently _____, and I have done so for more than 6 months.

6. I currently _____, and I have done so for more than 5 years.

Stage of change: (see Stages of Change list below) _____

Specific goal and date to be accomplished: _____

Principles of behavior modification to be used: _____

Stages of Change

1 = Precontemplation   4 = Action
2 = Contemplation   5 = Maintenance
3 = Preparation   6 = Termination/Adoption

Self-Reflection

In your own words, indicate barriers (what may keep you from changing) that you may encounter during the process of change and how can you best prepare to overcome these barriers.

_____

_____

_____

_____

_____

_____

_____

_____

© Fitness & Wellness, Inc.

Activity 1.2 Physical Activity Readiness Questionnaire (PAR-Q)

2015 PAR-Q+

The Physical Activity Readiness Questionnaire for Everyone

The health benefits of regular physical activity are clear; more people should engage in physical activity every day of the week. Participating in physical activity is very safe for MOST people. This questionnaire will tell you whether it is necessary for you to seek further advice from your doctor OR a qualified exercise professional before becoming more physically active.

GENERAL HEALTH QUESTIONS

Please read the 7 questions below carefully and answer each one honestly: check YES or NO.	YES	NO
1) Has your doctor ever said that you have a heart condition ☐ OR high blood pressure ☐?	☐	☐
2) Do you feel pain in your chest at rest, during your daily activities of living, **OR** when you do physical activity?	☐	☐
3) Do you lose balance because of dizziness **OR** have you lost consciousness in the last 12 months? Please answer **NO** if your dizziness was associated with over-breathing (including during vigorous exercise).	☐	☐
4) Have you ever been diagnosed with another chronic medical condition (other than heart disease or high blood pressure)? **PLEASE LIST CONDITION(S) HERE:** _____	☐	☐
5) Are you currently taking prescribed medications for a chronic medical condition? **PLEASE LIST CONDITION(S) AND MEDICATIONS HERE:** _____	☐	☐
6) Do you currently have (or have had within the past 12 months) a bone, joint, or soft tissue (muscle, ligament, or tendon) problem that could be made worse by becoming more physically active? Please answer **NO** if you had a problem in the past, but it *does not limit your current ability* to be physically active. **PLEASE LIST CONDITION(S) HERE:** _____	☐	☐
7) Has your doctor ever said that you should only do medically supervised physical activity?	☐	☐

✔ **If you answered NO to all of the questions above, you are cleared for physical activity.**
Go to Page 4 to sign the PARTICIPANT DECLARATION. You do not need to complete Pages 2 and 3.

▶ Start becoming much more physically active – start slowly and build up gradually.

▶ Follow International Physical Activity Guidelines for your age (www.who.int/dietphysicalactivity/en/).

▶ You may take part in a health and fitness appraisal.

▶ If you are over the age of 45 years and **NOT** accustomed to regular vigorous to maximal effort exercise, consult a qualified exercise professional before engaging in this intensity of exercise.

▶ If you have any further questions, contact a qualified exercise professional.

⬤ **If you answered YES to one or more of the questions above, COMPLETE PAGES 2 AND 3.**

⚠ **Delay becoming more active if:**

✓ You have a temporary illness such as a cold or fever; it is best to wait until you feel better.

✓ You are pregnant – talk to your health care practitioner, your physician, a qualified exercise professional, and/or complete the ePARmed-X+ at **www.eparmedx.com** before becoming more physically active.

✓ Your health changes – answer the questions on Pages 2 and 3 of this document and/or talk to your doctor or a qualified exercise professional before continuing with any physical activity program.

 OSHF
Ontario Society for Health and Fitness

Copyright © 2015 PAR-Q+ Collaboration 1 / 4
08-01-2014

Activity 1.2 **Physical Activity Readiness Questionnaire (PAR-Q)** *(continued)*

2015 PAR-Q+

FOLLOW-UP QUESTIONS ABOUT YOUR MEDICAL CONDITION(S)

1. Do you have Arthritis, Osteoporosis, or Back Problems?

If the above condition(s) is/are present, answer questions 1a-1c   If **NO** ☐ go to question 2

1a. Do you have difficulty controlling your condition with medications or other physician-prescribed therapies?   YES ☐ NO ☐
(Answer **NO** if you are not currently taking medications or other treatments)

1b. Do you have joint problems causing pain, a recent fracture or fracture caused by osteoporosis or cancer,   YES ☐ NO ☐
displaced vertebra (e.g., spondylolisthesis), and/or spondylolysis/pars defect (a crack in the bony ring on the
back of the spinal column)?

1c. Have you had steroid injections or taken steroid tablets regularly for more than 3 months?   YES ☐ NO ☐

2. Do you have Cancer of any kind?

If the above condition(s) is/are present, answer questions 2a-2b   If **NO** ☐ go to question 3

2a. Does your cancer diagnosis include any of the following types: lung/bronchogenic, multiple myeloma (cancer of   YES ☐ NO ☐
plasma cells), head, and neck?

2b. Are you currently receiving cancer therapy (such as chemotheraphy or radiotherapy)?   YES ☐ NO ☐

3. Do you have a Heart or Cardiovascular Condition? *This includes Coronary Artery Disease, Heart Failure,
Diagnosed Abnormality of Heart Rhythm*

If the above condition(s) is/are present, answer questions 3a-3d   If **NO** ☐ go to question 4

3a. Do you have difficulty controlling your condition with medications or other physician-prescribed therapies?   YES ☐ NO ☐
(Answer **NO** if you are not currently taking medications or other treatments)

3b. Do you have an irregular heart beat that requires medical management?   YES ☐ NO ☐
(e.g., atrial fibrillation, premature ventricular contraction)

3c. Do you have chronic heart failure?   YES ☐ NO ☐

3d. Do you have diagnosed coronary artery (cardiovascular) disease and have not participated in regular physical   YES ☐ NO ☐
activity in the last 2 months?

4. Do you have High Blood Pressure?

If the above condition(s) is/are present, answer questions 4a-4b   If **NO** ☐ go to question 5

4a. Do you have difficulty controlling your condition with medications or other physician-prescribed therapies?   YES ☐ NO ☐
(Answer **NO** if you are not currently taking medications or other treatments)

4b. Do you have a resting blood pressure equal to or greater than 160/90 mmHg with or without medication?   YES ☐ NO ☐
(Answer **YES** if you do not know your resting blood pressure)

5. Do you have any Metabolic Conditions? *This includes Type 1 Diabetes, Type 2 Diabetes, Pre-Diabetes*

If the above condition(s) is/are present, answer questions 5a-5e   If **NO** ☐ go to question 6

5a. Do you often have difficulty controlling your blood sugar levels with foods, medications, or other physician-   YES ☐ NO ☐
prescribed therapies?

5b. Do you often suffer from signs and symptoms of low blood sugar (hypoglycemia) following exercise and/or   YES ☐ NO ☐
during activities of daily living? Signs of hypoglycemia may include shakiness, nervousness, unusual irritability,
abnormal sweating, dizziness or light-headedness, mental confusion, difficulty speaking, weakness, or sleepiness.

5c. Do you have any signs or symptoms of diabetes complications such as heart or vascular disease and/or   YES ☐ NO ☐
complications affecting your eyes, kidneys, **OR** the sensation in your toes and feet?

5d. Do you have other metabolic conditions (such as current pregnancy-related diabetes, chronic kidney disease, or   YES ☐ NO ☐
liver problems)?

5e. Are you planning to engage in what for you is unusually high (or vigorous) intensity exercise in the near future?   YES ☐ NO ☐

OSHF
Ontario Society for Health and Fitness

Copyright © 2015 PAR-Q+ Collaboration 2 / 4
08-01-2014

SOURCE: Physical Activity Readiness Questionaire (PAR-Q) © 2015. Used with permission from the Canadian Society for Exercise
Physiology www.csep.ca.

Activity 1.2 **Physical Activity Readiness Questionnaire (PAR-Q)** *(continued)*

2015 PAR-Q+

6.   **Do you have any Mental Health Problems or Learning Difficulties?** *This includes Alzheimer's, Dementia, Depression, Anxiety Disorder, Eating Disorder, Psychotic Disorder, Intellectual Disability, Down Syndrome*

     If the above condition(s) is/are present, answer questions 6a-6b   If **NO** ☐ go to question 7

6a.   Do you have difficulty controlling your condition with medications or other physician-prescribed therapies? (Answer **NO** if you are not currently taking medications or other treatments)   YES☐ NO☐

6b.   Do you **ALSO** have back problems affecting nerves or muscles?   YES☐ NO☐

7.   **Do you have a Respiratory Disease?** *This includes Chronic Obstructive Pulmonary Disease, Asthma, Pulmonary High Blood Pressure*

     If the above condition(s) is/are present, answer questions 7a-7d   If **NO** ☐ go to question 8

7a.   Do you have difficulty controlling your condition with medications or other physician-prescribed therapies? (Answer **NO** if you are not currently taking medications or other treatments)   YES☐ NO☐

7b.   Has your doctor ever said your blood oxygen level is low at rest or during exercise and/or that you require supplemental oxygen therapy?   YES☐ NO☐

7c.   If asthmatic, do you currently have symptoms of chest tightness, wheezing, laboured breathing, consistent cough (more than 2 days/week), or have you used your rescue medication more than twice in the last week?   YES☐ NO☐

7d.   Has your doctor ever said you have high blood pressure in the blood vessels of your lungs?   YES☐ NO☐

8.   **Do you have a Spinal Cord Injury?** *This includes Tetraplegia and Paraplegia*

     If the above condition(s) is/are present, answer questions 8a-8c   If **NO** ☐ go to question 9

8a.   Do you have difficulty controlling your condition with medications or other physician-prescribed therapies? (Answer **NO** if you are not currently taking medications or other treatments)   YES☐ NO☐

8b.   Do you commonly exhibit low resting blood pressure significant enough to cause dizziness, light-headedness, and/or fainting?   YES☐ NO☐

8c.   Has your physician indicated that you exhibit sudden bouts of high blood pressure (known as Autonomic Dysreflexia)?   YES☐ NO☐

9.   **Have you had a Stroke?** *This includes Transient Ischemic Attack (TIA) or Cerebrovascular Event*

     If the above condition(s) is/are present, answer questions 9a-9c   If **NO** ☐ go to question 10

9a.   Do you have difficulty controlling your condition with medications or other physician-prescribed therapies? (Answer **NO** if you are not currently taking medications or other treatments)   YES☐ NO☐

9b.   Do you have any impairment in walking or mobility?   YES☐ NO☐

9c.   Have you experienced a stroke or impairment in nerves or muscles in the past 6 months?   YES☐ NO☐

10.   **Do you have any other medical condition not listed above or do you have two or more medical conditions?**

     If you have other medical conditions, answer questions 10a-10c   If **NO** ☐ read the Page 4 recommendations

10a.   Have you experienced a blackout, fainted, or lost consciousness as a result of a head injury within the last 12 months **OR** have you had a diagnosed concussion within the last 12 months?   YES☐ NO☐

10b.   Do you have a medical condition that is not listed (such as epilepsy, neurological conditions, kidney problems)?   YES☐ NO☐

10c.   Do you currently live with two or more medical conditions?   YES☐ NO☐

PLEASE LIST YOUR MEDICAL CONDITION(S) AND ANY RELATED MEDICATIONS HERE: _____

_____

GO to Page 4 for recommendations about your current medical condition(s) and sign the PARTICIPANT DECLARATION.

 OSHF
Ontario Society for Health and Fitness

Activity 1.2 Physical Activity Readiness Questionnaire (PAR-Q) *(continued)*

2015 PAR-Q+

☑ If you answered NO to all of the follow-up questions about your medical condition, you are ready to become more physically active - sign the PARTICIPANT DECLARATION below:

- ▶ It is advised that you consult a qualified exercise professional to help you develop a safe and effective physical activity plan to meet your health needs.

- ▶ You are encouraged to start slowly and build up gradually – 20 to 60 minutes of low to moderate intensity exercise, 3-5 days per week including aerobic and muscle strengthening exercises.

- ▶ As you progress, you should aim to accumulate 150 minutes or more of moderate intensity physical activity per week.

- ▶ If you are over the age of 45 years and **NOT** accustomed to regular vigorous to maximal effort exercise, consult a qualified exercise professional before engaging in this intensity of exercise.

⬤ If you answered YES to one or more of the follow-up questions about your medical condition:

You should seek further information before becoming more physically active or engaging in a fitness appraisal. You should complete the specially designed online screening and exercise recommendations program - the **ePARmed-X+ at www.eparmedx.com** and/or visit a qualified exercise professional to work through the ePARmed-X+ and for further information.

⚠ Delay becoming more active if:

- ✓ You have a temporary illness such as a cold or fever; it is best to wait until you feel better.

- ✓ You are pregnant – talk to your health care practitioner, your physician, a qualified exercise professional, and/or complete the ePARmed-X+ **at www.eparmedx.com** before becoming more physically active.

- ✓ Your health changes – talk to your doctor or a qualified exercise professional before continuing with any physical activity program.

- ⬤ You are encouraged to photocopy the PAR-Q+. You must use the entire questionnaire and NO changes are permitted.
- ⬤ The authors, the PAR-Q+ Collaboration, partner organizations, and their agents assume no liability for persons who undertake physical activity and/or make use of the PAR-Q+ or ePARmed-X+. If in doubt after completing the questionnaire, consult your doctor prior to physical activity.

PARTICIPANT DECLARATION

- ⬤ All persons who have completed the PAR-Q+ please read and sign the declaration below.

- ⬤ If you are less than the legal age required for consent or require the assent of a care provider, your parent, guardian or care provider must also sign this form.

I, the undersigned, have read, understood to my full satisfaction and completed this questionnaire. I acknowledge that this physical activity clearance is valid for a maximum of 12 months from the date it is completed and becomes invalid if my condition changes. I also acknowledge that a Trustee (such as my employer, community/fitness centre, health care provider, or other designate) may retain a copy of this form for their records. In these instances, the Trustee will be required to adhere to local, national, and international guidelines regarding the storage of personal health information ensuring that the Trustee maintains the privacy of the information and does not misuse or wrongfully disclose such information.

NAME _____   DATE _____

SIGNATURE _____   WITNESS _____

SIGNATURE OF PARENT/GUARDIAN/CARE PROVIDER _____

─── For more information, please contact ───
www.eparmedx.com
Email: eparmedx@gmail.com

Citation for PAR-Q+
Warburton DER, Jamnik VK, Bredin SSD, and Gledhill N on behalf of the PAR-Q+ Collaboration. The Physical Activity Readiness Questionnaire for Everyone (PAR-Q+) and Electronic Physical Activity Readiness Medical Examination (ePARmed-X+). Health & Fitness Journal of Canada 4(2):3-23, 2011.

Key References
1. Jamnik VK, Warburton DER, Makarski J, McKenzie DC, Shephard RJ, Stone J, and Gledhill N. Enhancing the effectiveness of clearance for physical activity participation; background and overall process. APNM 36(S1):S3-S13, 2011.
2. Warburton DER, Gledhill N, Jamnik VK, Bredin SSD, McKenzie DC, Stone J, Charlesworth S, and Shephard RJ. Evidence-based risk assessment and recommendations for physical activity clearance; Consensus Document. APNM 36(S1):S266-s298, 2011.

The PAR-Q+ was created using the evidence-based AGREE process (1) by the PAR-Q+ Collaboration chaired by Dr. Darren E. R. Warburton with Dr. Norman Gledhill, Dr. Veronica Jamnik, and Dr. Donald C. McKenzie (2). Production of this document has been made possible through financial contributions from the Public Health Agency of Canada and the BC Ministry of Health Services. The views expressed herein do not necessarily represent the views of the Public Health Agency of Canada or the BC Ministry of Health Services.

✝OSHF
Ontario Society for Health and Fitness

Copyright © 2015 PAR-Q+ Collaboration 4 / 4
08-01-2014

SOURCE: Physical Activity Readiness Questionnaire (PAR-Q) © 2015. Used with permission from the Canadian Society for Exercise Physiology www.csep.ca.

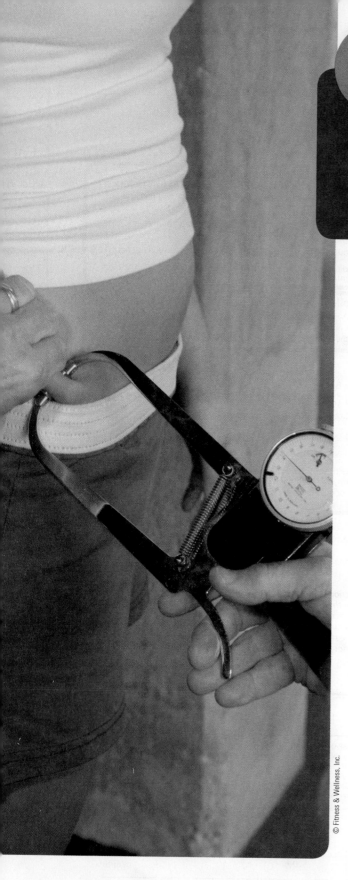

2

Assessment of Physical Fitness

"The assessment of physical fitness helps to determine your present fitness levels, serves as a starting point and provides an incentive to exercise, and allows you to evaluate progress and monitor changes throughout the years."

Objectives

> Identify the health-related components of physical fitness.

> Be able to assess cardiorespiratory fitness.

> Understand the difference between muscular strength and muscular endurance.

> Learn to assess muscular strength.

> Be able to assess muscular flexibility.

> Understand the components of body composition.

> Be able to assess body composition.

> Learn to determine recommended body weight.

> Learn to assess disease risk based on body mass index (BMI), waist circumference, and waist-to-height ratio.

REAL LIFE STORY | Jamie's Fitness Test Results

I didn't exercise a whole lot when I was in high school. I took a few years off from school to work and subsequently to get married. I always watched my weight and although not the athletic type, I felt that I was in shape. When I came back to school, I took a fitness class and the instructor required that we do all the health-related fitness tests. I couldn't run a mile-and-a-half, but it really surprised me that even for the 1-mile walk test I was only in the fair category. My strength and flexibility were fair and good, and although my BMI was in the acceptable category, my body fat was too high. The results of my fitness tests were an eye-opening experience and made sense based on my limited exercise time the last few years. I was determined to do something and started to exercise according to

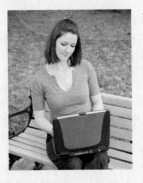
Allen/Shutterstock.com

what I learned in class. At the end of the term, I was proud of myself: My body fat was now better than the health fitness standard, and I was also able to do the mile-and-a-half test running the entire time and scoring in the good category. I am proud of my progress, and now in my second year, I still exercise regularly at the Student Rec Center.

Daily physical activity is the miracle medication that people are looking for. It makes you look and feel younger, boosts energy, provides lifetime weight management, improves self-confidence and self-esteem, and enhances independent living, health, and quality of life. It further allows you to enjoy a longer life by decreasing the risk of many chronic conditions, including heart disease, high blood pressure, stroke, diabetes, some cancers, and osteoporosis.

2.1 *The Value of Fitness Testing*

The health-related components of physical fitness—cardiorespiratory endurance, muscular fitness (strength and endurance), muscular flexibility, and body composition—are the topics of this chapter, along with basic techniques frequently used to assess these components. Through these assessment techniques you will be able to determine your level of physical fitness regularly as you engage in an exercise program. Fitness testing in a comprehensive program is important to:

1. Educate yourself regarding the various fitness components.
2. Assess your fitness level for each health-related fitness component and compare the results to health fitness and physical fitness standards.
3. Identify areas of weakness for training emphasis.
4. Motivate you to participate in exercise.
5. Use as a starting point for your personalized exercise prescriptions.

6. Evaluate the progress and effectiveness of your program.
7. Make adjustments in your exercise prescription, if necessary.
8. Reward yourself for complying with your exercise program (a change to a higher fitness level is a reward in and of itself).

You are encouraged to conduct at least pre- and post-exercise program fitness tests. A personal fitness profile is provided in Activity 2.1, page 55, for you to record the results of each fitness test in this chapter (pre-test). At the end of the term, you can use the post-test data form also provided in Activity 2.1 to record the results of your post-test.

In Chapter 3, you will learn to write personal fitness goals for this course (see Activity 3.4, page 98). You should base these goals on the actual results of your initial fitness assessments. As you proceed with your exercise program, you should allow a minimum of eight weeks before doing your post-fitness assessments.

As discussed in Chapter 1, exercise testing or exercise participation is not advised for individuals with certain medical or physical conditions. Therefore, before starting an exercise program or participating in any exercise testing, you should fill out the Physical Activity Readiness Questionnaire (PAR-Q) given in Chapter 1, Activity 1.2, page 26. A "yes" answer to any of the questions suggests that you consult a physician before initiating, continuing, or increasing your level of physical activity.

2.2 *Responders Versus Nonresponders*

Individuals who follow similar training programs show a wide variation in physiological responses. Heredity plays a crucial role in how each person responds to and improves after beginning an exercise program. Several studies have documented that following exercise training, most individuals, called **responders**, readily show improvements, but a few, **nonresponders**, exhibit small or no improvements at all. This concept is referred to as the **principle of individuality**.

After several months of cardiorespiratory endurance (aerobic) training, VO_{2max} increases are between 15 percent and 20 percent, on average, although individual responses can range from 0 percent (in a few selected cases) to more than 50 percent improvement, even when all participants follow exactly the same training program. Nonfitness and low-fitness participants, however, should not label themselves as nonresponders based on the previous discussion. Nonresponders constitute less than 5 percent of exercise participants. Some research indicates that lack of improvement in cardiorespiratory endurance among nonresponders might be related to low levels of leg strength. A lower body strength-training program has been shown to help these individuals improve VO_{2max} through aerobic exercise.[1]

Following assessment of cardiorespiratory endurance, if your fitness level is less than adequate, do not let that discourage you, but make it a priority to be physically active every day. In addition to regular exercise, lifestyle behaviors such as walking, taking stairs, cycling to work, parking farther from the office, doing household tasks, gardening, and doing yard work provide substantial benefits. In this regard, monitoring daily physical activity and exercise habits should be used in conjunction with fitness testing to evaluate compliance among nonresponders. After all, it is through increased daily activity that we reap the health benefits that improve quality of life.

2.3 *Fitness Assessment Battery*

No single test can provide a complete measure of physical fitness. Because health-related fitness has four components, a battery of tests is necessary to determine an individual's overall level of fitness. The next few pages include descriptions of several tests used to assess the health-related fitness components. When interpreting the results of fitness tests, two standards can be applied: health fitness and physical fitness.

Health Fitness Standard

As illustrated in Figure 2.1, although fitness (VO_{2max}—see discussion of cardiorespiratory endurance on page 33) improvements with a moderate aerobic activity program are not as notable, significant health benefits are reaped with such a program. Health benefits include a reduction in blood lipids; lower blood pressure; weight loss; stress release; and lower risk for type 2 diabetes and cardiovascular disease, certain cancers, and premature mortality.

More specifically, improvements in the **metabolic profile** (better insulin sensitivity and glucose tolerance and improved cholesterol levels) can be notable despite little or no improvement in aerobic capacity or weight loss. These improvements in the metabolic profile through an active lifestyle and moderate physical activity are referred to as **metabolic fitness**.

The health fitness (or criterion-referenced) standards used in this book are based on epidemiological data linking minimum fitness values to disease prevention and better health. Attaining the **health fitness standards** requires only moderate amounts of physical activity. For example, a 2-mile walk in less than 30 minutes, 5 to 6 times per week, seems to be sufficient to achieve the health fitness standard for cardiorespiratory endurance.

Figure 2.1 **Health and fitness benefits based on type of lifestyle and physical activity program.**

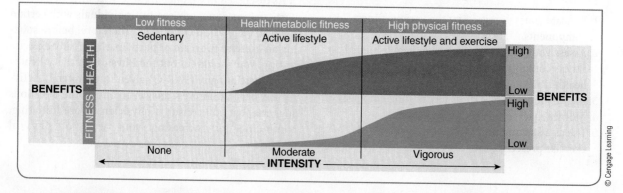

© Cengage Learning

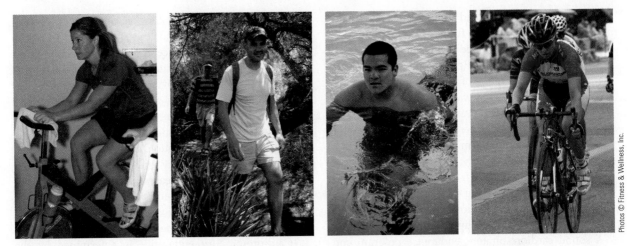

Aerobic activities promote cardiorespiratory development and help decrease the risk for chronic diseases.

Physical Fitness Standard

The **physical fitness standard** is set higher than the health fitness standard and requires a more vigorous exercise program. Whenever possible, participating in a vigorous exercise program is preferable because it provides even greater health and fitness benefits.[2] Such a program is recommended for individuals who wish to further improve personal fitness, reduce the risk for chronic disease and disabilities, prevent premature mortality, and prevent unhealthy weight gain.

By participating in vigorous exercise, physically fit people of all ages have the freedom to enjoy most of life's daily and recreational activities to their fullest potential. The current health fitness standards are not enough to achieve this goal.

Sound physical fitness gives the individual a level of independence throughout life that many people no longer enjoy. Most older people should be able to carry out activities similar to those they conducted in their youth, though not with the same intensity. Although a person does not have to be an elite athlete, activities such as changing a tire, chopping wood, climbing several flights of stairs, playing a game of basketball, mountain biking, playing soccer with grandchildren, walking several miles around a lake, and hiking through a national park require more than the "average fitness" level of the American people.

If the main objective of the fitness program is to lower the risk for disease, attaining the health fitness standards may be adequate to ensure better health. But if the individual wants to participate in moderate-to-vigorous fitness activities and further reduce the risk for chronic disease and premature mortality, achieving a high physical fitness standard is recommended. For the purposes of this book, both health fitness and physical fitness standards are given for each fitness test. You will have to decide your personal objectives for the fitness program.

2.4 *Cardiorespiratory Endurance*

Cardiorespiratory endurance is the single most important component of health-related physical fitness. The one possible exception occurs among older adults, for whom

---

GLOSSARY

Responders Individuals who exhibit improvements in fitness as a result of exercise training.

Nonresponders Individuals who exhibit small or no improvements in fitness as compared with others who undergo the same training program.

Principle of individuality Training concept that states that genetics plays a major role in individual responses to exercise training and that these differences must be considered when designing exercise programs for different people.

Metabolic profile Result of the assessment of diabetes and cardiovascular disease risk through plasma insulin, glucose, lipid, and lipoprotein levels.

Metabolic fitness Denotes improvements in the metabolic profile through a moderate-intensity exercise program despite little or no improvement in cardiorespiratory fitness.

Health fitness standard The lowest fitness requirements for maintaining good health, decreasing the risk for chronic diseases, and lowering the incidence of muscular/skeletal injuries.

Physical fitness standard Required criteria to achieve a high level of physical fitness; ability to do moderate-to-vigorous physical activity without undue fatigue.

Photos © Fitness & Wellness, Inc.

muscular fitness (strength and endurance) is particularly important to better maintain **functional independence**.

Aerobic exercise is viewed by scientists and sports medicine specialists as medicine of motion. We know that aerobic exercise is one of the most effective, affordable, and readily accessible "*medications*" available to all. Most chronic diseases improve and can be prevented through a daily routine of aerobic exercise. The myriad of immediate and long-term health benefits starts as soon as the individual begins the first exercise session. Aerobic exercise is especially important in preventing chronic conditions, including excessive body weight and obesity, diseases of the cardiovascular system, diabetes, some forms of cancer, and physical disability.

A sound cardiorespiratory endurance program contributes greatly to good health. The typical American is not exactly a good role model in terms of cardiorespiratory fitness. A poorly conditioned heart that has to pump more often just to keep a person alive is subject to more wear and tear than a well-conditioned heart. In situations that place strenuous demands on the heart, such as doing yard work, lifting heavy objects or weights, or running to catch a bus, the unconditioned heart may not be able to sustain the strain. Regular participation in aerobic activities also helps a person achieve and maintain recommended body weight—the fourth component of health-related physical fitness.

As a person breathes, part of the oxygen in the air is taken up in the lungs and transported in the blood to the heart. The heart then pumps the oxygenated blood through the circulatory system to all organs and tissues of the body. At the cellular level, oxygen is used to convert food substrates, primarily carbohydrates and fats, into the energy necessary to conduct body functions, maintain a constant internal equilibrium, and perform physical tasks.

Some examples of activities that promote **cardiorespiratory endurance**, or aerobic fitness, are brisk walking, jogging, elliptical training, cycling, spinning, rowing, swimming, cross-country skiing, aerobics, soccer, basketball, and racquetball. Guidelines to develop a lifetime cardiorespiratory endurance exercise program are given in Chapter 3, and an introduction and description of benefits of leading aerobic activities are given in Chapter 4.

Everyone who initiates a cardiorespiratory exercise program can expect a number of benefits from training. Among these are lower resting heart rate, blood pressure, low-grade body inflammation, blood lipids (cholesterol and triglycerides), recovery time following exercise, and risk for hypokinetic diseases (those associated with physical inactivity and sedentary living). Simultaneously, cardiac muscle strength, oxygen-carrying capacity, and aerobic capacity all increase.

Cardiorespiratory endurance is determined by the **maximal oxygen uptake**, or **VO_{2max}**, the maximum amount of oxygen the human body is able to utilize per minute of physical activity. This value can be expressed in liters per minute (L/min) or milliliters per kilogram (2.2 pounds) of body weight per minute (mL/kg/min). The relative value in mL/kg/min is used most often because it considers total body mass (weight) in kilograms. When comparing two individuals with the same absolute value, the one with the lesser body mass will have a higher relative value, indicating that more oxygen is available to each kilogram (2.2 pounds) of body weight. Because all tissues and organs of the body need oxygen to function, higher oxygen consumption indicates a more efficient cardiorespiratory system.

Critical Thinking

While your absolute maximal oxygen uptake remains unchanged, your relative maximal oxygen uptake can increase without engaging in an aerobic exercise program. • How can you accomplish this, and would you benefit from doing so?

Physical exertion requires more energy to perform the activity than sedentary living. As a result, the heart, lungs, and blood vessels have to deliver more oxygen to the cells to supply the required energy. During prolonged exercise, an individual with a high level of cardiorespiratory endurance is able to deliver the required amount of oxygen to the tissues with relative ease. The cardiorespiratory system of a person with a low level of endurance has to work much harder, as the heart has to pump more often to supply the same amount of oxygen to the tissues and consequently fatigues faster. Hence, a higher capacity to deliver and utilize oxygen (oxygen uptake) indicates a more efficient cardiorespiratory system.

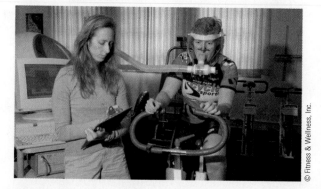

© Fitness & Wellness, Inc.

Maximal oxygen uptake (VO_{2max}) can be determined through direct gas analysis.

Oxygen uptake, expressed in L/min, is valuable in determining the caloric expenditure of physical activity. The human body burns about 5 calories for each liter of oxygen consumed, and oxygen uptake ranges from about .3 to .5 L/min during resting conditions to about 3 L/min during maximal exercise for moderately fit individuals and over 5 L/min in highly conditioned athletes. During aerobic exercise, the average person trains at between 50 and 75 percent of maximal oxygen uptake. Thus, we burn between 1.5 to 2.5 calories/min at rest to a range of 7 to 12 calories/min during vigorous-intensity aerobic exercise.

Let's use a practical illustration. A person with a maximal oxygen uptake of 3.5 L/min who trains at 60 percent of maximum uses 2.1 (3.5 × .60) liters of oxygen per minute of physical activity. This indicates that 10.5 calories are burned during each minute of exercise (2.1 × 5). If the activity is carried out for 30 minutes, 315 calories (10.5 × 30) have been burned. Because a pound of body fat represents 3,500 calories, the previous example indicates that this individual would have to exercise for a total of 333 minutes (3,500 ÷ 10.5) to burn the equivalent of a pound of body fat. At 30 minutes per exercise session, approximately 11 sessions would be required to expend the 3,500 calories, as long as there is no greater caloric intake (caloric compensation) as a result of the exercise program.

Assessing Cardiorespiratory Endurance

Even though most cardiorespiratory endurance tests probably are safe to administer to apparently healthy individuals (those with no heart disease risk factors or symptoms), the American College of Sports Medicine recommends that men over age 45 and women over age 55 with an additional heart disease risk factor have a physician present for all maximal exercise tests.[3]

A maximal test is any test that requires the participant's all-out or nearly all-out effort, such as the 1.5-Mile Run Test or a maximal exercise treadmill test (stress electrocardiogram). For submaximal exercise tests (such as a walking test), a physician should be present when testing higher-risk and symptomatic individuals, regardless of age.

1.5-Mile Run Test

The test used most often to determine cardiorespiratory endurance is the 1.5-Mile Run Test. The fitness category is determined according to the time a person takes to run or walk a 1.5-mile course. The only equipment necessary to conduct this test is a stopwatch and a track or a premeasured 1.5-mile course.

Although the 1.5-Mile Run Test is quite simple to administer, a note of caution is in order: As the objective is to cover the distance in the shortest time, it is considered a maximal exercise test. The 1.5-Mile Run Test should be limited to conditioned individuals who have been cleared for exercise. It is not recommended for unconditioned beginners, symptomatic individuals, those with known cardiovascular disease or risk factors for heart disease, and men over age 45 and women over age 55. Unconditioned beginners are encouraged to have at least 6 weeks of aerobic training before they take the test.

Prior to taking the 1.5-Mile Run Test, you should do a few warm-up exercises—some stretching exercises, some walking, and slow jogging. Next, time yourself during the 1.5-Mile Run to see how fast you cover the distance. If you notice any unusual symptoms during the test, do not continue. Stop immediately and see your physician, or retake the test after another six weeks of aerobic training. At the end of the test, cool down by walking or jogging slowly for another three to five minutes. Referring to your performance time, look up your estimated VO_{2max} in Table 2.1 and the corresponding fitness category in Table 2.2.

For example, a 20-year-old female runs the 1.5-mile course in 12 minutes and 40 seconds. Table 2.1 shows a VO_{2max} of 39.8 mL/kg/min for a time of 12:40. According to Table 2.2, this VO_{2max} places her in the good cardiorespiratory fitness category.

1.0-Mile Walk Test*

The 1.0-Mile Walk Test calls for a 440-yard track (four laps to a mile) or a premeasured 1.0-mile course. Body weight in pounds must be determined prior to the walk. A stopwatch is required to measure total walking time and exercise heart rate.

You can proceed to walk the 1-mile course at a brisk pace so the exercise heart rate at the end of the test is above 120 beats per minute. At the end of the 1.0-mile walk, check your walking time and immediately count your pulse for 10 seconds. You can take your pulse on the

---

*SOURCE: Dolgener, F.A., et al. "Validation of the Rockport Fitness Walking Test in College Males and Females," *Research Quarterly for Exercise and Sport*, 65 (1994): 152–158.

GLOSSARY

Functional independence The ability to carry out activities of daily living without assistance from other individuals.

Cardiorespiratory endurance Ability of the lungs, heart, and blood vessels to deliver adequate amounts of oxygen to the cells to meet the demands of prolonged physical activity.

Maximal oxygen uptake (VO_{2max}) Maximum amount of oxygen the human body is able to utilize per minute of physical activity.

Table 2.1 Estimated Maximal Oxygen Uptake (in mL/kg/min) for 1.5-Mile Run Test

Time	VO_{2max}	Time	VO_{2max}	Time	VO_{2max}
6:10	80.0	10:30	48.6	14:50	34.0
6:20	79.0	10:40	48.0	15:00	33.6
6:30	77.9	10:50	47.4	15:10	33.1
6:40	76.7	11:00	46.6	15:20	32.7
6:50	75.5	11:10	45.8	15:30	32.2
7:00	74.0	11:20	45.1	15:40	31.8
7:10	72.6	11:30	44.4	15:50	31.4
7:20	71.3	11:40	43.7	16:00	30.9
7:30	69.9	11:50	43.2	16:10	30.5
7:40	68.3	12:00	42.0	16:20	30.2
7:50	66.8	12:10	41.7	16:30	29.8
8:00	65.2	12:20	41.0	16:40	29.5
8:10	63.9	12:30	40.4	16:50	29.1
8:20	62.5	12:40	39.8	17:00	28.9
8:30	61.2	12:50	39.2	17:10	28.5
8:40	60.2	13:00	38.6	17:20	28.3
8:50	59.1	13:10	38.1	17:30	28.0
9:00	58.1	13:20	37.8	17:40	27.7
9:10	56.9	13:30	37.2	17:50	27.4
9:20	55.9	13:40	36.8	18:00	27.1
9:30	54.7	13:50	36.3	18:10	26.8
9:40	53.5	14:00	35.9	18:20	26.6
9:50	52.3	14:10	35.5	18:30	26.3
10:00	51.1	14:20	35.1	18:40	26.0
10:10	50.4	14:30	34.7	18:50	25.7
10:20	49.5	14:40	34.3	19:00	25.4

Adapted from "A Means of Assessing Maximal Oxygen Intake," by K. H. Cooper, Journal of the American Medical Association, 203 (1968), 201–204; Health and Fitness Through Physical Activity, by M. L. Pollock (New York: John Wiley and Sons, 1978); and Training for Sport Activity, by J. H. Wilmore (Boston: Allyn & Bacon, 1982).

wrist by placing two fingers over the radial artery (inside of the wrist on the side of the thumb) or over the carotid artery in the neck just below the jaw next to the voice box.

Next, multiply the 10-second pulse count by 6 to obtain the exercise heart rate in beats per minute. Now convert the walking time from minutes and seconds to minute units. Each minute has 60 seconds, so the seconds are divided by 60 to obtain the fraction of a minute. For instance, a walking time of 12 minutes and 15 seconds equals $12 + (15 \div 60)$, or 12.25 minutes. To obtain the estimated VO_{2max} in mL/kg/min for the 1.0-Mile Walk Test, plug your values into the following equation:

$$VO_{2max} = 88.768 - (0.0957 \times W) + (8.892 \times G) - (1.4537 \times T) - (0.1194 \times HR)$$

where:

W = weight in pounds
G = gender (use 0 for women and 1 for men)
T = total time for the mile walk in minutes
HR = exercise heart rate in beats per minute at the end of the mile walk

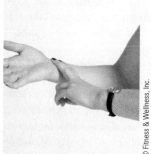

Taking the pulse at the radial artery.

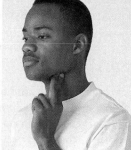

Taking the pulse at the cartoid artery.

Table 2.2 Cardiorespiratory Fitness Category According to Maximal Oxygen Uptake (in mL/kg/min)

Gender	Age	Fitness Category				
		Poor	Fair	Average	Good	Excellent
Men	≤29	≤24.9	25–33.9	34–43.9	44–52.9	≥53
	30–39	≤22.9	23–30.9	31–41.9	42–49.9	≥50
	40–49	≤19.9	20–26.9	27–38.9	39–44.9	≥45
	50–59	≤17.9	18–24.9	25–37.9	38–42.9	≥43
	60–69	≤15.9	16–22.9	23–35.9	36–40.9	≥41
Women	≤29	≤23.9	24–30.9	31–38.9	39–48.9	≥49
	30–39	≤19.9	20–27.9	28–36.9	37–44.9	≥45
	40–49	≤16.9	17–24.9	25–34.9	35–41.9	≥42
	50–59	≤14.9	15–21.9	22–33.9	34–39.9	≥40
	60–69	≤12.9	13–20.9	21–32.9	33–36.9	≥37

◻ High physical fitness standard   ◻ Health fitness or criterion-referenced standard

---

Behavior Modification Planning

Tips to Increase Daily Physical Activity

Adults need recess, too! There are 1,440 minutes in every day. Schedule a minimum of 30 of these minutes for physical activity. With a little creativity and planning, even the person with the busiest schedule can make room for physical activity. For many folks, before or after work or meals is often an available time to cycle, walk, or play. Think about your weekly or daily schedule and look for or make opportunities to be more active. Every little bit helps. Consider the following suggestions:

- Walk, cycle, jog, skate, etc., to school, work, the store, or place of worship.
- Use a pedometer to count your daily steps.
- Walk while doing errands.
- Get on or off the bus several blocks away.
- Park the car farther away from your destination.
- At work, walk to nearby offices instead of sending e-mails or using the phone.
- Walk or stretch a few minutes every hour that you are at your desk.
- Take fitness breaks—walking or doing desk exercises—instead of taking cigarette breaks or coffee breaks.
- Incorporate activity into your lunch break (walk to the restaurant).
- Take the stairs instead of the elevator or escalator.
- Play with children, grandchildren, or pets. Everybody wins. If you find it too difficult to be active after work, try it before work.

- Do household tasks.
- Work in the yard or garden.
- Avoid labor-saving devices. Turn off the self-propelled option on your lawnmower or vacuum cleaner.
- Use leg power. Take small trips on foot to get your body moving.
- Exercise while watching TV (for example, use hand weights, stationary bicycle/treadmill/stairclimber, or stretch).
- Spend more time playing sports than sitting in front of the TV or the computer.
- Dance to music.
- Keep a pair of comfortable walking or running shoes in your car and office. You'll be ready for activity wherever you go!
- Make a Saturday morning walk a group habit.
- Learn a new sport or join a sports team.
- Avoid carts when golfing.
- When out of town, stay in hotels with fitness centers.

Try It

Keep a three-day log of all your activities. List the activities performed, time of day, and how long you were engaged in these activities. You may be surprised by your findings.

SOURCE: Adapted from Centers for Disease Control and Prevention, Atlanta, 2013.

For example, a woman who weighs 140 pounds completed the mile walk in 14 minutes and 39 seconds with an exercise heart rate of 148 beats per minute. The estimated VO_{2max} is:

$$W = 140 \text{ lbs.}$$
$$G = 0 \text{ (female gender = 0)}$$
$$T = 14{:}39 = 14 + (39 \div 60) = 14.65 \text{ min}$$
$$HR = 148 \text{ bpm}$$
$$VO_{2max} = 88.768 - (0.0957 \times 140) + (8.892 \times 0) - (1.4537 \times 14.65) - (0.1194 \times 148)$$
$$VO_{2max} = 36.4 \text{ mL/kg/min}$$

As with the 1.5-Mile Run Test, the fitness categories based on VO_{2max} are found in Table 2.2. Record your cardiorespiratory fitness test results on your fitness profile in Activity 2.1, Pre-Test, page 55.

2.5 *Muscular Fitness*

Adequate levels of strength enhance a person's health and well-being throughout life. The need for good **muscular fitness** is not confined to highly trained athletes, fitness

---

GLOSSARY

Muscular fitness A term used to define good levels of both muscular strength and muscular endurance.

enthusiasts, or individuals who have jobs that require heavy muscular work. In fact, a well-planned strength-training program leads to increased muscle strength and endurance, muscle tone, tendon and ligament strength, and bone density—all of which help to improve and maintain everyday functional physical capacity.

Strength is crucial for top performance in daily activities such as sitting, walking, running, lifting and carrying objects, doing housework, and even enjoying recreational activities. Strength is also valuable in improving personal appearance and self-image, developing sports skills, promoting stability of joints, and meeting certain emergencies in life in which strength is necessary to cope effectively.

Good strength helps to increase or maintain muscle and a higher resting metabolic rate; encourages weight loss and maintenance, which prevents obesity; lessens the risk for injury; reduces chronic low back pain; reduces pressure on the joints, alleviating arthritic pain; aids in childbearing; improves bone density, which prevents osteoporosis; improves cholesterol levels, decreases triglyceride levels, and reduces high blood pressure, thus reducing the risk for cardiovascular disease and premature mortality; and promotes psychological well-being. Furthermore, it decreases the risk of developing physical function limitations and the overall risk of nonfatal disease. Muscular strength has also been shown to be inversely associated with all-cause mortality; the lower the strength level, the higher the risk for early mortality.[4]

Muscular strength also seems to be the most important health-related component of physical fitness in the older-adult population. Whereas proper cardiorespiratory endurance helps maintain a healthy heart, good strength levels do more to promote independent living than any other fitness component. More than anything else, older adults want to enjoy good health and function independently. Many, however, are confined to nursing homes because they lack sufficient strength to move about. They usually cannot walk very far, and some have to be helped in and out of beds, chairs, and tubs.

A common occurrence as people age is **sarcopenia** (the loss of muscle mass), a loss of strength and function. How much of this loss of muscle mass is related to the aging process itself or to actual physical inactivity and faulty nutrition is unknown. Sarcopenia leads to mobility disability and loss of independence. Estimates indicate that half of all adults 65 and older in the United States currently suffer from age-related muscle loss. Early muscle loss doesn't appear to bother them or hold them back. They think they are fine until they lose functional independence; at that point they realize the serious mistake made and subsequent loss of quality of life.

Regular strength training also helps control blood sugar. Much of the blood glucose from food consumption goes to the muscles, where it is stored as glycogen. When muscles are not used, muscle cells may become insulin resistant, and glucose cannot enter the cells, thereby increasing the risk for type 2 diabetes. Research data have clearly shown that a regular strength-training program improves blood glucose control in both diabetic men and women. Furthermore, across all ages, the greater the amount of muscle mass, relative to body size, the better the insulin sensitivity and the lower the risk for diabetes.

A strength-training program can have a tremendous impact on quality of life. Research has shown leg strength improvements as high as 200 percent in previously inactive adults over age 90.[5] As strength improves, so does the ability to move about, the capacity for independent living, and life enjoyment during the "golden years."

Because of the many health benefits provided by a regular muscular fitness training program, the American Medical Association (AMA), the American Heart Association (AHA), the American College of Sports Medicine, the American Diabetic Association (ADA), and the CDC have offered strong support of strength training as an exercise modality to promote health and prevent disease.

More specifically, good strength enhances quality of life in the following ways:

- It increases lean (muscle) tissue.
- It stresses the bones, preserves bone density, and decreases the risk for osteoporosis.
- It provides support and stability to the skeletal structure (bones and joints).
- It helps increase and maintain **resting metabolism**.
- It encourages weight loss and maintenance.
- It improves balance and restores mobility.
- It makes lifting and reaching easier.
- It decreases the risk for injuries and falls.
- It reduces chronic low back pain and alleviates arthritic pain.
- It lowers cholesterol, high blood pressure, and the risk for developing diabetes.
- It promotes psychological well-being.

Furthermore, with time, regular strength training decreases the heart rate and blood pressure response to lifting a heavy resistance (a weight). This adaptation reduces the demands on the cardiovascular system when performing activities such as carrying a child, the groceries, or a suitcase.

Muscular Strength and Muscular Endurance

Although **muscular strength** and **muscular endurance** are interrelated, the two have a basic difference. Muscular strength is the ability to exert maximum force against resistance. Muscular endurance (also called localized muscular endurance) is the ability of the muscle to exert submaximal force repeatedly over a period of time. Muscular endurance depends to a large extent on muscular strength and to a lesser extent on cardiorespiratory endurance. Weak muscles cannot repeat an action several times or sustain it for long. Keeping these concepts in mind, strength tests and training programs have been designed to measure and develop absolute muscular strength, muscular endurance, or a combination of the two.

Determining Strength

Muscular strength usually is determined using the **one repetition maximum (1 RM)** technique. Although this assessment gives a good measure of absolute strength, it does require a basic skill level and a considerable amount of time to administer. Muscular endurance commonly is established by the number of repetitions an individual can perform against a submaximal resistance or by the length of time a person can sustain a given contraction.

Muscular Endurance Test

We live in a world in which muscular strength and endurance are both required, and muscular endurance depends to a large extent on muscular strength. Accordingly, a muscular endurance test has been selected to determine the level of strength. Three exercises that help assess endurance of the upper body, lower body, and mid-body muscle groups have been selected for your muscular endurance test. To perform the test, you will need a stopwatch, a metronome, a bench or gymnasium bleacher 16¼" high, and a partner.

The exercises conducted for this test are the Bench Jump, Modified Dip (men) or Modified Push-Up (women), and Bent-Leg Curl-Up. Individuals who are susceptible to low back injury may do the Abdominal Crunch (see discussion on page 40) instead of the Bent-Leg Curl-Up test. All tests should be conducted with the aid of a partner. The correct procedures for performing these exercises follow.

Bench Jump For the Bench Jump, use a bench or gymnasium bleacher 16¼" high, and attempt to jump up and down on the bench as many times as you can in 1 minute. If you cannot jump the full minute, step up and down. A repetition is counted each time both feet return to the floor.

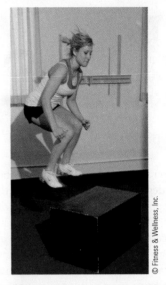

Bench jump.

Modified Dip The Modified Dip is an upper-body exercise that is done by men only. Using a bench or gymnasium bleacher, place your hands on the bench with the fingers pointing forward. Have a partner hold your feet in front of you. Bend your hips at approximately 90 degrees (you also may use three sturdy chairs; put your hands on two chairs placed by the sides of your body and your feet on the third chair in front of you).

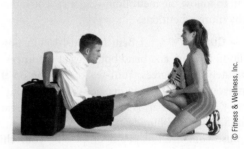

Modified dip.

GLOSSARY

Sarcopenia Age-related loss of lean body mass, strength, and function.

Resting metabolism The energy requirement to maintain the body's vital processes in the resting state.

Muscular strength Ability to exert maximum force against resistance.

Muscular endurance Ability of a muscle to exert submaximal force repeatedly over a period of time.

One repetition maximum (1 RM) The maximal amount of resistance a person is able to lift in a single effort.

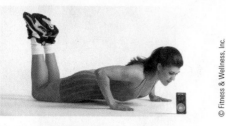

Modified push-up.

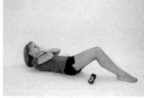

Bent-leg curl-up.

Next, lower your body by flexing your elbows until you reach a 90-degree angle at this joint, and then return to the starting position. The repetition does not count if you fail to reach 90 degrees. Perform the repetitions to a two-step cadence (down–up), regulated with a metronome set at 56 beats per minute. Perform as many continuous repetitions as possible. If you fail to follow the metronome cadence, you can no longer count the repetitions.

Modified Push-Up Women perform the Modified Push-Up instead of the Modified Dip. Lie down on the floor (face down), bend your knees (feet up in the air), and place your hands on the floor by your shoulders with the fingers pointing forward. Your lower body will be supported at the knees (rather than the feet) throughout the test. Your chest must touch the floor on each repetition.

Perform the repetitions to a two-step cadence (up–down) regulated with a metronome set at 56 beats per minute. Do as many continuous repetitions as possible. If you fail to follow the metronome cadence, you cannot count any more repetitions.

Bent-Leg Curl-Up For the Bent-Leg Curl-Up, lie down on the floor, face up, and bend both legs at the knees at approximately 100 degrees. Your feet should be on the floor, and you must hold them in place yourself throughout the test. Cross your arms in front of your chest, each hand on the opposite shoulder.

Now raise your head off the floor, placing your chin against your chest. This is the starting and finishing position for each curl-up. The back of the head may not come in contact with the floor, the hands cannot be removed from the shoulders, and neither the feet nor the hips can be raised off the floor at any time during the test. The test is terminated if any of these four conditions occur. When you curl up, your upper body must come to an upright position before going back down. The repetitions are performed to a two-step cadence (up–down) regulated with the metronome set at 40 beats per minute.

For this exercise, you should allow a brief practice period of 5 to 10 seconds to familiarize yourself with the cadence. (The up movement is initiated with the first beat, then you must wait for the next beat to initiate the down movement; one repetition is accomplished every two beats of the metronome.) Count as many repetitions as you are able to perform following the proper cadence. The test is terminated if you fail to maintain the appropriate cadence or if you accomplish 100 repetitions. Have your partner check the angle at the knees throughout the test to make sure that you maintain the 100-degree angle as closely as possible.

Abdominal Crunch The Abdominal Crunch is recommended only for individuals who are unable to perform the Bent-Leg Curl-Up because of susceptibility to low back injury. Exercise form must be monitored carefully during the test because many participants have difficulty maintaining proper form during this test. People often slide their bodies, bend their elbows, or shrug their shoulders during the test.

These actions make the test easier and misrepresent performance. Further, lack of spinal flexibility does not allow some individuals to move the required (3½″) range of motion. Others are unable to keep their heels on the floor during the test. Some research has questioned the validity of this test as an effective measure of abdominal strength or abdominal endurance.[6,7] With these caveats in mind, the procedure is as follows.

Tape a 3½″ × 30″ strip of cardboard onto the floor. Lie on the floor in a supine position (face up) with your knees bent at approximately 100 degrees and your legs slightly apart. Your feet should be on the floor, and you must hold them in place yourself throughout the test. Straighten your arms, and place them on the floor alongside your trunk with your palms down and fingers fully extended. The fingertips of both hands should barely touch the closest edge of the cardboard.

Bring your head off the floor until your chin is 1″ to 2″ away from your chest. Keep your head in this position during the entire test. (Do not move your head by flexing or extending the neck.) You now are ready to begin the test.

Perform the repetitions to a two-step cadence (up–down) regulated with a metronome set at 60 beats per minute. As you curl up, slide your fingers over the cardboard until your fingertips reach the far end (3½″) of the board, then return to the starting position.

Allow a brief practice period of about 10 seconds to familiarize yourself with the cadence. Initiate the up

Table 2.3 Muscular Endurance Scoring Table

	MEN					**WOMEN**			
	Repetitions					**Repetitions**			
Fitness Category	Bench Jumps	Modified Dips	Bent-Leg Curl-Ups	Abdominal Crunches	Fitness Category	Bench Jumps	Modified Push-Ups	Bent-Leg Curl-Ups	Abdominal Crunches
Excellent	≥59	≥33	≥52	≥67	Excellent	≥49	≥42	≥78	≥50
Good	57–58	28–32	32–51	39–66	Good	43–48	34–41	46–77	35–49
Average	52–56	24–27	26–31	30–38	Average	39–42	29–33	29–45	28–34
Fair	48–51	18–23	18–25	23–29	Fair	33–38	22–28	18–28	22–27
Poor	≤47	≤17	≤17	≤22	Poor	≤32	≤21	≤17	≤21

High physical fitness standard

Health fitness standard

(Adapted from W. W. K. Hoeger & S. A. Hoeger, Lifetime Physical Fitness & Wellness: A Personalized Program, Belmont, CA: Wadsworth Cengage Learning, 2015).

Table 2.4 Points for Each Test Item Based on Fitness Category

Fitness Category	Points
Excellent	5
Good	4
Average	3
Fair	2
Poor	1

© Cengage Learning

Table 2.5 Muscular Strength/Endurance Fitness Categories by Total Points

Total Points	Strength Endurance Category
≥13	Excellent
10–12	Good
7–9	Average
4–6	Fair
≤3	Poor

© Cengage Learning

movement with the first beat and the down movement with the next beat. Accomplish one repetition every two beats of the metronome. Count as many repetitions as you are able to perform while following the proper cadence. You may not count a repetition if your fingertips fail to reach the distant end of the cardboard.

Terminate the test if you (a) fail to maintain the appropriate cadence, (b) bend your elbows, (c) shrug your shoulders, (d) slide your body, (e) fail to keep your heels on the floor, (f) do not keep your chin close to your chest, (g) accomplish 100 repetitions, or (h) can no longer perform the test. Have your partner check the angle at the knees throughout the test to make sure you maintain the 100-degree angle as closely as possible. For this test you also may use a Crunch-Ster Curl-Up Tester, available from Novel Products.*

Interpreting the Strength Test

According to the number of repetitions you performed on each test item, look up the fitness category for each exercise in Table 2.3. Next, look up the number of points

*Novel Products Inc., Figure Finder Collection, P.O. Box 408, Rockton, IL 61072-0408; (800) 323-5143.

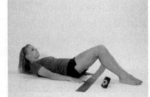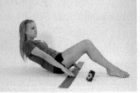

Abdominal crunch.

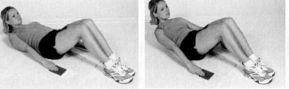

Abdominal crunch test using a Crunch-Ster Curl-Up Tester.

assigned for each test item's fitness category in Table 2.4. Now total the points and determine your overall strength endurance fitness category according to the ratings provided in Table 2.5.

Record the results of your strength tests in Activity 2.1, Pre-Test, page 55.

2.6 *Muscular Flexibility*

Flexibility refers to the achievable range of motion at a joint or group of joints without causing injury. Most people who exercise don't take the time to stretch. And many of those who do stretch don't stretch properly. When joints are not regularly moved through their full range of motion, muscles and ligaments shorten in time, and flexibility decreases.

Developing and maintaining some level of flexibility are important factors in all health enhancement programs, and even more so as we age. Good flexibility promotes healthy muscles and joints. Sports medicine specialists believe that many muscular/skeletal problems and injuries, especially in adults, are related to a lack of flexibility. At times in daily life we have to make rapid or strenuous movements we are not accustomed to making. A tight muscle that is abruptly forced beyond its normal range of motion often leads to injuries.

Improving elasticity of muscles and connective tissue around joints enables greater freedom of movement and the individual's ability to participate in many types of sports and recreational activities. Adequate flexibility also makes activities of daily living such as turning, lifting, and bending easier to perform. A person must take care, however, not to overstretch joints. Too much flexibility leads to unstable and loose joints, which may actually increase the injury rate.

A decline in flexibility can cause poor posture and subsequent aches and pains that lead to limited movement of joints. Inordinate tightness is uncomfortable and debilitating. Approximately 80 percent of all low back problems in the United States stem from improper alignment of the vertebral column and pelvic girdle, a direct result of inflexible and weak muscles. This backache syndrome costs U.S. industry billions of dollars each year in lost productivity, health services, and workers' compensation.

Muscular flexibility is highly specific and varies from one joint to the other (hip, trunk, and shoulder), as well as from one individual to the next. Muscular flexibility relates primarily to genetic factors and the index of physical activity. Beyond that, factors such as joint structure, ligaments, tendons, muscles, skin, tissue injury, adipose (fat) tissue, body temperature, age, and gender influence the range of motion about a joint.

On average, women are more flexible than men and seem to retain this advantage throughout life. Aging decreases the extensibility of soft tissue, decreasing flexibility in both genders. The most significant contributors to loss of flexibility, however, are sedentary living and lack of physical activity.

Most experts agree that participating in a regular flexibility program has the following benefits.

- It helps to maintain good joint mobility.
- It increases resistance to muscle injury and soreness.
- It prevents low back and other spinal column problems.
- It improves and maintains good postural alignment.
- It enhances proper and graceful body movement.
- It improves personal appearance and self-image.
- It facilitates the development of motor skills throughout life.

Flexibility exercises also have been prescribed successfully to treat **dysmenorrhea**[8] (painful menstruation), general neuromuscular tension (stress), and knots (trigger points) in muscles and fascia. Regular **stretching** helps decrease the aches and pains caused by psychological stress and contributes to a decrease in anxiety, blood pressure, and breathing rate.[9]

Further, mild stretching exercises, in conjunction with calisthenics, are helpful in warm-up routines to prepare the body for more vigorous aerobic or strength-training exercises, and as cool-down routines following exercise to help the person return to a normal resting state. Fatigued muscles tend to contract to a shorter-than-average resting length, and stretching exercises help fatigued muscles reestablish their normal resting length.

Similar to muscular strength, good range of motion is critical in older life. Because of decreased flexibility, older adults lose mobility and are unable to perform simple daily tasks such as bending forward and turning. Many older adults do not turn their head or rotate their trunk to look over their shoulder but, rather, step around 90 degrees to 180 degrees to see behind them.

Physical activity and exercise also can be hampered severely by restricted range of motion. Because of the pain involved during activity, older people who have tight hip flexors (muscles) cannot jog or walk very far. A vicious circle ensues, because the condition usually worsens with further inactivity. A simple stretching program can alleviate or prevent this problem and help people return to an exercise program.

Assessing Flexibility

Two flexibility tests are used to produce a flexibility profile: the Modified Sit-and-Reach Test and the Finger Touch Test.

Starting position for modified sit-and-reach test.

Modified sit-and-reach test.

Finger touch test.

© Fitness & Wellness, Inc.

Table 2.6 Modified Sit-and-Reach Scoring Table

Fitness Category	Score (inches)	
	Men	Women
Excellent	≥17.25	≥17.00
Good	15.25–17.00	16.00–16.75
Average	13.75–15.00	14.75–15.75
Fair	11.75–13.50	12.75–14.50
Poor	≤11.50	≤12.50

High physical fitness standard

Health fitness standard

(Adapted from W. W. K. Hoeger & S. A. Hoeger, Lifetime Physical Fitness & Wellness: A Personalized Program, Belmont, CA: Wadsworth Cengage Learning, 2015).

Modified Sit-and-Reach Test

To perform the Modified Sit-and-Reach Test, you will need the Acuflex I* sit-and-reach flexibility tester, or you may simply place a yardstick on top of a box approximately 12" high. The test is used to assess hamstring (back of the thighs) and low back flexibility. To administer this test:

1. Warm up properly before the first trial.
2. Remove your shoes for the test. Sit on the floor with your hips, back, and head against a wall, legs fully extended and the bottom of your feet against the Acuflex I or the sit-and-reach box.
3. Place your hands one on top of the other, and reach forward as far as possible without letting your hips, back, or head come off the wall.
4. Another person then should slide the reach indicator on the Acuflex I (or yardstick) along the top of the box until the end of the indicator touches the tips of your fingers. The indicator then must be held firmly in place throughout the rest of the test.
5. Your head and back now can come off the wall, and you may reach forward gradually three times, the third time stretching forward as far as possible on the indicator (or yardstick), holding the final position at least two seconds. Be sure to keep the back of your knees against the floor throughout the test.
6. Record to the nearest half inch the final number of inches you reached.
7. You are allowed two trials, and an average of the two scores is used as the final test score.

The fitness categories based on the number of inches reached are given in Table 2.6 and the number of points achieved for this test are found in Table 2.4.

Finger Touch Test

The Finger Touch Test is used to assess shoulder flexibility. The following procedure is used to administer the test:

1. Warm up properly by doing a few shoulder stretches before beginning this test.

2. Bring your right hand over your right shoulder and reach down the middle of your back as far down as possible with the fingers extended and pointing straight down to the ground.
3. Simultaneously as you are reaching down your back with the right hand, place your left hand behind your lower back with the palm facing out and gradually slide the hand with fingers extended as far up as possible.
4. The objective of the test is to bring the tips of the fingers as close together or overlap as much as possible behind your back, holding the final reached position for two seconds.
5. With the aid of a partner, measure to the nearest half inch the distance between the tips of the fingers or the amount of overlap between the fingers. If you are unable to touch or overlap your fingers, the distance between the fingers is recorded as a negative score. If your fingers touch but do not overlap, the score equals zero (0). If the fingers overlap, carefully measure the amount of overlap and report it as a positive score. Conduct the test twice and use an average of the two trials as the final score.
6. Now repeat the test on the left side (bring the left hand over the left shoulder and the right hand behind the lower back). Do two trials and average the final score.
7. Refer to Table 2.7 and Table 2.4 to determine the respective fitness categories and number of points for each side test.

*The Acuflex I flexibility tests can be obtained from Novel Products Inc., Figure Finder Collection, P.O. Box 408, Rockton, IL 61072-0408; (800) 323-5143.

GLOSSARY

Flexibility The achievable range of motion at a joint or group of joints without causing injury.

Dysmenorrhea Painful menstruation.

Stretching Moving the joints beyond the accustomed range of motion.

Table 2.7 Finger Touch Scoring Table

| | Score (inches) | | | | |
| | Men | | | Women | |
Fitness Category	Right	Left		Right	Left
Excellent	≥3.25	≥2.25		≥4.50	≥3.75
Good	1.75 to 3.00	0.25 to 2.00		3.25 to 4.25	1.75 to 3.50
Average	−0.75 to 1.50	−3.75 to 0.00		2.25 to 3.00	1.25 to 1.50
Fair	−2.75 to −1.00	−5.75 to −4.00		0.50 to 2.00	0.25 to 1.00
Poor	≤−3.00	≤−6.00		≤0.25	≤0.00

▨ High physical fitness standard

▨ Health fitness standard

SOURCE: W. W. K. Hoeger, Finger Touch Test, Data collected in the Department of Kinesiology, Boise State University, 2010.

Table 2.8 Muscular Flexibility Fitness Categories by Total Points

Total Points	Flexibility Category
≥9	Excellent
7–8	Good
5–6	Average
3–4	Fair
≤2	Poor

© Cengage Learning

Overall Flexibility Fitness

To obtain an overall flexibility fitness category, use the number of points given for the Modified Sit and Reach Test and the best result only (either right or left side) for the Finger Touch Test. Total the number of points obtained for these two tests (based on each fitness category—see Table 2.4) and determine the overall fitness category using the guidelines provided in Table 2.8. Record your flexibility test results in Activity 2.1, Pre-Test, page 55.

2.7 *Body Composition*

Obesity is a health hazard of epidemic proportions in the United States and most developed countries throughout the world. Trends indicate that adults in the United States gain 1 to 2 pounds of weight per year. Thus, during a span of 40 years, the average American will have gained 40 to 80 pounds. Because of the typical reduction in physical activity in our society, however, the average person also loses a half a pound of lean tissue each year. Therefore, this span of 40 years has produced an actual fat gain of 60 to 100 pounds accompanied by a 20-pound loss of lean body mass (Figure 2.2). These changes cannot be detected without assessing body composition periodically.

Body composition refers to the fat and nonfat components of the human body. The fat component of the body usually is called fat mass or **percent body fat**. The nonfat component of the body is termed **lean body mass**.

Total fat in the human body is classified into two types: essential fat and storage fat. **Essential fat** is the body fat needed for normal physiological functions. Essential fat constitutes about 3 percent of the total weight in men and 12 percent in women (see Figure 2.3). The percentage is higher in women because it includes gender-specific fat, such as that found in the breast

Figure 2.2 Typical body composition changes for adults in United States.

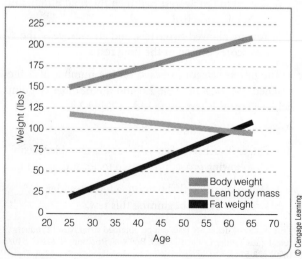

© Cengage Learning

Figure 2.3 Typical body composition of adult man and adult woman.

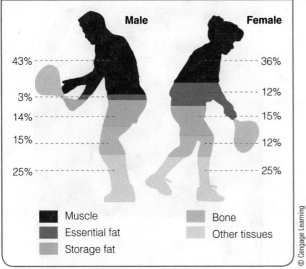

Male   Female

43% ----   ---- 36%

3% ----   ---- 12%

14% ----   ---- 15%

15% ----   ---- 12%

25% ----   ---- 25%

■ Muscle   ■ Bone
■ Essential fat   ■ Other tissues
■ Storage fat

© Cengage Learning

Figure 2.4 Percentage of the adult population (20 years and older) that is overweight (BMI ≥25) and obese (BMI ≥30) in the United States.

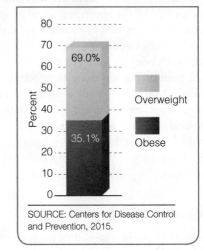

SOURCE: Centers for Disease Control and Prevention, 2015.

tissue, the uterus, and other gender-related fat deposits. Without it, human health deteriorates. **Storage fat**, the body fat stored in adipose tissue, is found mostly beneath the skin (subcutaneous fat) and around major organs in the body.

Obesity by itself has been associated with several serious health problems and accounts for 15 percent to 20 percent of the annual mortality rate in the United States. It is one of the six major risk factors for coronary heart disease. It also is a risk factor for other diseases of the cardiovascular system, including hypertension, congestive heart failure, elevated blood lipids, atherosclerosis, strokes, thromboembolitic disease, varicose veins, and intermittent claudication. Sixty-nine percent of the adult population in the United States is either overweight or obese (see Figure 2.4).

Underweight people, too, have health problems and a higher mortality rate. Although the social pressure to be thin has waned slightly in recent years, pressure to attain model-like thinness is still with us and contributes to the gradual increase in incidence of eating disorders (such as anorexia nervosa and bulimia nervosa, discussed in Chapter 5). Extreme weight loss can spawn medical conditions such as heart damage, gastrointestinal problems, shrinkage of internal organs, immune system abnormalities, disorders of the reproductive system, loss of muscle tissue, damage to the nervous system, and even death.

For many years, people relied on height/weight charts to determine **recommended body weight**, but we now know that these tables are highly inaccurate for many people. The standard height/weight tables, first published in 1912, were based on average weights (including shoes and clothing) for men and women who obtained life insurance policies between 1888 and 1905. The recommended weight on height/weight tables is obtained according to gender, height, and frame size. As no scientific guidelines are given to determine frame size, most people choose their frame size based on the column where the weight comes closest to their own!

The proper way to determine recommended weight is to find out what percent of total body weight is fat and what amount is lean tissue (body composition). Once the fat percentage is known, recommended weight can be calculated from recommended body fat.

Obesity is related to an excess of body fat. If body weight is the only criterion, an individual easily can be considered overweight according to height/weight charts, yet not be genuinely obese. Typical examples are football

GLOSSARY

Body composition The fat and nonfat components of the human body.

Percent body fat (fat mass) Fat component of the body.

Lean body mass Nonfat component of the body.

Essential fat Body fat needed for normal physiological functions.

Storage fat Body fat stored in adipose tissue.

Recommended body weight The weight at which there appears to be no harm to human health.

players, body builders, weight lifters, and other athletes with large muscle size. Some athletes who appear to be 20 or 30 pounds overweight really have little body fat.

At the other end of the spectrum, some people who weigh very little and are viewed by many as "skinny" or underweight actually can be classified as overweight because of their high body fat content. People who weigh as little as 120 pounds but are more than 30 percent fat (about a third of their total body weight) are not rare. These people often are sedentary or are dieting constantly. Physical inactivity and constant negative caloric balance both lead to a loss in lean body mass (see Chapter 6). Body weight alone clearly does not always tell the true story.

Assessing Body Composition

Body composition can be assessed through several procedures. The most common techniques are skinfold thickness; girth measurements; bioelectrical impedance; hydrostatic or underwater weighing; and to a lesser extent, air displacement, and dual energy X-ray absorptiometry (DXA). These procedures all yield estimates of body fat; thus, each technique may yield slightly different values. Therefore, when assessing body composition, the same technique should be used for pre- and post-test comparisons.

DXA is most frequently used in research and by medical facilities. A radiographic technique, DXA uses very low-dose beams of X-ray energy (hundreds of times lower than a typical body X-ray) to measure total body fat mass, fat distribution pattern (see "Waist Circumference" on page 48), and bone density. Many exercise scientists consider DXA to be the standard technique to assess body composition.

Hydrostatic or underwater weighing is commonly used in exercise physiology laboratories. In essence, a person's "regular" weight is compared with a weight taken underwater. Because fat is more buoyant than lean tissue, comparing the two weights can determine a person's percent of fat.

Air displacement uses computerized pressure sensors to determine the amount of air displaced by a person sitting inside an airtight chamber. Body volume is calculated by subtracting the air volume with the person inside the chamber from the volume of the empty chamber. This technique, however, tends to significantly overestimate percent body fat, and additional research is needed to make it an acceptable technique to determine body composition.

Bioelectrical impedance is much simpler to administer, but its accuracy is highly questionable. In this

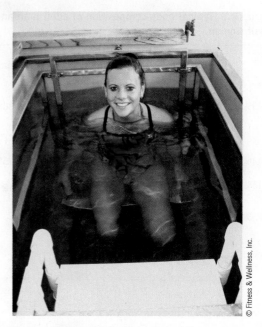

Hydrostatic weighing technique used for assessing body composition.

technique, sensors are applied to the skin and a weak (totally painless) electrical current is run through the body to estimate body fat, lean body mass, and body water. The technique is based on the principle that fat tissue is a less efficient conductor of electrical current than lean tissue is. The easier the conductance, the leaner the individual. Body weight scales with sensors on the surface are also available to perform this procedure, but again, the accuracy is highly questionable.

The technique discussed in this section is skinfold thickness, the most common and practical technique available to assess body composition. Three additional techniques, not used to assess body composition but used to determine excessive body weight, are body mass index, waist circumference, and waist-to-height ratio. These are also discussed in this section.

Skinfold Thickness

Assessment of body composition is done most frequently using skinfold thickness. This technique is based on the principle that approximately half of the body's fatty tissue is directly beneath the skin. Valid and reliable estimates of this tissue give a good indication of percent body fat.

The skinfold thickness test is performed with the aid of pressure calipers. To reflect the total percentage of fat, three sites are measured:

- For women: triceps, suprailium, and thigh
- For men: chest, abdomen, and thigh

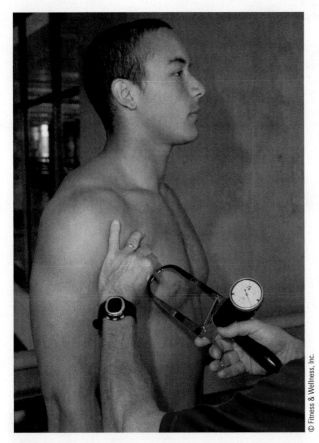

Skinfold thickness technique used for assessing body composition.

All measurements are taken on the right side of the body with the person standing. The correct anatomical landmarks for skinfolds are as follows and are also shown in Figure 2.5.

- Chest: a diagonal fold halfway between the shoulder crease and the nipple
- Abdomen: a vertical fold about one inch to the right of the umbilicus
- Triceps: a vertical fold on the back of the upper arm, halfway between the shoulder and the elbow
- Thigh: a vertical fold on the front of the thigh, midway between the knee and the hip
- Suprailium: a diagonal fold above the crest of the ilium (on the side of the hip)

Each site is measured by grasping a double thickness of skin firmly with the thumb and forefinger, pulling the fold slightly away from the muscle tissue. Hold the calipers perpendicular to the fold, and take the measurements half an inch below the finger hold. Measure each site three times, and read the values to the nearest .1 to .5 mm. Record the average of the two closest readings as the final value. Take the readings without delay to avoid excessive

compression of the skinfold. Releasing and refolding the skinfold is required between readings. Be sure to wear shorts, a loose-fitting T-shirt (no leotards), and do not use lotion on your skin the day when skinfolds are to be taken.

After determining the average value for each site, percent fat can be obtained by adding together all three skinfold measurements and looking up the respective values in Table 2.9 for women and Table 2.10 for men. You can record your results in Activity 2.1, Pre-Test, page 55. Then compute your recommended body weight using the range given in Table 2.11 and the computation form in Activity 2.2, page 57.

The recommended percent body fat values given in Table 2.11 include essential fat and storage fat, discussed previously. For example, the recommended body fat range for women under age 30 is 17 percent to 25 percent. This indicates that only 5 percent to 13 percent of the total recommended fat is storage fat and the other 12 percent is essential fat. The recommended range has been selected based on research indicating that some storage fat is required for optimal health and greater longevity.

The recommended body fat range selected in this book incorporates the recommendations of most health and fitness experts throughout the United States. If you desire to have just one target weight, you may select your body weight according to your personal preference, as long as it falls within the recommended range. The lower end of the range constitutes the physical fitness standard; the high end represents the health fitness standard.

Body Mass Index

Another technique scientists use to determine thinness and excessive fatness is the **body mass index (BMI)**. This index incorporates height and weight to estimate critical fat values at which the risk for disease increases. BMI is calculated by dividing the weight in kilograms by the square of the height in meters or multiplying your weight in pounds by 705 and dividing this figure by the square of the height in inches. For example, the BMI for an individual who weighs 172 pounds (78 kg) and is 67 inches (1.7 meters) tall would be 27 $[78 \div (1.7)^2]$ or $[172 \times 705 \div (67)^2]$.

Because of its simplicity and measurement consistency across populations, BMI is used almost exclusively to determine health risks and mortality rates associated with excessive body weight. You can compute and record

GLOSSARY

Body mass index (BMI) An index that incorporates height and weight to estimate critical fat values at which risk for disease increases.

Figure 2.5 Anatomical landmarks for skinfold measurements.

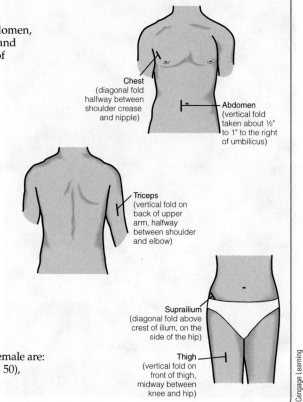

SKINFOLD MEASUREMENT

1. Select the proper anatomical sites. For men, use chest, abdomen, and thigh skinfolds. For women, use triceps, suprailium, and thigh skinfolds. Take all measurements on the right side of the body with the person standing.

2. Measure each site by grasping a double thickness of skin firmly with the thumb and forefinger, pulling the fold slightly away from the muscular tissue. Hold caliper perpendicular to the fold, and take the measurement one-half inch below the finger hold. Measure each site three times and read the values to the nearest .1 to .5 mm. Record the average of the two closest readings as the final value. Take the readings without delay to avoid excessive compression of the skinfold. Release and refold the skinfold between readings.

3. When doing pre- and post-assessments, conduct the measurement at the same time of day. The best time is early in the morning to avoid water hydration changes resulting from activity or exercise.

4. Obtain percent fat by adding the three skinfold measurements and looking up the respective values.

For example, if the skinfold measurements for an 18-year-old female are: (a) triceps = 16, (b) suprailium = 4, and (c) thigh = 30 (total = 50), the percent body fat is 20.6%.

Chest
(diagonal fold halfway between shoulder crease and nipple)

Abdomen
(vertical fold taken about ½" to 1" to the right of umbilicus)

Triceps
(vertical fold on back of upper arm, halfway between shoulder and elbow)

Suprailium
(diagonal fold above crest of ilium, on the side of the hip)

Thigh
(vertical fold on front of thigh, midway between knee and hip)

© Cengage Learning

your own BMI and recommended body weight according to BMI guidelines using the form provided in Activity 2.2 (pages 57–58). You also can obtain your BMI for selected weights and heights by looking it up in Table 2.12.

According to the BMI, the lowest risk for chronic disease is in the 22 to 25 range (see Table 2.13). Individuals are classified as overweight between 25 and 30. BMIs above 30 are defined as obesity and below 18.5 as underweight. Compared to individuals with a BMI between 22 and 25, people with a BMI between 25 and 30 (overweight) exhibit mortality rates up to 25 percent higher; rates for those with a BMI above 30 (obese) are 50 percent to 100 percent higher.[10] BMI is a useful tool to screen the general population, but, similar to height/weight charts, it fails to differentiate fat from lean body mass or where most of the fat is located. Using BMI, strength-trained individuals and athletes with a large amount of muscle mass (such as body builders and football players) easily can fall in the moderate- or even high-risk categories. Therefore, body composition and waist-to-hip ratios are better procedures to determine health risk and recommended body weight.

Waist Circumference

Scientific evidence suggests that the way people store fat affects their risk for disease. The total amount of body fat by itself is not the best predictor of increased risk for disease but rather the location of the fat. **Android obesity** is seen in individuals who tend to store fat in the trunk or abdominal area (which produces the "apple" shape). **Gynoid obesity** is seen in people who store fat primarily around the hips and thighs (which creates the "pear" shape).

Obese individuals with abdominal fat are clearly at higher risk for heart disease, hypertension, type 2

GLOSSARY

Android obesity Obesity pattern seen in individuals who tend to store fat in the trunk or abdominal area.

Gynoid obesity Obesity pattern seen in people who store fat primarily around the hips and thighs.

Table 2.9 **Percent Fat Estimates for Women, Calculated from Triceps, Suprailium, and Thigh Skinfold Thickness**

Sum of 3 Skinfolds	Under 22	23 to 27	28 to 32	33 to 37	38 to 42	43 to 47	48 to 52	53 to 57	Over 58
				Age					
23–25	9.7	9.9	10.2	10.4	10.7	10.9	11.2	11.4	11.7
26–28	11.0	11.2	11.5	11.7	12.0	12.3	12.5	12.7	13.0
29–31	12.3	12.5	12.8	13.0	13.3	13.5	13.8	14.0	14.3
32–34	13.6	13.8	14.0	14.3	14.5	14.8	15.0	15.3	15.5
35–37	14.8	15.0	15.3	15.5	15.8	16.0	16.3	16.5	16.8
38–40	16.0	16.3	16.5	16.7	17.0	17.2	17.5	17.7	18.0
41–43	17.2	17.4	17.7	17.9	18.2	18.4	18.7	18.9	19.2
44–46	18.3	18.6	18.8	19.1	19.3	19.6	19.8	20.1	20.3
47–49	19.5	19.7	20.0	20.2	20.5	20.7	21.0	21.2	21.5
50–52	20.6	20.8	21.1	21.3	21.6	21.8	22.1	22.3	22.6
53–55	21.7	21.9	22.1	22.4	22.6	22.9	23.1	23.4	23.6
56–58	22.7	23.0	23.2	23.4	23.7	23.9	24.2	24.4	24.7
59–61	23.7	24.0	24.2	24.5	24.7	25.0	25.2	25.5	25.7
62–64	24.7	25.0	25.2	25.5	25.7	26.0	26.2	26.4	26.7
65–67	25.7	25.9	26.2	26.4	26.7	26.9	27.2	27.4	27.7
68–70	26.6	26.9	27.1	27.4	27.6	27.9	28.1	28.4	28.6
71–73	27.5	27.8	28.0	28.3	28.5	28.8	29.0	29.3	29.5
74–76	28.4	28.7	28.9	29.2	29.4	29.7	29.9	30.2	30.4
77–79	29.3	29.5	29.8	30.0	30.3	30.5	30.8	31.0	31.3
80–82	30.1	30.4	30.6	30.9	31.1	31.4	31.6	31.9	32.1
83–85	30.9	31.2	31.4	31.7	31.9	32.2	32.4	32.7	32.9
86–88	31.7	32.0	32.2	32.5	32.7	32.9	33.2	33.4	33.7
89–91	32.5	32.7	33.0	33.2	33.5	33.7	33.9	34.2	34.4
92–94	33.2	33.4	33.7	33.9	34.2	34.4	34.7	34.9	35.2
95–97	33.9	34.1	34.4	34.6	34.9	35.1	35.4	35.6	35.9
98–100	34.6	34.8	35.1	35.3	35.5	35.8	36.0	36.3	36.5
101–103	35.2	35.4	35.7	35.9	36.2	36.4	36.7	36.9	37.2
104–106	35.8	36.1	36.3	36.6	36.8	37.1	37.3	37.5	37.8
107–109	36.4	36.7	36.9	37.1	37.4	37.6	37.9	38.1	38.4
110–112	37.0	37.2	37.5	37.7	38.0	38.2	38.5	38.7	38.9
113–115	37.5	37.8	38.0	38.2	38.5	38.7	39.0	39.2	39.5
116–118	38.0	38.3	38.5	38.8	39.0	39.3	39.5	39.7	40.0
119–121	38.5	38.7	39.0	39.2	39.5	39.7	40.0	40.2	40.5
122–124	39.0	39.2	39.4	39.7	39.9	40.2	40.4	40.7	40.9
125–127	39.4	39.6	39.9	40.1	40.4	40.6	40.9	41.1	41.4
128–130	39.8	40.0	40.3	40.5	40.8	41.0	41.3	41.5	41.8

Body density is calculated based on the generalized equation for predicting body density of women developed by A. S. Jackson, M. L. Pollock, and A. Ward, reported in *Medicine and Science in Sports and Exercise*, 12 (1980), 175–182. Percent body fat is determined from the calculated body density using the Siri formula.

Table 2.10 Percent Fat Estimates for Men Calculated from Chest, Abdomen, and Thigh Skinfold Thickness

Sum of 3 Skinfolds	Under 19	20 to 22	23 to 25	26 to 28	29 to 31	32 to 34	35 to 37	38 to 40	41 to 43	44 to 46	47 to 49	50 to 52	53 to 55	56 to 58	59 to 61	Over 62
8–10	.9	1.3	1.6	2.0	2.3	2.7	3.0	3.3	3.7	4.0	4.4	4.7	5.1	5.4	5.8	6.1
11–13	1.9	2.3	2.6	3.0	3.3	3.7	4.0	4.3	4.7	5.0	5.4	5.7	6.1	6.4	6.8	7.1
14–16	2.9	3.3	3.6	3.9	4.3	4.6	5.0	5.3	5.7	6.0	6.4	6.7	7.1	7.4	7.8	8.1
17–19	3.9	4.2	4.6	4.9	5.3	5.6	6.0	6.3	6.7	7.0	7.4	7.7	8.1	8.4	8.7	9.1
20–22	4.8	5.2	5.5	5.9	6.2	6.6	6.9	7.3	7.6	8.0	8.3	8.7	9.0	9.4	9.7	10.1
23–25	5.8	6.2	6.5	6.8	7.2	7.5	7.9	8.2	8.6	8.9	9.3	9.6	10.0	10.3	10.7	11.0
26–28	6.8	7.1	7.5	7.8	8.1	8.5	8.8	9.2	9.5	9.9	10.2	10.6	10.9	11.3	11.6	12.0
29–31	7.7	8.0	8.4	8.7	9.1	9.4	9.8	10.1	10.5	10.8	11.2	11.5	11.9	12.2	12.6	12.9
32–34	8.6	9.0	9.3	9.7	10.0	10.4	10.7	11.1	11.4	11.8	12.1	12.4	12.8	13.1	13.5	13.8
35–37	9.5	9.9	10.2	10.6	10.9	11.3	11.6	12.0	12.3	12.7	13.0	13.4	13.7	14.1	14.4	14.8
38–40	10.5	10.8	11.2	11.5	11.8	12.2	12.5	12.9	13.2	13.6	13.9	14.3	14.6	15.0	15.3	15.7
41–43	11.4	11.7	12.1	12.4	12.7	13.1	13.4	13.8	14.1	14.5	14.8	15.2	15.5	15.9	16.2	16.6
44–46	12.2	12.6	12.9	13.3	13.6	14.0	14.3	14.7	15.0	15.4	15.7	16.1	16.4	16.8	17.1	17.5
47–49	13.1	13.5	13.8	14.2	14.5	14.9	15.2	15.5	15.9	16.2	16.6	16.9	17.3	17.6	18.0	18.3
50–52	14.0	14.3	14.7	15.0	15.4	15.7	16.1	16.4	16.8	17.1	17.5	17.8	18.2	18.5	18.8	19.2
53–55	14.8	15.2	15.5	15.9	16.2	16.6	16.9	17.3	17.6	18.0	18.3	18.7	19.0	19.4	19.7	20.1
56–58	15.7	16.0	16.4	16.7	17.1	17.4	17.8	18.1	18.5	18.8	19.2	19.5	19.9	20.2	20.6	20.9
59–61	16.5	16.9	17.2	17.6	17.9	18.3	18.6	19.0	19.3	19.7	20.0	20.4	20.7	21.0	21.4	21.7
62–64	17.4	17.7	18.1	18.4	18.8	19.1	19.4	19.8	20.1	20.5	20.8	21.2	21.5	21.9	22.2	22.6
65–67	18.2	18.5	18.9	19.2	19.6	19.9	20.3	20.6	21.0	21.3	21.7	22.0	22.4	22.7	23.0	23.4
68–70	19.0	19.3	19.7	20.0	20.4	20.7	21.1	21.4	21.8	22.1	22.5	22.8	23.2	23.5	23.9	24.2
71–73	19.8	20.1	20.5	20.8	21.2	21.5	21.9	22.2	22.6	22.9	23.3	23.6	24.0	24.3	24.7	25.0
74–76	20.6	20.9	21.3	21.6	22.0	22.2	22.7	23.0	23.4	23.7	24.1	24.4	24.8	25.1	25.4	25.8
77–79	21.4	21.7	22.1	22.4	22.8	23.1	23.4	23.8	24.1	24.5	24.8	25.2	25.5	25.9	26.2	26.6
80–82	22.1	22.5	22.8	23.2	23.5	23.9	24.2	24.6	24.9	25.3	25.6	26.0	26.3	26.6	27.0	27.3
83–85	22.9	23.2	23.6	23.9	24.3	24.6	25.0	25.3	25.7	26.0	26.4	26.7	27.1	27.4	27.8	28.1
86–88	23.6	24.0	24.3	24.7	25.0	25.4	25.7	26.1	26.4	26.8	27.1	27.5	27.8	28.2	28.5	28.9
89–91	24.4	24.7	25.1	25.4	25.8	26.1	26.5	26.8	27.2	27.5	27.9	28.2	28.6	28.9	29.2	29.6
92–94	25.1	25.5	25.8	26.2	26.5	26.9	27.2	27.5	27.9	28.2	28.6	28.9	29.3	29.6	30.0	30.3
95–97	25.8	26.2	26.5	26.9	27.2	27.6	27.9	28.3	28.6	29.0	29.3	29.7	30.0	30.4	30.7	31.1
98–100	26.6	26.9	27.3	27.6	27.9	28.3	28.6	29.0	29.3	29.7	30.0	30.4	30.7	31.1	31.4	31.8
101–103	27.3	27.6	28.0	28.3	28.6	29.0	29.3	29.7	30.0	30.4	30.7	31.1	31.4	31.8	32.1	32.5
104–106	27.9	28.3	28.6	29.0	29.3	29.7	30.0	30.4	30.7	31.1	31.4	31.8	32.1	32.5	32.8	33.2
107–109	28.6	29.0	29.3	29.7	30.0	30.4	30.7	31.1	31.4	31.8	32.1	32.4	32.8	33.1	33.5	33.8
110–112	29.3	29.6	30.0	30.3	30.7	31.0	31.4	31.7	32.1	32.4	32.8	33.1	33.5	33.8	34.2	34.5
113–115	30.0	30.3	30.7	31.0	31.3	31.7	32.0	32.4	32.7	33.1	33.4	33.8	34.1	34.5	34.8	35.2
116–118	30.6	31.0	31.3	31.6	32.0	32.3	32.7	33.0	33.4	33.7	34.1	34.4	34.8	35.1	35.5	35.8
119–121	31.3	31.6	32.0	32.3	32.6	33.0	33.3	33.7	34.0	34.4	34.7	35.1	35.4	35.8	36.1	36.5
122–124	31.9	32.2	32.6	32.9	33.3	33.6	34.0	34.3	34.7	35.0	35.4	35.7	36.1	36.4	36.7	37.1
125–127	32.5	32.9	33.2	33.5	33.9	34.2	34.6	34.9	35.3	35.6	36.0	36.3	36.7	37.0	37.4	37.7
128–130	33.1	33.5	33.8	34.2	34.5	34.9	35.2	35.5	35.9	36.2	36.6	36.9	37.3	37.6	38.0	38.5

Body density is calculated based on the generalized equation for predicting body density of men developed by A. S. Jackson and M. L. Pollock, *British Journal of Nutrition*, 40 (1978), 497–504. Percent body fat is determined from the calculated body density using the Siri formula.

Table 2.11 Recommended Body Composition According to Percent Body Fat

Age	Males	Females
≤29	12–20%	17–25%
30–49	13–21%	18–26%
≥50	14–22%	19–27%

High physical fitness standard

Health fitness or criterion referenced standard

© Cengage Learning

diabetes ("non–insulin-dependent" diabetes), stroke, some types of cancer, dementia, migraines, and diminished lung function. Evidence also indicates that among individuals with a lot of abdominal fat, those whose fat deposits are located around internal organs (intra-abdominal or visceral fat) rather than subcutaneously or retroperitoneally (see Figure 2.6) have an even greater risk for disease than those with fat mainly just beneath the skin (subcutaneous fat).[11] Of even greater significance, the results of a recent study that followed more than 350,000 people over almost 10 years concluded that

Table 2.12 Body Mass Index

Height	Weight																												
	110	115	120	125	130	135	140	145	150	155	160	165	170	175	180	185	190	195	200	205	210	215	220	225	230	235	240	245	250
5'0"	21	22	23	24	25	26	27	28	29	30	31	32	33	34	35	36	37	38	39	40	41	42	43	44	45	46	47	48	49
5'1"	21	22	23	24	25	26	26	27	28	29	30	31	32	33	34	35	36	37	38	39	40	41	42	43	43	44	45	46	47
5'2"	20	21	22	23	24	25	26	27	27	28	29	30	31	32	33	34	35	36	37	37	38	39	40	41	42	43	44	45	46
5'3"	19	20	21	22	23	24	25	26	27	27	28	29	30	31	32	33	34	35	35	36	37	38	39	40	41	42	43	43	44
5'4"	19	20	21	21	22	23	24	25	26	27	27	28	29	30	31	32	33	33	34	35	36	37	38	39	39	40	41	42	43
5'5"	18	19	20	21	22	22	23	24	25	26	27	27	28	29	30	31	32	32	33	34	35	36	37	37	38	39	40	41	42
5'6"	18	19	19	20	21	22	23	23	24	25	26	27	27	28	29	30	31	31	32	33	34	35	36	36	37	38	39	40	40
5'7"	17	18	19	20	20	21	22	23	23	24	25	26	27	27	28	29	30	31	31	32	33	34	34	35	36	37	38	38	39
5'8"	17	17	18	19	20	21	21	22	23	24	24	25	26	27	27	28	29	30	30	31	32	33	33	34	35	36	36	37	38
5'9"	16	17	18	18	19	20	21	21	22	23	24	24	25	26	27	27	28	29	30	30	31	32	32	33	34	35	35	36	37
5'10"	16	17	17	18	19	19	20	21	22	22	23	24	24	25	26	27	27	28	29	29	30	31	32	32	33	34	34	35	36
5'11"	15	16	17	17	18	19	20	20	21	22	22	23	24	24	25	26	26	27	28	29	29	30	31	31	32	33	33	34	35
6'00"	15	16	16	17	18	18	19	20	20	21	22	22	23	24	24	25	26	26	27	28	28	29	30	31	31	32	33	33	34
6'1"	15	15	16	16	17	18	18	19	20	20	21	22	22	23	24	24	25	26	26	27	28	28	20	30	30	31	32	32	33
6'2"	14	15	15	16	17	17	18	19	19	20	21	21	22	22	23	24	24	25	26	26	27	28	28	29	30	30	31	31	32
6'3"	14	14	15	16	16	17	17	18	19	19	20	21	21	22	22	23	24	24	25	26	26	27	27	28	29	29	30	31	31
6'4"	13	14	15	15	16	16	17	18	18	19	19	20	21	21	22	23	23	24	24	25	26	26	27	27	28	29	29	30	30

© Cengage Learning

Table 2.13 Disease Risk According to Body Mass Index (BMI)

BMI	Disease Risk	Category
<18.5	Increased	Underweight
18.5–21.99	Low	Acceptable
22.0–24.99	Very low	Acceptable
25.0–29.99	Increased	Overweight
30.0–34.99	High	Obesity I
35.0–39.99	Very high	Obesity II
>40.0	Extremely high	Obesity III

© Cengage Learning

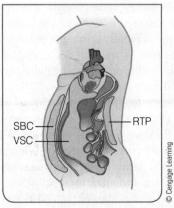

Figure 2.6 Visceral (VSC) fat is a greater risk factor for heart disease, stroke, hypertension, diabetes, and cancer than subcutaneous (SBC) or retroperitoneal (RTP) fat.

SBC
VSC
RTP

© Cengage Learning

Table 2.14 Disease Risk According to Waist Circumference (WC)

Men	Women	Disease Risk
>35.5	<32.5	Low
35.5–40.0	32.5–35.0	Moderate
>40.0	>35.0	High

© Cengage Learning

Table 2.15 Health Categories According to Waist-to-Height Ratio (WHtR)

Category	WHtR (Waist/Height)	Disease Risk
	<.4	Increased
Acceptable (OK)	.4–.5	Very low
Take Care	.5–.7	Increased
Take Action	>.7	Highest

Adapted from Expert Panel, "Executive Summary of the Clinical Guidelines on the Identification, Evaluation, and Treatment of Overweight and Obesity in Adults," Archives of Internal Medicine 158 (1998): 1855–1867.

even when body weight is viewed as "normal," individuals with a large waist circumference nearly double the risk for premature death.[12] Researchers believe that visceral fat secretes harmful inflammatory substances that contribute to chronic conditions.

Complex scanning techniques to identify individuals at risk because of high intra-abdominal fatness are costly, so a simple **waist circumference (WC)** measure, designed by the National Heart, Lung, and Blood Institute, is used to assess this risk. WC seems to predict abdominal visceral fat as accurately as DXA. A WC of more than 40 inches in men and 35 inches in women indicates a higher risk for cardiovascular disease, hypertension, and type 2 diabetes (see Table 2.14). Thus, weight loss is encouraged when individuals exceed these measurements.

> **! Critical Thinking**
>
> How do you feel about your current body weight? • What influence does society have on the way you perceive yourself in terms of your weight? • Do the results from your body composition measurements make you feel any different about the way you see your current body weight and image?

Waist-to-Height Ratio: "Keep your waist Circumference to Less Than Half Your Height."

The **waist-to-height ratio (WHtR)** is a new health risk assessment also used to ascertain the health risks of obesity. The ratio is rapidly gaining popularity in the scientific community as research indicates that it is better predictor of health outcomes, including multiple coronary heart disease risk factors, than BMI or WC.[13] While WC is superior to BMI, two individuals with a similar WC (e.g., 43) but of different heights, may not be at the same risk for disease, whereas the new WHtR method discriminates between individuals of different heights.

A systematic review of the literature that included 31 research studies, including more than 300,000 adults of several ethnic groups, showed that WHtR has significantly greater discriminatory power in predicting cardiac and metabolic complications as compared to BMI and WC.[14] Another study presented at the 2013 European Congress on Obesity compared the effect of abdominal obesity on life expectancy in terms of years of life lost. The data showed that a 30-year-old man with a BMI greater than 40 has a years-of-life-lost value of 10.5 years as compared to 16.7 years using the most severe category of the WHtR. A 30-year-old woman in these same categories loses 5.3 years of life using BMI as a calculator as compared to 9.5 years using WHtR.[15]

WHtR is determined by dividing the waist circumference in inches by the height in inches. As illustrated in Table 2.15, a ratio of .4 to .5 indicates the lowest risk for disease, whereas less than .4 or between .5 and .7 require "care" to decrease health risks, and a ratio of .7 or greater requires "action" to conform with the lowest health risk category of .4 to .5. An example of the WHtR for a person with a WC of 32 inches and a height of 68 inches (5'8") would be .47 (32 ÷ 68). The findings of many of these studies have prompted researchers to promote a public health message indicating that you should "keep your waist circumference to less than half your height."

2.8 *Effects of Exercise and Diet on Body Composition*

If you engage in a diet and exercise program, you should repeat body composition measurements about once a month to monitor changes in lean and fat tissue. This is

---GLOSSARY---

Waist circumference (WC) A waist girth measurement to assess potential risk for disease based on intra-abdominal fat content.

Waist-to-height ratio (WHtR) A ratio to determine health risks associated with obesity.

important because lean body mass is affected by weight-reduction programs as well as physical activity. A negative caloric balance does lead to a decrease in lean body mass. These effects will be explained in detail in Chapter 6. As lean body mass changes, so will your recommended body weight.

Changes in body composition resulting from a weight control/exercise program are illustrated by a coed aerobics course taught during a 6-week summer term. Students participated in aerobic dance routines 4 times a week, 60 minutes each time. On the first and the last days of class, several physiological parameters, including body composition, were assessed. Students also were given information on diet and nutrition and followed their own weight control program. At the end of the 6 weeks, the average weight loss for the entire class was only 3 pounds. When body composition was assessed, however, class members were surprised to find that the average fat loss was actually 6 pounds, accompanied by a 3-pound increase in lean body mass (see Figure 2.7).

Figure 2.7 Typical body composition changes as a result of a six- to eight-week exercise program without an increase in caloric intake.

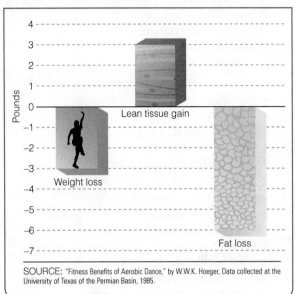

SOURCE: "Fitness Benefits of Aerobic Dance," by W.W.K. Hoeger, Data collected at the University of Texas of the Permian Basin, 1985.

Assess Your Behavior

1. Do you consciously attempt to incorporate as much physical activity as possible in your activities of daily living (walk, take stairs, cycle, participate in sports and recreational activities)?

2. Are your strength levels sufficient to perform tasks of daily living (climbing stairs, carrying a backpack, opening jars, doing housework, mowing the yard) without requiring additional assistance or feeling unusually fatigued?

3. Do you know what your percent body fat is according to a reliable body composition assessment technique administered by a qualified technician?

Assess Your Knowledge

1. The metabolic profile is used in reference to
   a. insulin sensitivity.
   b. glucose tolerance.
   c. cholesterol levels.
   d. cardiovascular disease.
   e. All of the above are correct choices.

2. Cardiorespiratory endurance is determined by
   a. the amount of oxygen the body is able to utilize per minute of physical activity.
   b. the length of time it takes the heart rate to return to 120 bpm following the 1.5-Mile Run Test.
   c. the difference between the maximal heart rate and the resting heart rate.
   d. the product of the heart rate and blood pressure at rest versus exercise.
   e. the time it takes a person to reach a heart rate between 120 and 170 bpm during the 1.0-Mile Walk Test.

3. An "excellent" cardiorespiratory fitness rating in mL/kg/min for young male adults is about
   a. 10.
   b. 20.
   c. 30.
   d. 40.
   e. 50.

4. Which of the following parameters is used to estimate maximal oxygen uptake according to the 1.0-Mile Walk Test?
   a. body weight
   b. gender
   c. total 1.0-mile walk time
   d. exercise heart rate
   e. All of the above are used to estimate VO_{2max}.

5. The ability of a muscle to exert submaximal force repeatedly over time is known as
   a. muscular strength.
   b. plyometric training.
   c. muscular endurance.
   d. isokinetic training.
   e. isometric training.

6. Indicate which of the following exercises is not used to assess muscular endurance in men.
   a. Bench jump
   b. Modified push-up
   c. Bent-leg curl-up
   d. All of the above are used by men.
   e. None of the above are used by men.

7. Muscular flexibility is defined as
   a. the capacity of joints and muscles to work in a synchronized manner.
   b. the achievable range of motion at a joint or group of joints without causing injury.
   c. the capability of muscles to stretch beyond their normal resting length without injury to the muscles.
   d. the capacity of muscles to return to their proper length following the application of a stretching force.
   e. the limitations placed on muscles as the joints move through their normal planes.

8. During the starting position of the Modified Sit-and-Reach Test
   a. the hips, back, and head are placed against a wall.
   b. you measure the distance from the hips to the feet.
   c. you make a fist with the hands.
   d. you stretch forward as far as possible over the reach indicator.
   e. All of the above are correct choices.

9. Essential fat in women is
   a. 3 percent.
   b. 5 percent.
   c. 10 percent.
   d. 12 percent.
   e. 17 percent.

10. Which of the following is not a technique used in the assessment of body fat?
    a. Hydrostatic weighing
    b. Skinfold thickness
    c. Body mass index
    d. Dual energy X-ray absorptiometry

Correct answers can be found on page 307.

Activity 2.1 Personal Fitness Profile: Pre-Test

Date		Course		Section	

Name _____ **Age** _____ ☐Male ☐Female

Body Weight _____

Fitness Component	Test Data	Test Results	Category	Goal
Cardiorespiratory Endurance	Time	VO_{2max}		VO_{2max}
1.5-Mile Run	____ : ____	____ . ____	_____	____ . ____
	Time			
1.0-Mile Walk	____ : ____			
	Heart Rate	VO_{2max}		VO_{2max}
	____ : ____	____ . ____	_____	____ . ____
Muscular Fitness (Strength/Endurance)		Reps		
Bench Jumps		_____	_____	_____
Chair Dips / Modified Push-Ups		_____	_____	_____
Bent-Leg Curl-Ups / Ab. Crunches		_____	_____	_____
Overall Fitness Category			_____	
Muscular Flexibility		Inches		
Modified Sit-and-Reach (MSR)		_____	_____	
Finger Touch (FT), Right		_____	_____	_____
Finger Touch (FT), Left		_____	_____	
Overall Fitness Category (use the MSR test plus only one of the FT tests)			_____	
BMI/Body Composition				
Body Mass Index (BMI)	_____		_____	_____
Waist Circumference (WC)	_____ inches		_____	_____
Waist-to-Height Ratio (WHtR)	_____		_____	_____
Chest / Triceps	_____ mm			
Abdominal / Suprailium	_____ mm			
Thigh	_____ mm			
Sum of Skinfolds	_____ mm			
Percent Body Fat		_____	_____	_____
Lean Body Mass		_____ lbs.		_____

_____ _____
Student Signature   Instructor Signature

Activity 2.1   Personal Fitness Profile: Post-Test

Date _____ Course _____ Section _____

Name _____ Age _____ ☐ Male ☐ Female

Body Weight _____

Fitness Component	Test Data	Test Results	Category	Goal
Cardiorespiratory Endurance	Time	VO$_2$max		VO$_2$max
1.5-Mile Run	____ : ____	____ . ____	_____	____ . ____
	Time			
1.0-Mile Walk	____ : ____			
	Heart Rate	VO$_2$max		VO$_2$max
	____ : ____	____ . ____	_____	____ . ____
Muscular Fitness (Strength/Endurance)		Reps		
Bench Jumps		_____	_____	_____
Chair Dips / Modified Push-Ups		_____	_____	_____
Bent-Leg Curl-Ups / Ab. Crunches		_____	_____	_____
Overall Fitness Category			_____	
Muscular Flexibility		Inches		
Modified Sit-and-Reach (MSR)		_____	_____	_____
Finger Touch (FT), Right		_____	_____	_____
Finger Touch (FT), Left		_____	_____	_____
Overall Fitness Category (use the MSR test plus only one of the FT tests)			_____	
BMI/Body Composition				
Body Mass Index (BMI)	_____		_____	_____
Waist Circumference (WC)	_____ inches		_____	_____
Waist-to-Height Ratio (WHtR)	_____		_____	_____
Chest / Triceps	_____ mm			
Abdominal / Suprailium	_____ mm			
Thigh	_____ mm			
Sum of Skinfolds	_____ mm			
Percent Body Fat		_____	_____	_____
Lean Body Mass		_____ lbs.		_____

_____   _____
Student Signature   Instructor Signature

Activity 2.2	Recommended Body Weight, Body Mass Index (BMI), Waist Circumference (WC), and Waist-to- Height Ratio (WHtR)

Name _____ **Date** _____

Course _____ **Section** _____

Recommended Body Weight According to Percent Body Fat

A. Current Body Weight (BW): _____ lbs.

B. Current Percent Fat (%F): _____ %

C. Fat Weight (FW) = BW × %F* = _____ × _____ = _____ lbs.

D. Lean Body Mass (LBM) = BW − FW = _____ − _____ = _____ lbs.

E. Age: _____

F. Recommended Fat Percent (RFP) Range (see Table 2.11, page 51):

Low End of Recommended Fat Percent Range (LRFP): _____ % (Physical Fitness Standard)

High End of Recommended Fat Percent Range (HRFP): _____ % (Health Fitness Standard)

G. Recommended Body Weight Range:

Low End of Recommended Body Weight Range (LRBW) = LBM ÷ (1.0 − LRFP*)

LRBW = _____ ÷ (1.0 − _____) = _____ lbs.

High End of Recommended Body Weight Range (HRBW) = LBM ÷ (1.0 − HRFP*)

HRBW = _____ ÷ (1.0 − _____) = _____ lbs.

Recommended Body Weight Range: _____ to _____ lbs.

*Express percentages in decimal form (e.g., 25% = .25)

Activity 2.2 Recommended Body Weight, Body Mass Index (BMI), Waist Circumference (WC), and Waist-to- Height Ratio (WHtR) *(continued)*

Body Mass Index (BMI)*

	Pre-test	Post-test
Date:	_____	_____
Weight (lbs.):	_____	_____
Height (inches):	_____	_____
BMI:*	_____	_____
Disease risk: (Table 2.13)	_____	_____

*BMI = [Weight in lbs. × 705 ÷ (Height in inches)^2] or [Weight in kgs ÷ (Height in meters)^2]

Waist Circumference (WC) and Waist-to-Height Ratio (WHtR)

	Pre-test	Post-test
Date:	_____	_____
Waist (inches):	_____	_____
Disease risk: (Table 2.14)	_____	_____
WHtR Disease risk: (Table 2.15)	_____	_____

Recommended Body Weight According to BMI

RBW based on BMI = Desired BMI × height (in.) × height (in.) ÷ 705

RBW at BMI of 25   =   25 × _____ × _____ ÷ 705 = [_____]

RBW at BMI of 22   =   22 × _____ × _____ ÷ 705 = [_____]

Body Composition Conclusions and Goals

Briefly state your feelings about your body composition results and your recommended body weight. Do you plan to reduce your percent body fat and increase your lean body mass? If so, indicate how you plan to achieve these goals.

_____

_____

_____

_____

_____

_____

_____

_____

_____

Exercise Prescription

*Daily physical activity should be a non-negotiable priority in life: It is the miracle medication that people are looking for. It makes you look and feel younger, boosts energy, provides lifetime weight management, improves self-confidence and self-esteem, and enhances independent living, health, and quality of life. It further allows you to enjoy a longer life by decreasing the risk of many chronic conditions, including heart disease, high blood pressure, stroke, diabetes, some cancers, and osteoporosis. Your attitude should be: **I do not fear nor will I avoid physical activity; bring it on!***

Objectives

> Determine your readiness to start an exercise program.

> Learn the factors that govern cardiorespiratory exercise prescription: intensity, mode, duration, and frequency.

> Understand the variables that govern development of muscular fitness (muscular strength and muscular endurance): mode, resistance, sets, and frequency.

> Understand the factors that contribute to the development of muscular flexibility: mode, intensity, repetitions, and frequency.

> Learn to write personalized cardiorespiratory, strength, and flexibility exercise programs.

> Be introduced to a program for the prevention and rehabilitation of low back pain.

> Learn some ways to enhance compliance with exercise.

> Be able to write fitness goals.

Andresr/Shutterstock.com

REAL LIFE STORY | Raul's Fitness Program

When I was in elementary school, I played a variety of sports, including basketball, baseball, soccer, and some football. Later in junior high and high school, I pretty much settled for football and baseball. We were required to run and lift weights for conditioning, and we got all the exercise we needed in our school sports' training program. I did have some back trouble on and off, but nothing I couldn't handle. My cardio and strength levels have always been good, and my percent body fat is excellent. I do know that my flexibility needs help; but then, us guys don't need to stretch.

Now in college during a basketball class, I came down with more back pain. I talked to my instructor and discovered that just playing basketball twice a week and doing only bench press, squat, arm curl, and curl-up exercises was not really a well-rounded program. Because I was really stiff, I started to stretch almost every day, added jogging two to three times per week on days when I didn't play sports, and included several

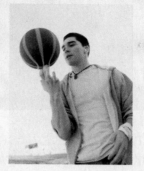

Fuse/Jupiter Images

additional exercises to my strength-training routine. For back health, I also added core training exercises and stability ball exercises. I do these exercises twice a week. It has been two years since I started this new exercise routine, and for the first time in my life I have been free of back pain. I am sleeping better, I have more energy, I am doing better in school, and I feel much better about myself. I don't know that it can get any better than that!

The inspiring story of George Snell from Sandy, Utah, illustrates what fitness can do for a person's health and well-being. At age 45, Snell weighed approximately 400 pounds, his blood pressure was 220/180, he was blind because of diabetes he did not know he had, and his blood glucose (sugar) level was 487. Determined to do something about his physical and medical condition, Snell started a walking/jogging program. After about 8 months of conditioning, he had lost almost 200 pounds, his eyesight had returned, his glucose level was down to 67, and he was taken off medication. Two months later—less than 10 months after initiating his personal exercise program—he completed his first marathon, running a course of 26.2 miles!

Research results have established that being physically active and participating in a lifetime exercise program contribute greatly to good health, physical fitness, and wellness. Nonetheless, too many individuals who exercise regularly are surprised to find when they take a battery of fitness tests that they are not as conditioned as they thought they were. Although these people may be exercising regularly, they most likely are not following the basic principles of exercise prescription. Therefore, they do not reap significant benefits.

To obtain optimal results, all programs must be individualized. Our bodies are not all alike, and fitness levels and needs vary among individuals. The information presented in this chapter provides you with the necessary

guidelines to write a personalized cardiorespiratory, strength, and flexibility exercise program to promote and maintain physical fitness and wellness. Information on weight management to achieve recommended body composition (the fourth component of physical fitness) is given in Chapter 6.

3.1 *Monitoring Daily Physical Activity*

Almost half of all adults in the United States do not achieve the recommended daily amount of physical activity. The first step toward becoming more active is to carefully monitor daily physical activity. Other than monitoring actual time engaged in activity with the use of a stopwatch and a daily log, activity trackers, smartphones, and **pedometers** are excellent tools to determine daily physical activity.

Both an **activity tracker** and the average smartphone contain a device called an accelerometer. The accelerometer measures gravity and changes in movement. Activity trackers add to that functionality an array of features. Popular activity trackers not only count your steps and monitor daily movement levels but also offer features like the ability to vibrate when you've been sedentary too long, to track your sleep, or to check your heart rate. Further, accompanying smartphone apps provide feedback on your progress, help set goals, and allow support through online social networks.

Activity trackers seem to be best at recording straightforward actions that are part of daily physical activity such as brisk walking or jogging. However, they tend to be inaccurate when recording less rhythmic activities, vigorous exercise, overall calories burned, sleep, or other metrics.

Pedometers are small mechanical devices that sense vertical body motion and are used to count footsteps. Wearing a pedometer throughout the day allows you to determine the total steps taken in a day. Although with less accuracy, some pedometer brands also record distance, calories burned, speeds, and actual time of activity each day. Before using a pedometer, be sure to verify its accuracy. Many of the free or low-cost pedometers provided by corporations for promotion and advertisement purposes are inaccurate, thus discouraging their use.

Both activity trackers and pedometers also tend to lose accuracy at very slow walking speeds (30 minutes per mile or less) because the movement of the wrist or vertical movement of the hip is too small to be accurately recorded by these devices. A good pedometer will offer the same information as an activity tracker for the price of about $25 as opposed to $100 or more. However, for some individuals the added features of an activity tracker are worth the added price. If you opt for an activity tracker, be sure to check reliable reviews and weigh the features that are most important to you before purchasing. Some companies offer different models depending on whether you are interested in tracking daily activity or vigorous exercise. Be sure to follow instructions to calibrate the device to your personal stride. In a category all its own is the Apple Watch, which has a higher price point but differentiates among how much you exercise, move, and stand during the day.

To test the accuracy of your device, reset the unit to zero and walk exactly 50 steps at your normal pace and look at the number of steps recorded. A reading within 10 percent of the actual steps taken (45 to 55 steps) is acceptable.

The typical American male takes about 6,000 steps per day, whereas women take about 5,300 steps. A general recommendation for adults is 10,000 steps per day, and Table 3.1 provides specific activity ratings based on the number of daily steps taken.

All daily steps count, but some of your steps should come in bouts of at least 10 minutes 3 times per day, so as to meet the national physical activity recommendation

Table 3.1 Adult Activity Levels Based on Total Number of Steps Taken per Day

Steps per Day	Category
<5,000	Sedentary lifestyle
5,000–7,499	Low active
7,500–9,999	Somewhat active
10,000–12,499	Active
≥12,500	Highly active

SOURCE: C. Tudor-Locke and D. R. Basset, "How Many Steps/Day Are Enough? Preliminary Pedometer Indices for Public Health," *Sports Medicine* 34 (2008): 1–8.

of accumulating 30 minutes of moderate-intensity physical activity in at least three 10-minute sessions 5 days per week. A 10-minute brisk walk (a distance of about 1,200 yards at a 15-minute-per-mile pace) is approximately 1,300 steps. A 15-minute mile (1,770 yards) walk is about 1,900 steps.[1] Some units have an "aerobic steps" function that records steps taken in excess of 60 steps per minute over a 10-minute period of time.

If you do not accumulate the recommended 10,000 daily steps, you can refer to Table 3.2 to determine the additional walking or jogging distance required to reach your goal. For example, if you are a 5'8" tall male, and you typically accumulate 5,200 steps per day, you would need an additional 4,800 daily steps to reach your 10,000-steps goal. You can do so by jogging 3 miles at a 10-minute-per-mile pace (1,602 steps × 3 miles = 4,806 steps) on some days and you can walk 2.5 miles at a 15-minute-per-mile pace (1,908 steps × 2.5 miles = 4,770 steps) on other days. If you do not find a particular speed (pace) that you typically walk or jog at in Table 3.2, you can estimate the number of steps at that speed using the prediction equations at the bottom of this table.

The first practical application that you can perform in this course is to determine your current level of daily activity. The log provided in Activity 3.1 (page 90) will help you keep a four-day log of all physical activities that you do on a daily basis. On this log, record the time of day,

GLOSSARY

Pedometer An activity tracker that counts footsteps. Some pedometers also record distance, calories burned, speeds, and time spent being physically active.

Activity tracker An electronic device that contains an accelerometer (a unit that measures gravity, changes in movement, and counts footsteps). These devices can also determine distance, calories burned, speeds, and time spent being physically active.

Table 3.2 **Estimated Number of Steps to Walk or Jog/Run a Mile Based on Gender, Height, and Pace**

	Pace (min/mile)							
	Walking				Jogging			
	20	18	16	15	12	10	8	6
Height								
Women								
5'0"	2,371	2,244	2,117	2,054	1,997	1,710	1,423	1,136
5'4"	2,315	2,188	2,061	1,998	1,943	1,656	1,369	1,082
5'8"	2,258	2,131	2,005	1,941	1,889	1,602	1,315	1,028
6'0"	2,202	2,075	1,948	1,885	1,835	1,548	1,261	974
Men								
5'2"	2,310	2,183	2,056	1,993	1,970	1,683	1,396	1,109
5'6"	2,253	2,127	2,000	1,937	1,916	1,629	1,342	1,055
5'10"	2,197	2,070	1,943	1,880	1,862	1,575	1,288	1,001
6'2"	2,141	2,014	1,887	1,824	1,808	1,521	1,234	947

Prediction Equations (pace in min/mile and height in inches):

Walking

Women: Steps/mile = 1,949 + [(63.4 × pace) − (14.1 × height)]

Men: Steps/mile = 1,916 + [(63.4 × pace) − (14.1 × height)]

Running

Women and Men: Steps/mile = 1,084 + [(143.6 × pace) − (13.5 × height)]

Adapted from W. W. K. Hoeger et al., "One-Mile Step Count at Walking and Running Speeds," *ACSM's Health & Fitness Journal* 12, no. 1 (2008): 14–19.

type and duration of the activity/exercise, and, if possible, steps taken while engaged in the activity. The results will provide an indication of how active you are and will serve to monitor changes in the next few months and years.

3.2 *Readiness for Exercise*

The research data on the benefits of regular physical activity and exercise are far too impressive to be ignored. All of the benefits of being active, however, do not help unless people carry out a lifetime program of physical activity. Of greater concern, the majority of the population does not exercise regularly, and of those who exercise, only about 20 percent are able to achieve a high physical fitness standard. More than half of those who start exercising drop out during the first few months of the program.

If you are not exercising now, are you willing to give exercise a try? The first step is to decide positively that you will try. To help you make this decision, look at Activity 3.2 (page 92). Make a list of the advantages and disadvantages of incorporating exercise into your lifestyle. Your list of advantages may include things such as:

It will make me feel better.
My self-esteem will improve.
I will lose weight.
I will have more energy.
It will lower my risk for chronic diseases.

Your list of disadvantages may include:

I don't want to take the time.
I'm too out of shape.

There's no good place to exercise.
I don't have the willpower to do it.

When the reasons for exercise outweigh the reasons for not exercising, it will become easier to try.

A questionnaire that may provide answers about your readiness to start an exercise program is also included in Activity 3.2, page 93. Read each statement carefully and circle the number that best describes your feelings. Be completely honest in your answers. You are evaluated in four categories: mastery (self-control), attitude, health, and commitment. The higher you score in any

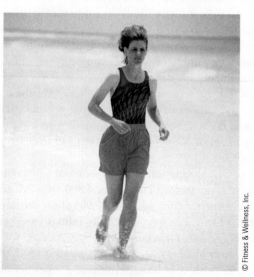

© Fitness & Wellness, Inc.

Good cardiorespiratory fitness is essential to enjoy a good quality of life.

category—mastery, for example—the more important that reason is for you to exercise.

Scores can vary from 4 to 16. A score of 12 and above is a strong indicator that that factor is important to you, whereas 8 and below is low. If you score 12 or more points in each category, your chances of initiating and sticking to an exercise program are good. If you do not score at least 12 points in three categories, your chances of succeeding at exercise may be slim. You need to be better informed about the benefits of exercise, and retraining may be helpful. Tips on how to enhance commitment to exercise are provided later in the chapter on page 88.

3.3 *Exercise Prescriptions*

To better understand how overall fitness can be developed, we have to be familiar with the guidelines that govern exercise prescriptions for cardiovascular endurance, muscular fitness (strength and endurance), and body flexibility.[2] A brief summary of these guidelines is provided in the Physical Activity Pyramid given in Figure 3.1, and they will be explained in detail in the next few sections of this chapter.

3.4 *Cardiorespiratory Endurance*

A sound cardiorespiratory (CR) endurance program contributes greatly to enhancing and maintaining good health. Of the four health-related physical fitness components, CR endurance is the single most important—except during older age, when strength seems to be more critical. Even though certain levels of muscular strength and flexibility are necessary to perform **activities of daily living**, a person can get by without a lot of strength and flexibility. A person cannot do without a good CR system, though.

GLOSSARY

Activities of daily living Everyday behaviors that people normally do to function in life (cross the street, carry groceries, lift objects, do laundry, and sweep floors).

Figure 3.1 **Physical activity pyramid.**

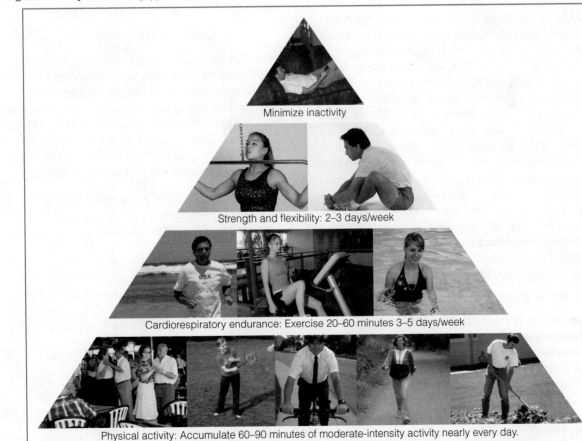

Minimize inactivity

Strength and flexibility: 2–3 days/week

Cardiorespiratory endurance: Exercise 20–60 minutes 3–5 days/week

Physical activity: Accumulate 60–90 minutes of moderate-intensity activity nearly every day.

© Fitness & Wellness, Inc.

Despite the fact that regular moderate physical activity provides substantial health benefits and the overwhelming scientific evidence validating the benefits of exercise on health, longevity, and quality of life, the majority of adults in the United States still do not meet the minimum recommendations for the improvement and maintenance of CR fitness. According to the most recent survey released in 2013 by the Centers for Disease Control and Prevention (CDC), overall, only 46.1 percent of adults (50.4 percent of men and 42.1 percent of women) in the United States meet the 2008 federal guidelines for aerobic physical activity. Furthermore, almost 34 percent do not engage in any leisure-time physical activities.

Cardiorespiratory Exercise Prescription

As far back as 380 BC, Plato, the renowned Greek philosopher stated: *"Lack of activity destroys the good condition of every human being, while movement and methodical physical exercise save it and preserve it."* This statement is more applicable than ever in our modern-day technologically driven culture.

The objective of aerobic exercise is to improve the capacity of the CR system. To accomplish this, the heart muscle has to be overloaded like any other muscle in the human body. Just as the biceps muscle in the upper arm is developed through strength training, the heart muscle is exercised to increase in size, strength, and efficiency.

To better understand how the CR system can be developed, we have to be familiar with four factors involved in aerobic exercise: intensity, mode, duration, and frequency of exercise. First, however, you should be aware that the ACSM recommends that individuals with two or more risk factors for cardiovascular disease (men 45 or older and women 55 or older, family history, cigarette smoking, sedentary lifestyle, obesity, high blood pressure, high LDL cholesterol, low HDL cholesterol, or prediabetes) get a medical exam prior to **vigorous exercise**.[3] They may, however, initiate a light-to-moderate intensity exercise program without medical clearance. The ACSM has defined vigorous exercise as exercise intensity greater than 60 percent of maximal capacity.

Intensity of Exercise

Muscles have to be overloaded for them to develop. Just as the training stimulus to develop the biceps muscle can be accomplished with curl-up exercises, the stimulus for the CR system is provided by making the heart pump at a higher rate for a certain period of time.

CR development occurs when the heart is working between 30 percent and 90 percent of **heart rate reserve (HRR)**.[4,5] Health benefits are achieved when training at a lower exercise intensity, that is, between 30 percent and 60 percent of the person's HRR. Even greater health and cardioprotective benefits, and higher and faster improvements in CR fitness (VO_{2max}), however, are achieved primarily through vigorous-intensity programs, that is, at an intensity greater than 60 percent.[6] For this reason, many experts prescribe exercise between 60 percent and 90 percent. **Intensity of exercise** can be calculated easily, and training can be monitored by checking your pulse. To determine the intensity of exercise or **cardiorespiratory training zone**, follow these steps:

1. Estimate your maximal heart rate (MHR) according to the following formula[7]:

$$MHR = 207 - (.7 \times age)$$

2. Check your resting heart rate (RHR) sometime in the evening after you have been sitting quietly for 15 to 20 minutes. You may take your pulse for 30 seconds and multiply it by 2, or take it for a full minute. As explained in Chapter 2, you can check your pulse on the wrist by placing two or three fingers over the radial artery or on the neck by placing your fingers over the carotid artery.

3. Determine the heart rate reserve (HRR) by subtracting the resting heart rate from the maximal heart rate

$$(HRR = MHR - RHR).$$

4. Calculate the training intensities (TIs) at 30, 40, 50, 60, 70, and 90 percent. Multiply the heart rate reserve by the respective .30, .40, .50, .60, .70, and .90, and then add the resting heart rate to all 4 of these figures (for example, 70% TI = HRR $\times$ .70 + RHR).

    Example. The 30, 40, 50, 60, 70, and 90 percent TIs for a 20-year-old with a resting heart rate of 68 beats per minute (bpm) would be as follows:

    MHR: $207 - (.70 \times 20) = 193$ bpm
    RHR: $= 68$ bpm
    HRR: $193 - 68 = 125$ beats
    30% TI = $(125 \times .30) + 68 = 106$ bpm
    40% TI = $(125 \times .40) + 68 = 118$ bpm
    50% TI = $(125 \times .50) + 68 = 131$ bpm
    60% TI = $(125 \times .60) + 68 = 143$ bpm
    70% TI = $(125 \times .70) + 68 = 155$ bpm
    90% TI = $(125 \times .90) + 68 = 181$ bpm

    Light-intensity CR training zone: 106 to 118 bpm
    Moderate-intensity CR training zone: 118 to 143 bpm
    Vigorous-intensity CR training zone: 143 to 181 bpm

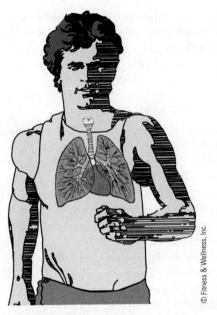

© Fitness & Wellness, Inc.

Cardiorespiratory endurance is the ability of the heart, lungs, and blood vessels to deliver adequate amounts of oxygen to the cells to meet the demands of prolonged physical activity.

When you exercise to improve the CR system, ideally you should maintain the heart rate between the 60 and 90 percent training intensities to obtain the best development. If you have been physically inactive, you should train at around the 30 to 40 percent intensity during the first 2 to 4 weeks of the exercise program. You may then increase to a 40 percent to 60 percent training intensity for the next four weeks. Thereafter you should exercise between the 60 percent and 90 percent training intensities.

When determining the training intensity for your own program, you need to consider your personal fitness goals. Individuals who exercise at around the 50 percent training intensity will reap significant health benefits—in particular, improvements in the metabolic profile (see "Health Fitness Standard," page 32). Training at this lower percentage, however, may place you in only the "average" or moderately fit category (see Table 2.2, page 36). Exercising at this lower intensity does lower the risk for cardiovascular mortality (health fitness) but will not allow you to achieve a "good" or "excellent" CR fitness rating (the physical fitness standard). The latter ratings are obtained by exercising closer to the 90 percent threshold.

Following a few weeks of training, you may have a considerably lower resting heart rate (10 to 20 beats fewer in 8 to 12 weeks). Therefore, you should recompute your target zone periodically. You can compute your own CR training zone by using the form in Activity 3.3,

page 94. Once you have reached an ideal level of CR endurance, training in the 60 to 90 percent range will allow you to maintain your fitness level.

Moderate- Versus Vigorous-Intensity Exercise As fitness programs became popular in the 1970s, vigorous-intensity exercise was routinely prescribed for all fitness participants. Following extensive research in the late 1980s and 1990s, we learned that moderate-intensity physical activity provided substantial health benefits— including decreased risk for cardiovascular mortality, a statement endorsed by the U.S. Surgeon General in 1996.[8] Thus, the emphasis switched from vigorous- to moderate-intensity training in the mid-1990s. In the 1996 report, the surgeon general also stated that vigorous-intensity exercise would provide even greater benefits than moderate-intensity activity. Limited attention, however, has been paid to this recommendation since the publication of the report.

Vigorous-intensity programs yield higher improvements in VO_{2max} than moderate-intensity programs. And higher levels of aerobic fitness are associated with lower cardiovascular mortality, even when the duration of moderate-intensity activity is prolonged to match the energy expenditure performed during a shorter vigorous-intensity effort.[9] A recent review of several clinical studies substantiated that vigorous intensity, as compared to moderate-intensity activity, leads to better improvements in coronary heart disease risk factors, including aerobic endurance, blood pressure, and blood glucose control.[10]

A 2007 joint report by the American College of Sports Medicine and the American Heart Association indicated that, when feasible, vigorous-intensity physical activity is preferable over moderate-intensity physical activity because it provides greater benefits in terms of personal fitness, chronic disease and disability prevention, decreased risk of premature mortality, and lifetime weight management.[11] As a result, the pendulum is again swinging toward vigorous-intensity activity because of the extra benefits and increased chronic disease protection.

GLOSSARY

Vigorous exercise An exercise intensity that is either above 6 METs, 60 percent of maximal oxygen uptake, or one that provides a "substantial" challenge to the individual.

Heart rate reserve (HRR) The difference between the maximal heart rate (MHR) and resting heart rate (RHR).

Intensity of exercise How hard a person has to exercise to improve cardiorespiratory endurance.

Cardiorespiratory training zone The range of intensity at which a person should exercise to develop the cardiorespiratory system.

Monitoring Exercise Heart Rate During the first few weeks of an exercise program, you should monitor your exercise heart rate regularly to make sure you are training in the proper zone. Wait until you are about 5 minutes into your exercise session before taking your first reading. When you check your heart rate, count your pulse for 10 seconds and then multiply by 6 to get the per-minute pulse rate. Exercise heart rate will remain at the same level for about 15 seconds following exercise. After 15 seconds, your heart rate will drop rapidly. Do not hesitate to stop during your exercise bout to check your pulse. If the rate is too low, increase the intensity of exercise. If the rate is too high, slow down.

To develop the CR system, you do not have to exercise above the 90 percent rate. From a fitness standpoint, training above this percentage will not give extra benefits and actually may be unsafe for some individuals. For unconditioned people and older adults, CR training should be conducted around the 50 percent rate to discourage potential problems associated with vigorous-intensity exercise.

Mode of Exercise

The **mode of exercise** that develops the CR system has to be aerobic in nature. **Aerobic exercise** involves the major muscle groups of the body, and it must be rhythmic and continuous. As the amount of muscle mass involved during exercise increases, so does the effectiveness of the activity in providing CR development.

Once you have established your CR training zone, any activity or combination of activities that will get your heart rate up to that training zone and keep it there for as long as you exercise will give you adequate development. Examples of these activities are walking, jogging, swimming, water aerobics, cross-country skiing, rope skipping, cycling, racquetball, elliptical training, and stationary running or cycling.

The activity you choose should be based on your personal preferences—what you enjoy doing most—and your physical limitations. Low-impact activities greatly decrease the risk for injuries. Most injuries to beginners are related to vigorous-impact activities. For individuals who have been inactive, general strength conditioning also is recommended prior to initiating an aerobic exercise program. Strength conditioning will reduce the incidence of injuries significantly.

The amount of strength or flexibility a person develops through various activities differs, but in terms of CR development, the heart doesn't know whether you are walking, swimming, or cycling. All the heart knows is that it has to pump at a certain rate, and as long as that rate is in the desired range, your CR fitness will improve.

From a health fitness point of view, training in the lower end of the CR zone will yield optimal health benefits. The closer the heart rate is to the higher end of the CR training zone, however, the greater will be the improvements in VO_{2max} (high physical fitness).

Duration of Exercise

The general recommendation is that a person exercise between 20 and 60 minutes per session. For vigorous-intensity exercise, a minimum of 75 total minutes per week is recommended, while those in a moderate-intensity program should accumulate at least 150 minutes per week.

The **duration of exercise** is based on how hard a person trains. The variables are inversely related. If the training is done at around 90 percent, 20 minutes of exercise is sufficient. At about 50 percent intensity, the individual should train close to 60 minutes. As mentioned in the discussion of intensity of exercise previously, unconditioned people and older adults should train at lower percentages; therefore, the activity should be carried out over a longer time.

Although most experts traditionally have recommended 20 to 60 minutes of continuous aerobic exercise per session, evidence suggests that accumulating 30 minutes or more of moderate-intensity physical activity provides substantial health benefits. Research further indicates that three 10-minute exercise sessions per day (separated by at least 4 hours), at approximately 70 percent of maximal heart rate, also produce fitness benefits.[12] Although the increases in VO_{2max} with this program were only 57 percent of those in a group performing one continuous 30-minute bout of exercise per day, the researchers concluded that moderate-intensity exercise conducted for 10 minutes three times per day benefits the CR system significantly.

Results of this study are meaningful because people often mention lack of time as the reason for not taking part in an exercise program. Many think they have to exercise at least 20 continuous minutes to get any benefits at all. Even though 20 to 60 minutes are recommended, short, intermittent exercise bouts also are helpful to the CR system.

The 2008 Federal Guidelines for Physical Activity measure duration of exercise in terms of the total quantity of physical activity performed on a weekly basis. Two hours and 30 minutes of moderate-intensity aerobic activity, 1 hour and 15 minutes of vigorous-intensity aerobic activity per week, or an equivalent combination of the two are recommended (30 minutes of moderate-intensity twice per week combined with 20 minutes of vigorous-intensity another 2 times per week).

Two hours and 30 minutes per week represents the accumulation of 30 minutes of moderate-intensity aerobic activity (done in bouts of at least 10 minutes long each) per session/day performed 5 days per week, whereas 1 hour and 15 minutes is approximately 25 minutes of vigorous-intensity aerobic activity done three times per week. The federal guidelines also indicate that 5 hours of moderate-intensity activity or 2 hours and 30 minutes of vigorous-intensity activity per week provide additional benefits. Thus, when possible, people are encouraged to go beyond the minimum recommendation.

For people whose goal is weight management, the Institute of Medicine of the National Academy of Sciences recommends accumulating 60 minutes of moderate-intensity physical activity per day,[13] whereas 60 to 90 minutes of daily moderate-intensity activity is necessary to prevent weight regain.[14] These recommendations are based on evidence that people who maintain healthy weight typically accumulate between 1 and 1½ hours of daily physical activity. Exercise duration should be increased gradually to avoid undue fatigue and exercise-related injuries.

If lack of time is a concern, you should exercise daily at a vigorous intensity for 30 minutes, which can burn as many calories as 60 minutes of moderate-intensity exercise (see "The Role of Exercise Intensity and Duration in Weight Management," Chapter 6, pages 164–166)—but only 15 percent of adults in the United States typically exercise at a vigorous-intensity level. Novice and overweight exercisers also need proper conditioning prior to vigorous-intensity exercise to avoid injuries or cardiovascular-related problems.

Exercise sessions always should be preceded by a 5- to 10-minute **warm-up** and followed by a 10-minute **cool-down**. The purpose of warm-up is to aid in the transition from rest to exercise. A good warm-up increases muscle and connective tissue extensibility and joint range of motion and enhances muscular activity. A warm-up consists of general calisthenics, mild stretching exercises, and walking/jogging/cycling for a few minutes at a lower intensity level than the actual target zone. The concluding phase of the warm-up is a gradual increase in exercise intensity to the lower end of the target training zone.

In the cool-down, the intensity of exercise is decreased gradually to help the body return to near resting levels, followed by stretching and relaxation activities. Stopping abruptly causes blood to pool in the exercised body parts, diminishing the return of blood to the heart. The pressure in the veins of the limbs is too low to effectively pump the blood back to the heart against gravity. Immediately following exercise, the veins in the limbs depend on the contraction of the surrounding muscles to squeeze the large amount of blood used during physical activity back to the heart, also known as the skeletal muscle pump. Less blood return can cause a sudden drop in blood pressure, dizziness, and faintness, or it can bring on cardiac abnormalities. The cool-down phase also helps dissipate body heat and aids in removing the lactic acid produced during high-intensity exercise.

Frequency of Exercise

The recommended **frequency of exercise** for aerobic exercise is 3 to 5 days per week. When exercising at 60 percent to 90 percent of HRR, three 20- to 30-minute exercise sessions per week, performed on nonconsecutive days, are sufficient to improve or maintain VO_{2max}. When training at lower intensities, exercising 30 to 60 minutes more than 3 days per week is required. If training is conducted more than 5 days a week, further improvements in VO_{2max} are minimal. Although endurance athletes often train 6 to 7 days per week (often twice per day), their training programs are designed to increase training mileage so they can endure long-distance races (6 to 100 miles) at a high percentage of VO_{2max}.

For individuals on a weight loss program, the recommendation is 60 to 90 minutes of light-to-moderate intensity activity on most days of the week. Longer exercise sessions increase caloric expenditure for faster weight reduction (also see Chapter 6).

Although three exercise sessions per week will maintain CR fitness, the importance of regular physical activity in preventing disease and enhancing quality of life has been pointed out clearly by the American College of Sports Medicine, by the U.S. Centers for Disease Control and Prevention, and by the President's Council on Physical Fitness and Sports. These organizations advocate at least 30 minutes of moderate-intensity physical activity at least 5 days per week. This routine has been promoted as an effective way to improve health.

These recommendations were subsequently upheld by the U.S. Surgeon General in the 1996 "Report on Physical Activity and Health." The Surgeon General's report states that people can improve their health and quality of life substantially by including moderate amounts of

---

GLOSSARY

Mode of exercise Form of exercise (e.g., aerobic).

Aerobic exercise Activity that requires oxygen to produce the necessary energy to carry out the activity.

Duration of exercise Time exercising per session.

Warm-up A period preceding exercise when exercise begins slowly.

Cool-down A period at the end of an exercise session when exercise is tapered off.

Frequency of exercise How often a person engages in an exercise session.

physical activity on most, preferably all, days of the week. Further, it states that no one, including older adults, is too old to enjoy the benefits of regular physical activity.

To enjoy better health and fitness, physical activity must be pursued regularly. According to Dr. William Haskell from Stanford University: *"Physical activity should be viewed as medication, and, therefore, should be taken on a daily basis."* Many of the benefits of exercise and activity diminish within two weeks of substantially decreased physical activity. These benefits are completely lost within two to eight months of inactivity.

Daily Active Lifestyle

New research indicates that excessive sitting throughout most days of the week is a "deadly proposition," also known as "the sitting disease." People who spend most of the day sitting are canceling out the health benefits obtained through physical activity and exercise. The human body was created for movement and activity. Our society, however, is primarily a sedentary society that lulls people into physical inactivity. Most Americans spend more than half their waking hours sitting: driving to and from work, working at a desk, sitting at the computer, and watching television. Studies indicate that people who spend most of their day sitting have as much as a 50 percent greater risk of dying prematurely from all causes and an 80 percent greater risk of dying from cardiovascular disease.[15] The data further indicate that death rates are still high for people who spend most of their day sitting, even though they meet the current minimum moderate-physical activity recommendations (30 minutes at least 5 times per week).[16]

If you are physically active or exercise seven times per week for 30 minutes a day, you will accumulate 210 weekly minutes of intentional activity. Even though you perceive yourself as being physically active because of the daily 30 minutes of activity, the issue at hand is the physical stillness the rest of the day. Two hundred and ten minutes translates into just 2 percent of the total 10,080 minutes available to you on a weekly basis. Thus the difference between a regular exerciser and a sedentary individual is 30 minutes of activity per day. The other 98 percent of the time, most exercisers and sedentary people spend their time in very similar non-moving activities.

Among many other conditions, excessive sitting leads to weaker muscles, a sluggish central nervous system, increased fatigue, decreased insulin sensitivity, higher blood pressure, decreased activity of lipoprotein lipase (an enzyme that breaks down fats in the blood), and increased cholesterol, LDL cholesterol, and triglycerides. Even if you are meeting the exercise guidelines of physical activity on most days of the week, you should not spend most of the remainder of your day being sedentary. Thus, people are strongly encouraged to incorporate as many physical activities throughout the day, at least 10 minutes every waking hour of the day.

To minimize inactivity, look to enhance daily **non-exercise activity thermogenesis (NEAT)**, or the energy expended doing daily activities not related to exercise. Examples of such activities include the following:

1. Walk instead of drive when you only need to go short distances.
2. Park farther away or get off the subway, train, or bus several blocks from the campus or office.
3. Take a short walk right after each meal or snack.
4. Walk faster than usual.
5. Move about whenever you take a break.
6. Take the stairs as often as you can. Walk up and down the escalators when you don't have a choice of stairs.
7. When watching TV, stand up and move during each commercial break, or even better, stretch or work out during TV time. When working or watching TV, drink plenty of water, which is not only healthy on its own but will give you extra reasons to take a walk for refills and bathroom breaks.
8. Do not shy away from housecleaning chores or yard work, even for a minute or two at a time.
9. Stand more while working/studying. Place your computer on an elevated stand or shelf and stand while doing work, writing emails, or surfing the Internet. Standing triples the energy requirement of doing a similar activity sitting. For extended periods of work or study adopt a rotating pattern of standing and sitting roughly every 20 minutes.
10. Always stand or pace while talking on the phone.
11. When reading a book, get up and move after every 6-10 pages of the book.
12. Use a stability ball for a chair. Such use enhances body stability, balance, and abdominal, low back, and leg strength.
13. Whenever feasible, walk while conversing or holding meetings. If meetings are in a conference room, take the initiative to stand.
14. Walk to classmates' homes or coworkers' offices to study or discuss matters with them instead of using the phone, email, or computer.

Exercise Volume

A relatively new concept, volume of exercise is the product of frequency, intensity, and duration. The recommended absolute minimum volume is an energy expenditure of 1,000 calories per week or the equivalent of 150 minutes of moderate-intensity exercise each week. Volume can also be measured using a pedometer and achieving 10,000 or more steps each day. This minimal amount of volume is essential to achieve health benefits. A minimum of 75 minutes of vigorous-intensity aerobic activity per week (conducted over three nonconsecutive days), along with at least 2 additional days of 30 minutes each of moderate-intensity physical activity are required for substantial fitness benefits.

Training volume is also used as an indicator of excessive exercise. Too much exercise and physical activity lead to overtraining, muscle soreness, undue fatigue, shortness of breath, and an increase in the risk for injury. Should you experience any adverse effects as a result of your physical activity/exercise program, downward adjustments are recommended to the exercise prescription, including the rate of exercise progression (discussed next).

Rate of Progression

How quickly an individual progresses through an exercise program depends on the person's health status, exercise tolerance, and exercise program goals.[17] Initially, only 3 weekly training sessions of 15 to 20 minutes are recommended to avoid musculoskeletal injuries. You may then increase the duration by 5 to 10 minutes per week and the

frequency so that by the fourth or fifth week you are exercising 5 times per week. Thereafter, progressively increase frequency, duration, and intensity of exercise until you reach your fitness maintenance goal. All increases in the exercise prescription variables should be gradual to minimize the risk of overtraining and injuries.

A summary of the CR exercise prescription guidelines according to the American College of Sports Medicine is provided in Figure 3.2. Ideally, to reap both the high fitness and the health fitness benefits of exercise, a person needs to exercise a minimum of three times per week in the appropriate target zone for high fitness maintenance and three to four additional times per week in moderate-intensity activities to enjoy the full benefits of health fitness. Preferably, all exercise/physical activity sessions should last a minimum of 30 minutes. The form in Activity 3.4, page 98, is provided to help you keep a daily log of your CR (aerobic) activities.

GLOSSARY

Non-exercise activity thermogenesis (NEAT) Energy expended doing everyday activities not related to exercise.

Figure 3.2 **Cardiorespiratory exercise prescription guidelines.**

Mode:	Moderate- or vigorous-intensity aerobic activity (examples: walking, jogging, stair climbing, elliptical activity, aerobics, water aerobics, cycling, stair climbing, swimming, cross-country skiing, racquetball, basketball, and soccer)
Intensity:	30% to 90% of heart rate reserve (the training intensity is based on age, health status, initial fitness level, exercise tolerance, and exercise program goals)
Duration:	At least 20 minutes of continuous vigorous-intensity or 30 minutes of moderate-intensity aerobic activity (the latter may be accumulated in segments of at least 10 minutes in duration each over the course of the day)
Frequency:	3 to 5 days per week for vigorous-intensity aerobic activity to accumulate at least 75 minutes per week, or 5 days per week of moderate-intensity aerobic activity for a minimum total of 150 minutes weekly
Volume of exercise:	Accumulate at least 150 minutes of moderate intensity or 75 minutes of vigorous-intensity aerobic activity per week. You may also accumulate a minimum of 10,000 steps per day, each day of the week (at least 70,000 steps per week)
Rate of progression:	Start with three training sessions per week of 15 to 20 minutes Increase the duration by 5 to 10 minutes per week and the frequency so that by the fourth or fifth week you are exercising five times per week Progressively increase frequency, duration, and intensity of exercise until you reach your fitness goal prior to exercise maintenance

SOURCE: Adapted from American College of Sports Medicine, ACSM's Guidelines for Exercise Testing and Prescription (Philadelphia: Wolters Kluwer/Lippincott Williams & Wilkins, 2014) and U.S. Department of Health and Human Services, 2008 Physical Activity Guidelines for Americans, http://health. gov/paguidelines, downloaded October 15, 2014.

3.5 *Muscular Fitness (Muscular Strength and Muscular Endurance)*

The capacity of muscle cells to exert force increases and decreases according to demands placed upon the muscular system. If specific muscle cells are overloaded beyond their normal use, such as in strength-training programs, the cells increase in size (hypertrophy), strength, or endurance, or some combination of these. If the demands on the muscle cells decrease, such as in sedentary living or required rest because of illness or injury, the cells decrease in size (atrophy) and lose strength.

Two types of muscular hypertrophy are known: **myofibrillar hypertrophy** and **sarcoplasmic hypertrophy**. Myofibrils are composed of the myosin and actin filaments, the contractile portion of the muscle. Myofibrillar hypertrophy is the result of increased synthesis of the protein filaments myosin and actin that slide past one another to produce muscle contraction. With this type of hypertrophy the area density (size) of the myofibrils increases and results in a greater ability of the muscle to generate tension (exert muscle strength). This type of hypertrophy is achieved by training with heavy resistances and low repetitions (1 to 6). Strength and power athletes use this training method because it results in greater strength increases.

Sarcoplasmic hypertrophy is achieved primarily through an increase in sarcoplasm. The sarcoplasm in muscle is comparable to the cytoplasm in other cells. This semifluid substance in muscle contains primarily myosin and actin myofibrils, but also large amounts of glycosomes (organelles that store glycogen and enzymes) and myoglobin (the oxygen binding protein in muscle). Training for sarcoplasmic hypertrophy is conducted with lower resistances but performing a larger number of repetitions (8 to 15). This type of training results in greater muscle size than observed in myofibrillar hypertrophy, but lower increases in strength. Muscular strength is primarily dependent on the amount and the density of the muscle fibers. Adding more muscle fluid (sarcoplasm) does not increase strength to the same extent. Bodybuilders typically rely on training that leads to sarcoplasmic hypertrophy as they are judged by appearance and not by the amount of resistance lifted.

All people need adequate muscular fitness for good health, improved functional capacity, and a better quality of life. Unfortunately, according to the 2013 survey by the CDC, only 27 percent of men and 19 percent of women meet the 2008 Federal Physical Activity Guidelines for muscular fitness. Worse yet, almost 74 percent or nearly 3 out of every 4 American adults do not participate in any type of muscular fitness activity; that is, they do not strength train or take a class that requires some sort of muscular strength activity such as cardio/strength training, Pilates, boot camp, PX90, CrossFit, or even a single push-up during their available leisure time.

Overload Principle

The **overload principle** states that for strength or endurance to improve, demands placed on the muscle must be increased systematically and progressively over time, and the **resistance** (weight lifted) must be of a magnitude significant enough to produce development. In simpler terms, just like all other organs and systems of the human body, muscles have to be taxed beyond their accustomed loads to increase in physical capacity.

Specificity of Training

Muscular strength is the ability to exert maximum force against resistance. Muscular endurance (also referred to as localized muscular endurance) is the ability of a muscle to exert submaximal force repeatedly over time. Both of these components require **specificity of training**.

As discussed later in this section, a person attempting to increase muscular strength needs a program of few repetitions and near-maximum resistance. To increase muscular endurance, the strength-training program consists primarily of many repetitions at a lower resistance. In like manner, to increase isometric (static) versus dynamic strength (see the section "Mode of Training" that follows), an individual must use the corresponding static or dynamic training procedures to achieve the appropriate results.

In like manner, if a person is trying to improve a specific movement or skill through strength gains, the selected strength-training exercises must resemble the actual movement or skill as closely as possible.

Periodization

The concept of **periodization** (variation) entails systematically altering training variables over time to keep the program challenging and lead to greater strength development. Periodization means cycling one's training objectives (hypertrophy, strength, and endurance), with each phase of the program lasting anywhere from 2 to 12 weeks. Training variables altered include resistance (weight lifted), number of repetitions, number of sets, and/or number of exercises performed.

Periodization is popular among fitness participants who wish to achieve maximal strength gains. Over the long run, for intermediate and advanced participants, the periodized approach has been shown to be superior to nonperiodized training where participants always use the same exercises, sets, and repetitions.

Three types of periodized training, based on program design and objectives, are commonly used.[18] These are:

1. Classical periodization. Used primarily by individuals seeking maximal strength development. It starts with an initial high volume of training using low resistances and then gradually switches to a lower volume and higher resistances in subsequent cycles.
2. Reverse periodization. This model is used by individuals seeking greater muscular endurance. Unlike the classical model, individuals start with high resistances and low volume and subsequently follow it with progressive decreases in resistances and increases in training volume.
3. Undulating periodization. This model uses a combination of volumes and resistances within a cycle by alternating randomly or systematically among the muscular fitness components: strength, hypertrophy, power, and endurance. This model compares favorably, and in some cases is superior, to the classical and reverse models.

Muscular Strength-Training Prescription

Similar to the prescription of CR exercise, several factors or variables have to be taken into account to improve muscular fitness. These are mode, resistance, sets, and frequency of training.

Mode of Training

Two basic training methods are used to improve strength: isometric and dynamic. **Isometric exercise** involves pushing or pulling against immovable objects. **Dynamic exercise** involves movement at the joints, such as extending the knees with resistance (weight) on the ankles.

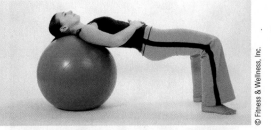

Isometric strength training.

Although isometric training does not require much equipment, it is not a very popular mode of training. Strength gains with isometric training are specific to the angle of muscle contraction; this type of training remains beneficial in sports such as gymnastics that require regular static contractions during routines. Isometric training, however, is a critical component of health conditioning programs for the lower back (see "Preventing and Rehabilitating Low Back Pain," pages 82–86).

Dynamic exercise (previously referred to as **isotonic exercise**) can be conducted without weights or with **free weights** (barbells and dumbbells), **fixed-resistance**

GLOSSARY

Myofibrillar hypertrophy Muscle hypertrophy as a result of increased protein synthesis in the myosin and actin myofibrils.

Sarcoplasmic hypertrophy Muscle hypertrophy as a result of an increase in sarcoplasm.

Overload principle Training concept holding that the demands placed on a body system must be increased systematically and progressively over time to cause physiologic adaptation.

Resistance Amount of weight lifted.

Specificity of training A principle holding that, for a muscle to increase in strength or endurance, the training program must be specific to obtain the desired effects.

Periodization A training approach that divides the season into cycles using a systematic variation in intensity and volume of training to enhance fitness and performance.

Isometric exercise Strength training with muscle contraction that produces little or no movement.

Dynamic exercise Strength training with muscle contraction that produces movement.

Isotonic exercise See Dynamic exercise.

Free weights Barbells and dumbbells.

Fixed-resistance Exercise with strength-training equipment that provides a constant amount of resistance through the range of motion.

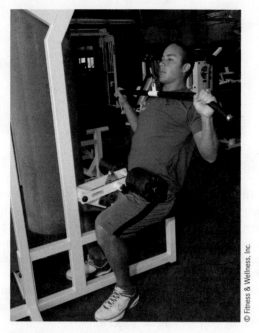

Dynamic strength training.

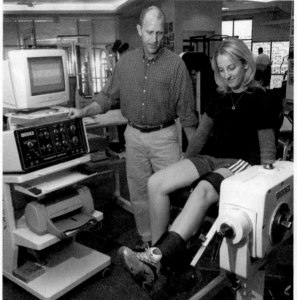

Isokinetic strength training.

machines, **variable-resistance** machines, and isokinetic equipment. When performing dynamic exercises without weights (for example, pull-ups, push-ups), with free weights, or with fixed-resistance machines, a constant resistance (weight) is moved through a joint's full range of motion. The greatest resistance that can be lifted equals the maximum weight that can be moved at the weakest angle of the joint, because of changes in muscle length and angle of pull as the joint moves through its range of motion.

As strength training became more popular, new strength-training machines were developed. This technology brought about isokinetic and variable-resistance training. These training programs require special machines equipped with mechanical devices that provide differing amounts of resistance, with the intent of overloading the muscle group maximally through the entire range of motion. A distinction of **isokinetic exercise** is that the speed of the muscle contraction is kept constant because the machine provides resistance to match the user's force through the range of motion. Because of the expense of the equipment needed for isokinetic training, this type of program usually is reserved for clinical settings (physical therapy), research laboratories, and certain professional sports.

Dynamic training has two action phases: **concentric,** or **positive resistance**, and **eccentric,** or **negative resistance**. In the concentric phase, the muscle shortens as it contracts to overcome the resistance. For example, during the bench press exercise, when the resistance is lifted from the chest to full arm extension, the triceps muscle on the back of the upper arm contracts and shortens to extend the elbow. During the eccentric phase, the muscle lengthens as it contracts. In the case of the bench press exercise, the same triceps muscle contracts to lower the resistance during elbow flexion, but it lengthens to avoid dropping the resistance.

Eccentric muscle contractions allow us to lower weights in a smooth, gradual, and controlled manner. Without eccentric contractions, weights would be dropped on the way down. Because the same muscles work when you lift and lower a resistance, you should be sure to always execute both actions in a controlled manner. Failure to do so diminishes the benefits of the training program and increases the risk for injuries.

The mode of training depends mainly on the type of equipment available and the specific objective of the training program. Dynamic training is the most popular mode for strength training. Its primary advantage is that strength is gained through the full range of motion. Most daily activities are dynamic in nature. We constantly lift, push, and pull objects, which requires strength through a given range of motion. Another advantage of dynamic exercise is that improvements are measured easily by the amount lifted.

Benefits of isokinetic and variable-resistance training are similar to those of the other dynamic training methods. Theoretically, strength gains should be better because maximum resistance is applied through the entire range of motion. Research, however, has not shown this type of training to be more effective than other modes of dynamic training. A possible advantage is that specific speeds for a small number of selected sport skills can be duplicated more closely with isokinetic strength training, which may enhance performance (specificity of training). A disadvantage is that the equipment is not readily available to everyone.

Plate-loaded barbells (free weights) were the most popular weight-training equipment available during the first half of the 20th century. Strength-training machines were developed in the middle of the century but did not become popular until the 1970s. With the advent of, and subsequent technological improvements to, these machines, a stirring debate surfaced over which of the two training modalities was better.

Free weights require that the individual balance the resistance through the entire lifting motion. Thus, a logical assumption could be made that free weights are a better training modality because of the involvement of additional stabilizing muscles needed to balance the resistance as it is moved through its range of motion. Research, however, has not shown any differences in strength development between the two exercise modalities. Although each modality has pros and cons, the muscles do not know whether the source of a resistance is a barbell, a dumbbell, a Universal Gym machine, a Nautilus machine, or a simple cinder block. What determines the level of a person's strength development is the quality of the program and the individual's effort during the training program itself—not the type of equipment used.

Two additional modes of strength training that have gained extensive popularity in recent years are stability ball exercises and elastic-band resistive exercises. Stability exercises are specifically designed to develop abdominal, hip, chest, and spinal muscles by addressing core stabilization while the exerciser maintains a balanced position over the ball. Although the primary objective is core strength and stability, many stability exercises can be performed to strengthen other body areas as well. Elastic

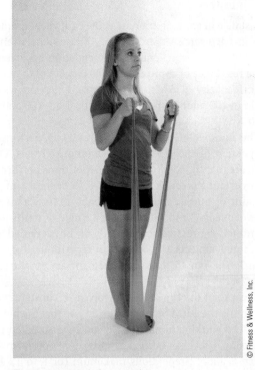

Elastic-band resistive exercise.

bands and tubing can also be used for strength training. This type of constant-resistance training has been shown to help increase strength, mobility, and functional ability (particularly in older adults) and aid in the rehab of many types of injuries. Some of the advantages of this type of training include low cost, versatility, and use of a large number of exercises to work all joints of the body; it also provides a great way to work out while traveling.

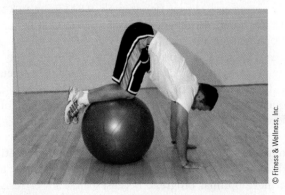

Stability ball exercises help improve core strength and stability.

GLOSSARY

Variable-resistance Exercise that utilizes special equipment with mechanical devices that provide differing amounts of resistance through the range of motion.

Isokinetic exercise Strength training method in which the speed of the muscle contraction is kept constant because the equipment (machine) provides an accommodating resistance to match the user's force through the full range of motion.

Concentric Shortening of a muscle during muscle contraction.

Positive resistance The lifting, pushing, or concentric phase of a repetition during the performance of a strength-training exercise.

Eccentric Lengthening of a muscle during muscle contraction.

Negative resistance The lowering or eccentric phase of a repetition during the performance of a strength-training exercise.

Resistance

Resistance in strength training is the equivalent of intensity in CR exercise prescription. To stimulate strength development, the general recommendation has been to use a resistance of approximately 80 percent of the maximum capacity (1 RM). For example, a person with a 1 RM of 150 pounds should work with about 120 pounds (150 × .80).

The number of repetitions that one can perform at 80 percent of the 1 RM varies among exercises. Data indicate that the total number of repetitions performed at a certain percentage of the 1 RM depends on the amount of muscle mass used (bench press versus triceps extension) and whether it is a single or multi-joint exercise (leg press versus leg curl). In both trained and untrained subjects, the number of repetitions is greater with larger muscle mass involvement and multi-joint exercises.[19]

Because of the time factor involved in constantly determining the 1 RM on each lift to ensure that the person is indeed working around 80 percent, the accepted rule for many years has been that individuals perform between 8 and 12 repetitions maximum (or 8 to 12 **RM zone**) for adequate strength gains. For example, if a person is training with a resistance of 120 pounds and cannot lift it more than 12 times—that is, the person reaches volitional fatigue at or before 12 repetitions—the training stimulus (weight used) is adequate for strength development. Once the person can lift the resistance more than 12 times, the resistance is increased by 5 to 10 pounds and the person again should build up to 12 repetitions. This is referred to as **progressive resistance training**.

Strength development, however, can also occur when working with less than 80 percent of the 1 RM. Although 8 to 12 RM is the most commonly prescribed resistance, benefits do occur when working below 8 or above 12 RM. If the main objective of the training program is muscular endurance, 15 to 25 repetitions per set are recommended. Older adults and individuals susceptible to musculoskeletal injuries are encouraged to work with 10 to 15 repetitions using moderate resistances (about 50 percent to 60 percent of the 1 RM).

In both young and older individuals, all repetitions should be performed at a moderate velocity (about 1 second concentric and 1 second eccentric), as such yields the greatest strength gains. For advanced training, varying training velocity between sets, from very slow to fast, is recommended.

Elite strength athletes typically work using a 1 to 6 RM zone but often shuffle training with different numbers of repetitions for selected periods (weeks) of time. Body builders tend to work with moderate resistance levels (60 percent to 90 percent of the 1 RM) and work in an 8 to 20 RM zone. A foremost objective of body building is to increase muscle size. Moderate resistance promotes blood flow to the muscles, "pumping up the muscles" (also known as "the pump") and making them look much larger than they do in a resting state.

From a general fitness point of view, working near a 10-repetition threshold seems to improve overall performance most effectively. We live in a dynamic world in which muscular strength and endurance are both required to lead an enjoyable life. Working in an 8 to 12 RM zone produces good results in terms of strength, endurance, and **muscular hypertrophy**. For older and more frail individuals (50 to 60 years of age and above), 10 to 15 repetitions of moderate to high intensity of effort are recommended.

We must mention here that a certain resistance (for example, 50 pounds) is seldom the same on two different weight machines, or between free weights and weight machines. The industry has no standard calibration procedure for strength equipment. Consequently, if you lift a certain weight with free weights or a given machine, you may or may not be able to lift the same amount on a different piece of equipment.

Sets

Strength training is done in **sets**. For example, a person lifting 120 pounds 8 times performs one set of 8 **repetitions** (1/8/120). For general fitness, the recommendation is one to three sets per exercise. Some evidence suggests greater strength gains using multiple sets as opposed to a single set for a given exercise. Other research, however, concludes that similar increases in strength, endurance, and hypertrophy are derived between single- and multiple-set strength training, as long as the single set, or at least one of the multiple sets, is a heavy (maximum) set performed to volitional exhaustion using an RM zone (for example, 9 RM using an 8 to 12 RM zone).[20] Strength gains may be lessened by performing too many sets.

A recommended program for beginners is 1 or 2 light warm-up sets per exercise using about 50 percent of the 1 RM (no warm-up sets are necessary for subsequent exercises that use the same muscle group) followed by 1 to 3 sets per exercise. Maintaining a resistance and effort that will temporarily fatigue the muscle (volitional exhaustion) in the number of repetitions selected in at least one of the sets is critical to achieve optimal progress. Because of the lower resistances used in body building, four to eight sets can be done for each exercise.

To avoid muscle soreness and stiffness, new participants ought to build up gradually to the three sets of maximal repetitions. This can be done by performing only one set of each exercise with a lighter resistance on the first day. During the second session, two sets of each exercise can be done: the first light and the second with the regular resistance. During the third session, three sets could be performed—one light and two heavy sets. After that, a person should be able to do all three heavy sets.

The time necessary to recover between sets depends mainly on the resistance used during each set. In strength training, the energy to lift heavy weights is derived primarily from the system involving adenosine triphosphate (ATP) and creatine phosphate (CP) stored in muscle, also known as the phosphagen system. Ten seconds of maximal exercise nearly depletes the CP stores in the exercised muscle(s). These stores are replenished in about three to five minutes of recovery.

Based on this principle, rest intervals between sets vary in length depending on the program goals and are dictated by the amount of resistance used in training. Short rest intervals of less than two minutes are commonly used when one is trying to develop local muscular endurance. Moderate rest intervals of two to four minutes are used for strength development. Long intervals of more than four minutes are used when one is training for power development.[21] Using these guidelines, individuals training for health fitness purposes might allow two minutes of rest between sets. Body builders, who use lower resistances, should rest no more than one minute to maximize the "pumping" effect.

> **!**
> ## Critical Thinking
>
> What role should strength training have in a fitness program? • Should people be motivated for the health fitness benefits, or should they participate to enhance their body image? • What are your feelings about individuals (male or female) with large body musculature?

You can also work out smarter to save time. The exercise program will be more time-effective if two or three exercises are alternated that require different muscle groups. In this way you can go directly from one exercise to another and will not have to wait two to three minutes before proceeding to a new set on a different exercise. For example, the bench press, leg extension, and abdominal curl-up exercises may be combined so that the person can go almost directly from one exercise set to the next.

Frequency of Training

Strength training should be done either with a total body workout two or three times per week, or more frequently if using a split-body routine (upper body one day and lower body the next). Strength training two times per week produces about 80 percent of the strength gains seen in a traditional three times per week program.

After a maximum strength workout, the muscles should be rested for about 48 hours to allow adequate recovery. If not recovered completely in 2 or 3 days, the person most likely is overtraining and therefore not reaping the full benefits of the program. In that case, a decrease in the total number of sets or exercises, or both, performed during the previous workout is recommended.

A summary of strength-training guidelines for health fitness purposes is provided in Figure 3.3. Significant strength gains require a minimum of eight weeks of consecutive training. After achieving the recommended strength level, one training session per week will be sufficient to maintain the new strength level.

Frequency of strength training for body builders varies from person to person. Because body builders use moderate resistances, daily or even two-a-day workouts are common. The frequency depends on the amount of resistance, number of sets performed per session, and the person's ability to recover from the previous exercise bout (see Table 3.3). The latter often is dictated by level of conditioning.

Strength-Training Exercises

Two strength-training programs, presented in Appendix A, have been developed to provide a complete body workout. Only a minimum of equipment is required for the

---

GLOSSARY

RM zone A range of repetitions that are to be performed maximally during one set. For example, an 8 to 12 RM zone implies that the individual will perform anywhere from 8 to 12 repetitions, but cannot perform any more following the completion of the final repetition (e.g., 9 RM and could not perform a 10th repetition).

Progressive resistance training A gradual increase of resistance over a period of time.

Muscular hypertrophy An increase in muscle mass or size.

Set The number of repetitions performed for a given exercise.

Repetitions The number of times a movement is performed.

Figure 3.3 Strength-training guidelines.

Mode:	Select 8 to 10 dynamic strength-training exercises that involve the body's major muscle groups and include opposing muscle groups (chest and upper back, abdomen and lower back, front and back of the legs)
Resistance:	Sufficient resistance to perform 8 to 12 repetitions maximum for muscular strength and 15 to 25 repetitions to near fatigue for muscular endurance. Older adults and injury prone individuals should use 10 to 15 repetitions with moderate resistance (50% to 60% of their 1 RM)
Sets:	2 to 4 sets per exercise with 2 to 3 minutes recovery between sets for optimal strength development. 30 seconds to 2 minutes recovery per set if exercises are alternated that require different muscle groups (chest and upper back) or between muscular endurance sets
Frequency:	2 to 3 days per week on nonconsecutive days. More frequent training can be done if different muscle groups are exercised on different days (allow at least 48 hours between strength-training sessions of the same muscle group)

SOURCE: Adapted from American College of Sports Medicine, ACSM's Guidelines for Exercise Testing and Prescription (Philadelphia: Wolters Kluwer/ Lippincott Williams & Wilkins, 2014).

Table 3.3 Guidelines for Various Strength-Training Programs

Strength-Training Program	Resistance	Sets	Rest Between Sets*	Frequency (workouts per week)**
General fitness	8–12 reps max	2–4	2–3 min	2–3
Muscular endurance	15–25 reps	2–4	1–2 min	2–3
Maximal strength	1–6 reps max	2–5	3 min	2–3
Body building	8–20 reps near max	3–8	Up to 1 min	4–12

© Cengage Learning

*Recovery between sets can be decreased by alternating exercises that use different muscle groups.
**Weekly training sessions can be increased by using a split-body routine.

first program, "Strength-Training Exercises without Weights" (Exercise 1 through Exercise 15). This program can be conducted within the walls of your own home. Your body weight is used as the primary resistance for most exercises. A few exercises call for a friend's help or basic implements from around your home to provide greater resistance.

"Strength-Training Exercises with Weights" (Exercise 16 through Exercise 27) requires machines such as those shown in the various photographs. Some of these exercises can also be performed with free weights.

Strength-Training Exercise Guidelines

As you prepare to design your strength-training program, you should keep several guidelines in mind.

1. Select exercises that will involve all major muscle groups: chest, shoulders, back, legs, arms, hips, and trunk.
2. Select exercises that will strengthen the core. Use controlled movements and start with light-to-moderate resistances (later, athletes may use explosive movements with heavier resistances).
3. Never lift weights alone. Always have someone work out with you in case you need a spotter or help with an injury. When you use free weights, one to two spotters are recommended for certain exercises (e.g., bench press, squats, and overhead press).
4. Prior to lifting weights, warm up properly by performing a light- to moderate-intensity aerobic activity (five to seven minutes) and some gentle stretches for a few minutes.
5. Use proper lifting technique for each exercise. The correct lifting technique will involve only those muscles and joints intended for a specific exercise. Involving other muscles and joints to "cheat" during the exercise to complete a repetition or to be able to lift a greater resistance decreases the long-term effectiveness of the exercise and can lead to injury (such as arching the back during the push-up, squat, or bench press exercises). Proper lifting technique also implies performing the exercises in a controlled manner and throughout the entire range of motion. Perform each repetition

in a rhythmic manner and at a moderate speed. Avoid fast and jerky movements, and do not throw the entire body into the lifting motion. Do not arch the back when lifting a weight.

6. Maintain proper body balance while lifting. Proper balance involves good posture, a stable body position, and correct seat and arm/leg settings on exercise machines. Loss of balance places undue strain on smaller muscles and leads to injuries because of the heavy resistances suddenly placed on them. In the early stages of a program, first-time lifters often struggle with bar control and balance when using free weights. This problem is overcome quickly with practice following a few training sessions.

7. Exercise larger muscle groups (such as those in the chest, back, and legs) before exercising smaller muscle groups (arms, abdominals, ankles, neck). For example, the bench press exercise works the chest, shoulders, and back of the upper arms (triceps), whereas the triceps extension works the back of the upper arms only.

8. Exercise opposing muscle groups for a balanced workout. When you work the chest (bench press), also work the back (rowing torso). If you work the biceps (arm curl), also work the triceps (triceps extension).

9. Breathe naturally. Inhale during the eccentric phase (bringing the weight down), and exhale during the concentric phase (lifting or pushing the weight up). Practice proper breathing with lighter weights when you are learning a new exercise.

10. Avoid holding your breath while straining to lift a weight. Holding your breath increases the pressure inside the chest and abdominal cavity greatly, making it nearly impossible for the blood in the veins to return to the heart. Although rare, a sudden high intrathoracic pressure may lead to dizziness, a blackout, a stroke, a heart attack, or a hernia.

11. Based on the program selected, allow adequate recovery time between sets of exercises (see Table 3.3).

12. If you experience unusual discomfort or pain, discontinue training. The high-tension loads used in strength training can exacerbate potential injuries. Discomfort and pain are signals to stop and determine what's wrong. Be sure to evaluate your condition properly before you continue training.

13. Use common sense on days when you feel fatigued or when you are performing sets to complete fatigue. Excessive fatigue affects lifting technique, body balance, muscles involved, and range of motion—all of which increase the risk for injury. A spotter is recommended when sets are performed to complete

fatigue. The spotter's help through the most difficult part of the repetition will relieve undue stress on muscles, ligaments, and tendons—and help ensure that you perform the exercise correctly.

14. At the end of each strength-training workout, stretch out for a few minutes to help your muscles return to their normal resting length and to minimize muscle soreness and risk for injury.

Core Strength Training

The trunk (spine) and pelvis are referred to as the "core" of the body. Core muscles include the abdominal muscles (rectus, transversus, and internal and external obliques), hip muscles (front and back), and spinal muscles (lower and upper back muscles). These muscle groups are responsible for maintaining the stability of the spine and pelvis.

Many of the major muscle groups of the legs, shoulders, and arms attach to the core. A strong core allows a person to perform activities of daily living with greater ease, improve sports performance through a more effective energy transfer from large to small body parts, and decrease the incidence of low back pain.

Interest in core strength-training programs has increased recently. A major objective of core training is to exercise the abdominal and lower back muscles in unison. Furthermore, individuals should spend as much time training the back muscles as they do the abdominal muscles. Besides enhancing stability, core training improves dynamic balance, which is often required during participation in physical activity and sports.

Key core-training exercises include the abdominal crunch and bent-leg curl-up, reverse crunch, pelvic tilt, lateral plank, prone plank, supine plank, leg press, lat pull-down, seated back, and back extension (Exercises 4, 11, 12, 13, 14, 15, 19, 21, 25, and 27 in Appendix A) and pelvic clock (Exercise 51 in Appendix C, page 286).

When core training is used in athletic conditioning programs, athletes attempt to mimic the dynamic skills used in their sport. To do so, they use special equipment such as balance boards, stability balls, and foam pads. The use of this equipment allows the athletes to train the core while seeking balance and stability in a sport-specific manner.

Designing Your Own Strength-Training Program

The pre-exercise guidelines outlined in the Physical Activity Readiness Questionaire (see Activity 1.2, page 26–29) also apply to strength training. If you have any concerns about whether your present health status will allow you to safely participate in strength training, consult a physician before you start. Strength training is not advised for people with advanced heart disease.

Depending on the facilities available to you, choose one of the two training programs outlined in Appendix A. Once you begin your strength training, you may use the form provided in Activity 3.4, page 98, to keep a record of your training program.

The resistance, the number of repetitions, and the sets you use with your program should be based on your current strength-fitness level and the amount of time that you have for your strength workout. If you are training for reasons other than general health fitness, review Table 3.3, page 76, for a summary of the guidelines.

Dietary Recommendations for Strength Development

Individuals who wish to enhance muscle growth and strength during periods of intense strength training should increase protein to 1.2 to 2.0 grams per kilogram of body weight per day. The selected amount should be based on the volume of the undertaken strength-training program. Adequate dietary protein (at least 1.2 g per kilogram of body weight per day) distributed throughout the day is particularly important for older adults. Unless protein intake is adequate, even strength-training is associated with lower muscle mass. For a 140-pound older adult, 1.2 g per kilogram of body weight translates into 76 total g of protein per day or 25 g per meal.

The timing, dose, and type of protein are all important in promoting muscle growth. Studies suggest that consuming a pre-exercise snack consisting of a combination of carbohydrates and protein leads to greater amino acid (the building blocks of protein) uptake by the muscle cells. The carbohydrates supply energy for training, and the availability of amino acids in the blood during training enhances muscle building. A peanut butter, turkey, or tuna sandwich; milk or yogurt and fruit; or nuts and fruit consumed 20 to 60 minutes before training are excellent choices for a pre-workout snack. As an added benefit, research showed that a whey protein (18 grams) supplement ingested 20 minutes prior to strength training resulted in a greater increase in resting energy expenditure during the 24 hours following the exercise session as compared to a carbohydrate (19 grams) only supplement.[22] Consuming a carbohydrate/protein snack immediately following strength training and a meal or second snack an hour thereafter further promotes muscle growth and strength development. Post-exercise carbohydrates help restore muscle glycogen depleted during training and, in combination with protein, induce an increase in blood insulin and growth hormone levels. These hormones are essential to the muscle-building process.

The higher level of circulating amino acids in the bloodstream immediately following training is believed to increase protein synthesis to a greater extent than amino acids made available later in the day. People who consume a carbohydrate/protein pre-exercise/post-exercise supplement gain significantly more muscle mass than those who consume a similar supplement morning and evening.[23] A ratio of 4 to 1 grams of carbohydrates to protein is recommended—such as a snack containing 40 grams of carbohydrates (160 calories) and 10 grams of protein (40 calories).

The type of protein you consume is also important for optimal development. Whey protein, found in milk, has been shown to be the most effective type of protein for strength development and myofibrillar hypertrophy. Milk contains two major types of proteins: whey and casein. Whey can be separated from the casein or formed as a by-product of cheese production. Whey protein has been reported to be superior to casein, soy, or egg proteins for muscular development.

The relatively immediate preexercise/postexercise carbohydrate/protein consumption is critical, but muscle fibers do continue to absorb a greater amount of amino acids up to 48 hours following strength training. Thus, while attempting to increase muscular strength and size, proper distribution of protein intake at regular intervals throughout the day is important. Research indicates that further myofibrillar protein synthesis and muscle development are best accomplished with a 20-gram-dose of whey protein taken every three hours throughout the day.[24] The latter has proven to be more effective than taking a similar total amount of protein with morning and evening meals.

Once you have reached your strength and hypertrophy goals, do not neglect your daily protein intake. Spreading the intake over three meals (about 20 to 40 grams of high-quality protein per meal based on your body size and level of activity) is most effective in keeping you satisfied, maintaining your muscle tissue, and helping reduce your caloric intake the rest of the day.

3.6 Flexibility

Improving and maintaining good joint range of motion throughout life is important in enhancing health and quality of life. Nevertheless, fitness participants generally have underestimated and overlooked flexibility fitness.

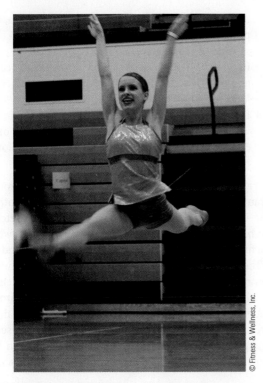

Performance of complex motor skills improves with good flexibility.

The most significant detriments to flexibility are sedentary living and lack of physical activity. As physical activity decreases, muscles lose elasticity, and tendons and ligaments tighten and shorten. Aging also reduces the extensibility of soft tissue, decreasing flexibility.

Generally, flexibility exercises to improve range of motion around the joints are conducted following an aerobic workout. Stretching exercises seem to be most effective when a person is warmed up properly. Cool muscle temperatures decrease joint range of motion. Changes in muscle temperature can increase or decrease flexibility by as much as 20 percent. Because of the effects of muscular temperature on flexibility, many people prefer to do their stretching exercises after the aerobic phase of their workout.

Muscular Flexibility Prescription

Because range of motion is highly specific to each body part (ankle, trunk, shoulder, and so on), a comprehensive stretching program should include all body parts and follow the basic guidelines for development of flexibility. To increase the total range of motion of a joint, the specific muscles surrounding that joint have to be stretched progressively beyond their accustomed length. The factors of mode, intensity, repetitions, and frequency of exercise also can be applied to flexibility programs.

Mode of Exercise

There are several modes of stretching that promote flexibility:

1. Static (slow-sustained stretching)
2. Ballistic stretching
3. Dynamic stretching
4. Controlled ballistic stretching
5. Proprioceptive neuromuscular facilitation (PNF) stretching

Although all five modes of stretching are effective in developing better flexibility, each has certain advantages.

Static Stretching With **static stretching** or **slow-sustained stretching**, muscles are lengthened gradually through a joint's complete range of motion and the final position is held for a few seconds. A slow-sustained stretch causes the muscles to relax and thereby achieve greater length. This type of stretch causes little pain and has a low risk for injury. In flexibility-development programs, slow-sustained stretching exercises are the most frequently used and recommended. Static stretching can be active or passive. In an **active static stretch** the position is held by the strength of the muscle being stretched, as is performed in many yoga poses. Although similar to active static stretching, in a **passive static stretch** the muscles are relaxed, (i.e., they are in a passive state), and an external force, provided by another person or apparatus (for example, a ballet barre or an elastic band), is applied to increase the range of motion.

Ballistic Stretching **Ballistic stretching** requires the impetus of a moving body or body part to force a joint or group of joints beyond the normal range of motion. This type of stretching requires a fast and repetitive bouncing motion to achieve a greater degree of stretch. An example would be repeatedly bouncing down and up to touch the toes. Ballistic stretching is the least recommended form of

---GLOSSARY---

Static stretching (slow-sustained stretching) Exercises in which the muscles are lengthened gradually through a joint's complete range of motion.

Active static stretch Stretching exercise wherein the position is held by the strength of the muscle being stretched.

Passive static stretch Stretching exercise performed with the aid of an external force applied by either another individual or an external apparatus.

Ballistic stretching Stretching exercises performed with jerky, rapid, and bouncy movements.

stretching. Fitness professionals feel that it causes muscle soreness and increases the risk of injuries to muscles and nerves. Limited data, however, are available to corroborate such effects. This form of stretching should never be performed without a previous mild aerobic warm-up and only gentle bouncing actions are recommended for those who wish to use this mode of stretching.

Dynamic Stretching Speed of movement, momentum, and active muscular effort are used in **dynamic stretching** to increase the range of motion about a joint or group of joints. Unlike ballistic stretching, it does not require bouncing motions. Exaggerating a kicking action, walking lunges, and arm circles are all examples of dynamic stretching. Research indicates that dynamic stretches are preferable to static stretches before athletic competition because dynamic stretching does not seem to have a negative effect on the athlete's strength and power. Dynamic stretching is beneficial for athletes such as gymnasts, dancers, figure skaters, divers, and hurdlers, whose sports activities require ballistic actions.

Precautions must be taken not to overstretch ligaments with ballistic and dynamic stretching. Ligaments undergo plastic or permanent elongation. If the stretching force cannot be controlled—as often occurs in fast, jerky movements—ligaments can easily be overstretched. This, in turn, leads to excessively loose joints, increasing the risk for injuries.

Controlled Ballistic Stretching **Controlled ballistic stretching**—that is, exercises that are performed through slow, gentle, and controlled ballistic movements (instead of jerky, rapid, and bouncy movements)—is quite effective in developing flexibility. Properly performed, this type of stretching can be done safely by most individuals, and is more commonly used by those participating in sports and activities that involve ballistic movements, like basketball.

Proprioceptive Neuromuscular Facilitation **Proprioceptive neuromuscular facilitation (PNF)** stretching is based on a "contract-and-relax" method and requires the assistance of another person. The procedure is as follows:

1. The person assisting with the exercise provides initial force by pushing slowly in the direction of the desired stretch. This first stretch does not cover the entire range of motion.
2. The person being stretched then applies force in the opposite direction of the stretch, against the assistant, who tries to hold the initial degree of stretch as closely as possible. This results in an isometric contraction at the angle of the stretch. The force of the isometric contraction can be anywhere from 20 to 75 percent of the person's maximum contraction.

3. After 3 to 6 seconds of isometric contraction, the person being stretched relaxes the target muscle(s) completely. The assistant then increases the degree of stretch slowly to a greater angle and for the PNF technique the stretch is held for 10 to 30 seconds.
4. If a greater degree of stretch is achievable, the isometric contraction is repeated for another 5 or 6 seconds, after which the degree of stretch is slowly increased again and held for 10 to 30 seconds.

If a progressive degree of stretch is used, steps 1 through 4 can be repeated up to five times. Each isometric contraction is held for 3 to 6 seconds. The progressive stretches are held for about 10 seconds—until the last trial, when the final stretched position is held for up to 30 seconds.

Theoretically, with the PNF technique, the isometric contraction helps relax the muscle being stretched, which results in lengthening the muscle. Some fitness leaders believe PNF is more effective than slow-sustained stretching. Another benefit of PNF is an increase in strength of the muscle(s) being stretched. Research has shown increases in absolute strength and muscular

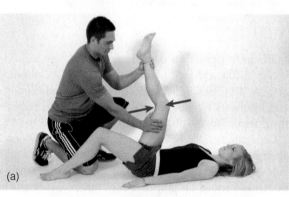

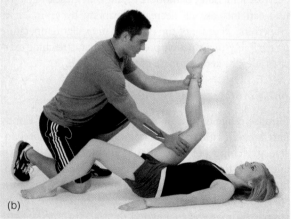

Proprioceptive neuromuscular facilitation (PNF) stretching technique: (A) isometric phase, (B) stretching phase.

endurance when the PNF technique is used. The results are consistent in both men and women and are attributed to the isometric contractions performed during PNF. Disadvantages of PNF are (1) more pain, (2) the need for a second person to assist, and (3) the need for more time to conduct each session.

Intensity of Exercise

When you do flexibility exercises, the **intensity** of each stretch should be only to the point of mild discomfort or mild tension at the end of the range of motion. Excessive pain is an indication that the load is too high and may lead to injury. All stretching should be done to slightly below the pain threshold. As participants reach this point, they should try to relax the muscle being stretched as much as possible. After completing the stretch, the body part is brought back gradually to the starting point.

Repetitions

The time required for an exercise session for development of flexibility is based on the number of repetitions and the length of time each repetition is held in the final stretched position. As a general recommendation, about at least 15 minutes in duration that include the major muscle/tendon units of the body should be performed. Four or more repetitions per exercise should be done, holding the final position each time for 10 to 30 seconds.[25] The goal is to achieve 60 seconds of total stretching per exercise by adjusting the duration and repetitions. Older adults may derive greater improvements when the final stretched position is held for 30 to 60 seconds.

As flexibility increases, a person can gradually increase the time each repetition is held from 10 to about 30 seconds. Data indicate that stretching for 10 to 30 seconds is better to increase range of motion than stretching for shorter periods of time and is just as effective as stretching for longer durations.[26] Individuals who are susceptible to flexibility injuries should limit each stretch to 20 seconds.

Frequency of Exercise

Flexibility exercises should be conducted a minimum of 2 or 3 days per week, but ideally 5 to 7 days per week. After 6 to 8 weeks of almost daily stretching, flexibility can be maintained with 2 to 3 sessions per week, involving the major muscle/tendon groups of the body and doing 2 to 4 repetitions for up to a total of 60 seconds for each exercise performed. Figure 3.4 summarizes the flexibility development guidelines.

When to Stretch?

Many people do not differentiate a warm-up from stretching. Warming up means starting a workout slowly with walking, cycling, or slow jogging, followed by gentle stretching (not through the entire range of motion). Stretching implies movement of joints through their full range of motion and holding the final degree of stretch according to recommended guidelines.

A warm-up that progressively increases muscle temperature and mimics movement that will occur during training enhances performance. For some activities, gentle stretching is recommended in conjunction with warm-up routines. Before steady activities (walking, jogging, cycling), a warm-up of 3 to 5 minutes is recommended. The recommendation is up to 10 minutes before stop-and-go activities (e.g., racquet sports, basketball, and soccer) and athletic participation in general (e.g., football and gymnastics). Activities that require abrupt changes in direction are more likely to cause muscle strains if they are performed without proper warm-up that includes mild stretching.

Sports-specific pre-exercise stretching can improve performance in sports that require a greater-than-average

Figure 3.4 Flexibility development guidelines.

Mode:	Slow-sustained (static), ballistic (dynamic), or proprioceptive neuromuscular facilitation (PNF) stretching to include all major muscle/tendon groups of the body
Intensity:	To the point of mild tension or limits of discomfort
Repetitions:	Repeat each exercise 2 to 4 times, holding the final position between 10 and 30 seconds
Frequency:	At least 2 or 3 days per week Ideally 5 to 7 days per week

SOURCE: Adapted from American College of Sports Medicine, ACSM's Guidelines for Exercise Testing and Prescription (Philadelphia: Wolters Kluwer/ Lippincott Williams & Wilkins, 2014).

GLOSSARY

Dynamic stretching Stretching exercises that require speed of movement, momentum, and active muscular effort to help increase the range of motion about a joint or group of joints.

Controlled ballistic stretching Exercises done with slow, short, gentle, and sustained movements.

Proprioceptive neuromuscular facilitation (PNF) Mode of stretching that uses reflexes and neuromuscular principles to relax the muscles being stretched.

Intensity (for flexibility exercises) Degree of stretch when doing flexibility exercises.

range of motion, such as gymnastics, dance, diving, and figure skating. Intense stretching conducted prior to participating in sports that rely on force and power for peak performance is not recommended, as data suggest that acute stretching during warm-up can lead to a temporary short-term (up to 60 minutes) decrease in strength and power.[27]

In terms of preventing injuries, the best time to stretch is controversial. In limited studies on athletic populations, the evidence is unclear as to whether stretching before or after exercise is more beneficial in preventing injury. Additional research is necessary to clarify this issue.

In general, unless the activity requires extensive range of motion, a good time to stretch is after aerobic workouts. Higher body temperature in itself helps to increase the joint range of motion. Muscles also are fatigued following exercise, and a fatigued muscle tends to shorten, which can lead to soreness and spasms. Stretching exercises help fatigued muscles reestablish their normal resting length and prevent unnecessary pain. Whether performed before or after exercise, studies show that overall, those who stretch either before or after a workout report a relative decrease in discomfort felt from delayed-onset muscle soreness that typically peaks 24 to 48 hours after physical activity.[28]

Designing a Flexibility Program

To improve body flexibility, each major muscle group should be subjected to at least one stretching exercise. A complete set of exercises for developing muscular flexibility is presented in Appendix B.

You may not be able to hold a final stretched position with some of these exercises (such as lateral head tilts and arm circles), but you still should perform the exercise through the joint's full range of motion. Depending on the number and the length of repetitions, a complete workout will last between 15 and 30 minutes.

Critical Thinking

Carefully consider the relevance of stretching exercises in your personal fitness program throughout the years.
• How much importance do you place on these exercises?
• Have any conditions improved through your stretching program or have any specific exercises contributed to your health and well-being?

3.7 *Preventing and Rehabilitating Low Back Pain*

Few people make it through life without having low back pain at some point. An estimated 60 percent to 80 percent of the population has been afflicted by back pain or injury. When it comes to back pain, prevention and treatment through physical exercise is by far the best medicine.

Back pain is caused by (a) physical inactivity, (b) poor postural habits and body mechanics, (c) excessive body weight, and/or (d) psychological stress and is preventable more than 80 percent of the time. Back injuries are also more common among smokers because smoking reduces blood flow to the spine, increasing back pain susceptibility.

More than 95 percent of all back pain is related to muscle/tendon injury, and only 1 percent to 5 percent is related to intervertebral disk damage.[29] Usually, back pain is the result of repeated micro-injuries that occur over an extended time (sometimes years) until a certain movement, activity, or excessive overload causes a significant injury to the tissues.[30]

People tend to think of back pain as a problem with the skeleton. Actually, the spine's curvature, alignment, and movement are controlled by surrounding muscles. The most common reason for chronic low back pain is a lack of physical activity. In particular, a major contributor to back pain is excessive sitting, which causes back muscles to shorten, stiffen, and become weaker.

Deterioration or weakening of the abdominal and gluteal muscles, along with tightening of the lower back (erector spinae) muscles, brings about an unnatural forward tilt of the pelvis (Figure 3.5). This tilt puts extra pressure on the spinal vertebrae, causing pain in the lower back. Accumulation of fat around the midsection of the body contributes to the forward tilt of the pelvis, which further aggravates the condition.

Low back pain frequently is associated with faulty posture and improper body mechanics, or body positions. Incorrect posture and poor mechanics, such as prolonged static postures, repetitive bending and pushing, twisting a loaded spine, and prolonged (more than an hour) sitting with little movement increase strain on the lower back and many other bones, joints, muscles, and ligaments. Figure 3.6 provides a summary of proper body mechanics that promote back health.

Data recently published in 2013 indicate that between 40 percent and 80 percent of long-term back pain due to a herniated or slipped disk may be related to a bacterial infection caused by *Propionibacterium acnes*.[31,32] This infection can lead to swelling and tissue damage in the

Figure 3.5 Incorrect (left) and correct (right) pelvic alignment.

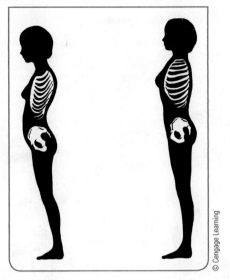

© Cengage Learning

spine. Long-term (100 days) treatment with antibiotics provided significant relief of pain and disability for up to a year later in most of these patients. Additional clinical studies are still required to confirm these findings, but people who suffer from persistent back pain should request a blood test to check for such a bacterial infection.

In the majority of back injuries, pain is present only with movement and physical activity. According to the National Institutes of Health (NIH), most back pain goes away on its own in a few weeks. A physician should be consulted if any of the following conditions are present:

- Numbness in the legs
- Trouble urinating
- Leg weakness
- Fever
- Unintentional weight loss
- Persistent severe pain even at rest

A physician can rule out any disk damage, arthritis, osteoporosis, a slipped vertebra, spinal stenosis (narrowing of the spinal canal), or other serious condition. For common back pain, he or she may prescribe proper bed rest using several pillows under the knees for leg support (Figure 3.6). This position helps relieve muscle spasms by stretching the muscles involved. He or she may also prescribe a muscle relaxant or anti-inflammatory medication (or both) and some type of physical therapy.

In most cases, an X-ray and MRI are not required unless pain lingers for more than four to six weeks. In the early stages of back pain, tight muscles and muscle spasms tend to compress the vertebrae, squeezing the intervertebral disks and revealing apparent disk

problems on an X-ray. In these cases, the real problem is the tight muscles and subsequent muscle spasms. A daily physical activity and stretching program helps to decompress the spine, stretch tight muscles, strengthen weak muscles, and increase blood flow (promoting healing) to the back muscles.

Time is often the best treatment approach. Even with severe pain, most people feel better within days or weeks without being treated by health care professionals. Up to 90 percent of people heal on their own. To relieve symptoms, you may use over-the-counter pain relievers and hot or cold packs. You also should stay active to avoid further weakening of the back muscles. Low-impact activities such as walking, swimming, water aerobics, and cycling are recommended. Once you are pain free in the resting state, you need to start correcting the muscular imbalance by stretching the tight muscles and strengthening the weak ones. Stretching exercises always are performed first.

If there is no indication of disease or injury (such as leg numbness or pain), a herniated disk, or fractures, spinal manipulation by a chiropractor or other health care professional can provide pain relief. Spinal manipulation as a treatment modality for low back pain has been endorsed by the federal Agency for Health Care Policy and Research. The guidelines suggest that spinal manipulation may help to alleviate discomfort and pain during the first few weeks of an acute episode of low back pain. Generally, benefits are seen in fewer than 10 treatments. People who have had chronic pain for more than 6 months should avoid spinal manipulation until they have been thoroughly examined by a physician.

Acute or short-term low back pain is most often the result of trauma or injury to the lower back and typically lasts a few days or weeks. Back pain is considered chronic if it persists longer than 3 months. Surgery is seldom the best option, as it often weakens the spine. Scar tissue and surgical alterations also decrease the success rate of a subsequent surgery. Only about 10 percent of people with chronic pain are candidates for surgery. If surgery is recommended, always seek a second opinion. And consider all other options. In many cases, pushing beyond the pain and participating in aggressive physical therapy ("exercise boot camps" for back pain) aimed at strengthening the muscles that support the spine are what's needed to overcome the condition. Data from the Physicians Neck & Back Clinic in Minneapolis showed that only 3 in 38 patients recommended for surgery needed it upon completion of a 10-week aggressive physical therapy program.[33]

Back pain can be reduced greatly through aerobic exercise, muscular flexibility exercise, and muscular fitness

Figure 3.6 **Proper back care.**

Low back pain is caused by (a) physical inactivity, (b) poor postural habits and body mechanics, (c) excessive body weight, and/or (d) psychological stress. To protect your back and avoid debilitating low-back strain, you need to use proper body mechanics and correct improper body posture. Using appropriate body positions and actions in all daily activities is vital for back health. The following guidelines help avoid unnecessary back strain and protect and support your back.

Correct standing position

To learn the correct standing posture, stand a foot away from a wall and place your upper body completely straight against the wall. You will need to tighten the abdominal and gluteal muscles to do so. Next, walk around for a few minutes holding this same position and at the end return to the wall to evaluate how well you maintained the posture.

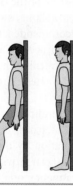

Standing, lifting, and carrying positions

Incorrect: **Correct:**

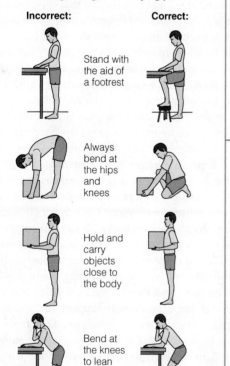

Stand with the aid of a footrest

Always bend at the hips and knees

Hold and carry objects close to the body

Bend at the knees to lean forward

Correct sitting position

Most people spend many daily hours sitting. Proper sitting and preventing a forward slump is essential for back health. To straighten your back (a) put your head back, (b) pull in your chin toward your chest, (c) tighten your abdominal muscles, and (d) raise your chest. You should always sit in this manner. The following guidelines will also help correct improper sitting throughout the day.

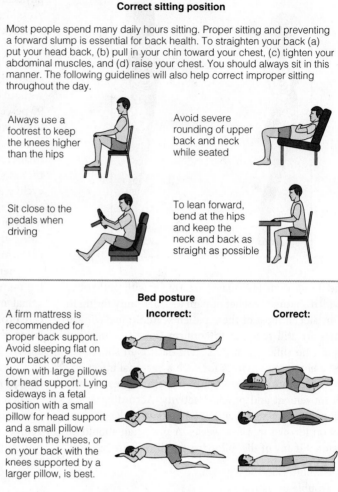

Always use a footrest to keep the knees higher than the hips

Avoid severe rounding of upper back and neck while seated

Sit close to the pedals when driving

To lean forward, bend at the hips and keep the neck and back as straight as possible

Bed posture

A firm mattress is recommended for proper back support. Avoid sleeping flat on your back or face down with large pillows for head support. Lying sideways in a fetal position with a small pillow for head support and a small pillow between the knees, or on your back with the knees supported by a larger pillow, is best.

Incorrect: **Correct:**

When resting, do it right

When at home resting or relaxing, lie flat on your back with a small pillow under your neck and with pillows under the knees for support. You may also place the lower legs on a chair with your knees bent at 90 degrees. This position is also good to relieve back spasms when suffering from back pain.

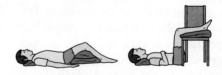

When watching TV or sitting on the floor, do so by lying on a straight-back chair covered with a firm pillow and a second large pillow under the knees.

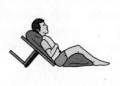

© Cengage Learning

training that includes specific exercises to strengthen the spine-stabilizing muscles, often referred to as the "core." The core consists of many distinctive muscles running the length of the torso, including the back, abdominals, hips, chest, and inner and outer thighs. Because having a strong core is the best defense against injury to the spine, a good core-strengthening program can also help reduce back pain or prevent recurring pain. Exercise requires effort by the patient, and it may create discomfort initially, but exercise promotes circulation, healing, muscle size, and muscle strength and endurance. Many patients abstain from aggressive physical therapy because they are unwilling to commit the time required for the program.

In terms of alleviating back pain, *exercise is medicine*, but it needs to be the right type of exercise. Aerobic exercise is beneficial because it helps decrease body fat and psychological stress. During an episode of back pain, however, people often avoid activity and cope by getting more rest. In most cases, this restriction on physical activity has been shown in studies to be exactly the opposite of what people need to do to reduce low back pain.[34] Patients who continued daily work and physical activity experienced faster recoveries than those treated with bed rest. Rest is recommended if the pain is associated with a herniated disk, but if your physician rules out a serious problem, exercise is a better choice of treatment. Exercise helps restore physical function, and individuals who start and maintain an aerobic exercise program have back pain less frequently. Individuals who exercise also are less likely to require surgery or other invasive treatments.

Regular stretching exercises that help the hip and trunk go through a functional range of motion, rather than increasing the range of motion, are recommended. That is, for proper back care, stretching exercises should not be performed to the extreme range of motion. Individuals with a greater spinal range of motion also have a higher incidence of back injury. Spinal stability, instead of mobility, is desirable for back health.

A strengthening program for a healthy back should be conducted around the endurance threshold—15 or more repetitions to near fatigue. Muscular endurance of the muscles that support the spine is more important than absolute strength because these muscles perform their work during the course of an entire day.

Critical Thinking

Consider your own low back health. • Have you ever had episodes of low back pain? If so, how long did it take you to recover, and what helped you recover from this condition?

DESK ERGONOMICS
8 Tips for Improving Your Computer Workspace

1 Center your monitor and keyboard in front of you with the top of the monitor at or below eye level. Be sure your monitor viewing distance is at about an arm's length away to prevent eye strain.

2 Rest your feet flat on the floor and position your knees at or below hip height. Use a footrest if your feet don't comfortably reach the floor or lower the keyboard and chair.

3 Adjust the height of your chair so your elbows are at about keyboard level with your wrists positioned straight and in-line with your forearms. Use a wrist rest if needed to ensure minimal bend at the wrists.

4 Place the mouse next to the keyboard to keep your arms and elbows close to your body as you work. Use a mouse pad to protect your hands and forearms from pressing against the hard surface of the desk.

5 Adjust the incline of your chair to provide good support for your lower back. Use a small pillow or lumbar support cushion if needed.

6 Reduce screen glare. Tilt or reposition the monitor as needed, and clean the screen regularly. Set the screen contrast and brightness for comfortable viewing.

7 Take frequent short breaks, 10 minutes per hour of sitting. Breaks can include stretching, walking around, or standing/walking while talking to others.

8 Be mindful to correct your sitting posture often.

© Fitness & Wellness, Inc.

Several exercises for preventing and rehabilitating the backache syndrome are given in Appendix C, pages 284–286. These exercises can be done twice or more daily when a person has back pain. Under normal circumstances, doing these exercises three or four times a week is enough to prevent the syndrome. Using additional core exercises will further enhance your low back management program. Back pain recurs more often in people who rely solely on medication, compared with people who use both medication and exercise therapy to recover.[35]

Effects of Posture

Good posture enhances personal appearance, self-image, and confidence; improves balance and endurance; protects against misalignment-related pains and aches; prevents falls; and enhances your overall sense of well-being.[36] The relationship among different body parts is the essence of posture.

Poor posture is a risk factor for musculoskeletal problems of the neck, shoulders, and lower back. Incorrect posture also strains hips and knees. Faulty posture and weak and inelastic muscles are also a leading cause of chronic low back problems.

Adequate body mechanics also aid in reducing chronic low back pain. Proper body mechanics means using correct positions in all the activities of daily life, including sleeping, sitting, standing, walking, driving, working, and exercising. Because of the high incidence of low back pain, illustrations of proper body mechanics are shown in Figure 3.6. Besides engaging in the recommended exercises, you need to continuously strive to maintain good posture. As posture improves, you frequently become motivated to change other aspects, such as muscular strength and flexibility and decreasing body fat.

Effects of Stress

Psychological stress, too, may lead to back pain.[37] The brain is "hardwired" to the back muscles. Excessive stress causes muscles to contract. Frequent tightening of the back muscles can throw the back out of alignment and constrict blood vessels that supply oxygen and nutrients to the back. Chronic stress also increases the release of hormones that have been linked to muscle and tendon injuries. Furthermore, people under stress tend to forget proper body mechanics, placing themselves at unnecessary risk for injury. If you are undergoing excessive stress and back pain at the same time, proper stress management (see Chapter 7) should be a part of your comprehensive back-care program.

3.9 Contraindicated Exercises

Most strength and flexibility exercises are relatively safe to perform, but even safe exercises can be hazardous if they are done incorrectly. Some exercises may be safe for you to perform occasionally but, when executed repeatedly, could cause trauma and injury. Preexisting muscle or joint conditions (old sprains or injuries) can further increase the risk of harm when performing certain exercises. As you develop your exercise program, you are encouraged to follow the exercise descriptions and guidelines given in this book.

A few exercises are not recommended because they pose a potentially high risk for injury. These exercises are sometimes performed in videotaped workouts and some fitness classes. **Contraindicated exercises** may cause harm because of the excessive strain placed on muscles and joints—in particular, the spine, lower back, knees, neck, or shoulders.

Illustrations of contraindicated exercises are presented in Appendix D, pages 287–290. Safe alternative exercises are listed below each contraindicated exercise and are illustrated in Appendix A (strength exercises), pages 272–280, and Appendix B (flexibility exercises), pages 281–283. In isolated instances a qualified physical therapist may select one or a few of the contraindicated exercises to treat a certain injury or disability in a carefully supervised setting. Unless you are instructed specifically to use one of these exercises, it is best that you select safe exercises from this book.

3.10 Getting Started

Introducing new behaviors into one's daily routine takes most people months or longer to accomplish. A fitness program is no exception. Adding exercise to a person's lifestyle may require retraining (behavior modification).

Different things motivate different people to start and remain in a fitness program. Regardless of your initial reason for initiating an exercise program, you now need to plan for ways to make your workout fun. The psychology behind it is simple: If you enjoy an activity, you will continue to do it.

The first few weeks probably will be the most difficult, but where there's a will, there's a way. Once you begin to see positive changes, it won't be as hard. Soon you will develop a habit for exercise that will be deeply satisfying and will bring about a sense of self-accomplishment. The suggestions in the box on the next page have been used by people to help them change behavior and adhere to a lifetime exercise program.

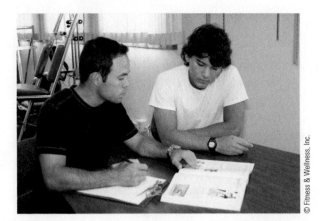

Setting realistic goals will help you design and guide your fitness program.

While fitness evaluation is important to assess changes in physical capacity, attention must be given to actual program compliance. Regular physical activity is the key to better health and quality of life (see "Health Fitness Standard" in Chapter 2, page 32). Exercise logs provide the means to carefully document your participation in fitness programs and allow you to monitor your progress and compare it against previous months and years. Activity 3.4, pages 98–101, contains exercise log sheets to monitor your CR endurance and muscular strength programs. You are strongly encouraged to keep a detailed record of all of your activities.

3.11 *Setting Fitness Goals*

Before you leave this chapter, consider your fitness goals. In the last few decades we have become accustomed to "quick fixes" with everything from super-fast foods to one-hour dry cleaning. Fitness, however, has no quick fix. Fitness takes time and dedication, and only those who are committed and persistent will reap the rewards. As described in Chapter 1, setting realistic fitness goals will guide your program. Activity 3.4, page 98, offers a goal-setting form that will help you determine your fitness goals. Take the time, either by yourself or with your instructor's help, to fill it out.

As you prepare to write realistic fitness goals, base these goals on the results of your initial fitness test (pre-test). For instance, if your CR fitness category was "poor" on the pre-test, you should not expect to improve to the "excellent" category in a little more than 3 months. Whenever possible, your fitness goals should be measurable and time-specific. A goal that simply states "to improve my CR endurance" is not as good as a goal that states "to improve to the 'good' fitness category in CR endurance by April 15" or "to run the 1.5-mile course in less than 11 minutes the week of final exams."

After determining each goal, monitor your progress toward your goal regularly. You also will need to write measurable actions to accomplish that goal. These actions provide the actual plan to accomplish your goal. A sample of actions to accomplish the previously stated goal for development of CR endurance could be:

1. Use jogging as the mode of exercise.
2. Jog at 10:00 a.m. five times per week.
3. Jog around the track in the field house.
4. Jog for 30 minutes each exercise session.
5. Monitor heart rate regularly during exercise.
6. Take the 1.5-Mile Run Test once a month.

You will not always meet your specific actions. If so, your goal may be out of reach. Reevaluate your actions and make adjustments accordingly. If you set unrealistic goals at the beginning of your exercise program, be flexible with yourself and reconsider your plan of action, but do not quit. Reconsidering your plan of action does not mean that you have failed. Failure comes only to those who stop trying, and success comes to those who are committed and persistent.

GLOSSARY

Contraindicated exercises Exercises that are not recommended because they pose potentially high risk for injury.

Behavior Modification Planning

Tips to Enhance Compliance with Your Fitness Program

Adults need recess, too! There are 1,440 minutes in every day. Schedule a minimum of 30 of these minutes for physical activity. With a little creativity and planning, even the person with the busiest schedule can make room for physical activity. For many folks, before or after work or meals is often an available time to cycle, walk, or play. Think about your weekly or daily schedule and look for or make opportunities to be more active. Every little bit helps. Consider the following suggestions:

1. Set aside a regular time for exercise. If you don't plan ahead, it is a lot easier to skip. On a weekly basis, using red ink, schedule your exercise time into your day planner. Next, hold your exercise hour "sacred." Give exercise priority equal to the most important school or business activity of the day.

2. If you are too busy, attempt to accumulate 30 to 60 minutes of daily activity by doing separate 10-minute sessions throughout the day. Try reading the mail while you walk, taking stairs instead of elevators, walking the dog, or riding the stationary bike as you watch the evening news.

3. Exercise early in the day, when you will be less tired and the chances of something interfering with your workout are minimal; thus, you will be less likely to skip your exercise session.

4. Select aerobic activities you enjoy. Exercise should be as much fun as your favorite hobby. If you pick an activity you don't enjoy, you will be unmotivated and less likely to keep exercising. Don't be afraid to try out a new activity, even if that means learning new skills.

5. Combine different activities. You can train by doing two or three different activities the same week. This cross-training may reduce the monotony of repeating the same activity every day. Try lifetime sports. Many endurance sports, such as racquetball, basketball, soccer, badminton, roller skating, cross-country skiing, and body surfing (paddling the board), provide a nice break from regular workouts.

6. Use the proper clothing and equipment for exercise. A poor pair of shoes, for example, can make you more prone to injury, discouraging you from the beginning.

7. Find a friend or group of friends to exercise with. Social interaction will make exercise more fulfilling. Besides, exercise is harder to skip if someone is waiting to go with you.

8. Set goals and share them with others. Quitting is tougher when someone else knows what you are trying to accomplish. When you reach a targeted goal, reward yourself with a new pair of shoes or a jogging suit.

9. Purchase a pedometer (step counter) and build up to 10,000 steps per day. These 10,000 steps may include all forms of daily physical activity combined. Pedometers motivate people toward activity because they track daily activity, provide feedback on activity level, and remind the participant to enhance daily activity.

10. Don't become a chronic exerciser. Overexercising can lead to chronic fatigue and injuries. Exercise should be enjoyable, and in the process you should stop and smell the roses.

11. Exercise in different places and facilities. This will add variety to your workouts.

12. Exercise to music. People who listen to fast-tempo music tend to exercise more vigorously and longer. Using headphones when exercising outdoors, however, can be dangerous. Even indoors, it is preferable not to use headphones so you still can be aware of your surroundings.

13. Keep a regular record of your activities. Keeping a record allows you to monitor your progress and compare it against previous months and years (see Activity 3.4, page 98).

14. Conduct periodic assessments. Improving to a higher fitness category is often a reward in itself, and creating your own rewards is even more motivating.

15. Listen to your body. If you experience pain or unusual discomfort, stop exercising. Pain and aches are an indication of potential injury. If you do suffer an injury, don't return to your regular workouts until you are fully recovered. You may cross-train using activities that don't aggravate your injury (for instance, swimming instead of jogging).

16. If a health problem arises, see a physician. When in doubt, it's better to be safe than sorry.

Try It

The most difficult challenge about exercise is to keep going once you start. The above behavioral change tips will enhance your chances for exercise adherence. In your Online Journal or class notebook, describe which suggestions were most useful in helping you stick to your exercise program and why they are so effective for you.

© Cengage Learning

Assess Your Behavior

1. Do you accumulate at least 30 minutes of moderate-intensity physical activity (or higher intensity) a minimum of five days per week?

2. Do you participate in a vigorous-intensity aerobic exercise program for a minimum of 20 minutes at least three times per week?

3. Do you engage in an overall strength-training program where you perform at least one set of 8 to 12 repetitions to near fatigue, using 8 to 10 dynamic exercises that involve the major-muscle groups of the body, a minimum of two times per week?

4. Does your exercise program include stretching all major joints of the body a minimum of two times per week?

Assess Your Knowledge

1. The vigorous-intensity cardiorespiratory training zone for a 22-year-old individual with a resting heart rate of 68 bpm is
   a. 120 to 148.
   b. 132 to 156.
   c. 138 to 164.
   d. 142 to 179.
   e. 154 to 188.

2. Which of the following activities does not contribute to the development of cardiorespiratory endurance?
   a. low-impact aerobics
   b. jogging
   c. 400-yard dash
   d. racquetball
   e. All of the activities contribute to its development.

3. The recommended duration for each cardiorespiratory training session is
   a. 10 to 20 minutes.
   b. 15 to 30 minutes.
   c. 20 to 60 minutes.
   d. 45 to 70 minutes.
   e. 60 to 120 minutes.

4. During an eccentric muscle contraction,
   a. the muscle shortens as it overcomes the resistance.
   b. there is little or no movement during the contraction.
   c. a joint has to move through the entire range of motion.
   d. the muscle lengthens as it contracts.
   e. the speed is kept constant throughout the range of motion.

5. The training concept that states that the demands placed on a system must be increased systematically and progressively over time to cause physiological adaptation is referred to as
   a. the overload principle.
   b. positive resistance training.
   c. specificity of training.

   d. variable-resistance training.
   e. progressive resistance.

6. For general fitness, during strength training each set should be performed between
   a. 1 and 6 reps maximum.
   b. 4 and 8 reps maximum.
   c. 8 and 12 reps maximum.
   d. 8 and 20 reps maximum.
   e. 15 and 25 reps maximum.

7. Which of the following is not a mode of stretching?
   a. proprioceptive neuromuscular facilitation
   b. elastic elongation
   c. ballistic stretching
   d. slow-sustained stretching
   e. All are modes of stretching.

8. When you perform stretching exercises, the degree of stretch should be
   a. through the entire arc of movement.
   b. to about 80 percent of capacity.
   c. to the point of mild tension.
   d. applied until the muscle(s) start shaking.
   e. progressively increased until the desired stretch is attained.

9. Low back pain is associated with
   a. physical inactivity.
   b. faulty posture.
   c. excessive body weight.
   d. improper body mechanics.
   e. All are correct choices.

10. A goal is effective when it is
   a. written.
   b. measurable.
   c. time-specific.
   d. monitored.
   e. All are correct choices.

Correct answers can be found on page 307.

Activity 3.1 Daily Physical Activity Log

Name _____ **Date** _____

Course _____ **Section** _____

Date: [_____] Day of the Week: [_____]

Time of Day	Exercise/Activity	Duration	Number of Steps	Comments
[ ]	[ ]	[ ]	[ ]	[ ]
[ ]	[ ]	[ ]	[ ]	[ ]
[ ]	[ ]	[ ]	[ ]	[ ]
[ ]	[ ]	[ ]	[ ]	[ ]
[ ]	[ ]	[ ]	[ ]	[ ]
[ ]	[ ]	[ ]	[ ]	[ ]
[ ]	[ ]	[ ]	[ ]	[ ]
		Totals:	[ ]	[ ]

Activity category based on steps per day (use Table 3.1, page 61): [_____]

Date: [_____] Day of the Week: [_____]

Time of Day	Exercise/Activity	Duration	Number of Steps	Comments
[ ]	[ ]	[ ]	[ ]	[ ]
[ ]	[ ]	[ ]	[ ]	[ ]
[ ]	[ ]	[ ]	[ ]	[ ]
[ ]	[ ]	[ ]	[ ]	[ ]
[ ]	[ ]	[ ]	[ ]	[ ]
[ ]	[ ]	[ ]	[ ]	[ ]
[ ]	[ ]	[ ]	[ ]	[ ]
		Totals:	[ ]	[ ]

Activity category based on steps per day (use Table 3.1, page 61): [_____]

Activity 3.1 **Daily Physical Activity Log** *(continued)*

Date: [   ]   Day of the Week: [   ]

Time of Day	Exercise/Activity	Duration	Number of Steps	Comments
[ ]	[ ]	[ ]	[ ]	[ ]
[ ]	[ ]	[ ]	[ ]	[ ]
[ ]	[ ]	[ ]	[ ]	[ ]
[ ]	[ ]	[ ]	[ ]	[ ]
[ ]	[ ]	[ ]	[ ]	[ ]
[ ]	[ ]	[ ]	[ ]	[ ]
[ ]	[ ]	[ ]	[ ]	[ ]
		Totals:	[ ]	[ ]

Activity category based on steps per day (use Table 3.1, page 61): [   ]

Date: [   ]   Day of the Week: [   ]

Time of Day	Exercise/Activity	Duration	Number of Steps	Comments
[ ]	[ ]	[ ]	[ ]	[ ]
[ ]	[ ]	[ ]	[ ]	[ ]
[ ]	[ ]	[ ]	[ ]	[ ]
[ ]	[ ]	[ ]	[ ]	[ ]
[ ]	[ ]	[ ]	[ ]	[ ]
[ ]	[ ]	[ ]	[ ]	[ ]
[ ]	[ ]	[ ]	[ ]	[ ]
		Totals:	[ ]	[ ]

Activity category based on steps per day (use Table 3.1, page 61): [   ]

Briefly evaluate your current activity patterns, discuss your feelings about the results, and provide a goal for the weeks ahead.

_____

_____

_____

_____

Activity 3.2 Exercise Readiness

Name _____ **Date** _____

Course _____ **Section** _____

List advantages of starting an exercise program.

1. _____
2. _____
3. _____
4. _____
5. _____
6. _____
7. _____
8. _____
9. _____
10. _____

List disadvantages of starting an exercise program.

1. _____
2. _____
3. _____
4. _____
5. _____
6. _____
7. _____
8. _____
9. _____
10. _____

Activity 3.2 Exercise Readiness *(continued)*

Instructions

Carefully read each statement and circle the number that best describes your feelings in each statement. Please be completely honest with your answers.

	Strongly Agree	Mildly Agree	Mildly Disagree	Strongly Disagree
1. I can walk, ride a bike (or use a wheelchair), swim, or walk in a shallow pool.	4	3	2	1
2. I enjoy exercise.	4	3	2	1
3. I believe exercise can help decrease the risk for disease and premature mortality.	4	3	2	1
4. I believe exercise contributes to better health.	4	3	2	1
5. I have previously participated in an exercise program.	4	3	2	1
6. I have experienced the feeling of being physically fit.	4	3	2	1
7. I can envision myself exercising.	4	3	2	1
8. I am contemplating an exercise program.	4	3	2	1
9. I am willing to stop contemplating and give exercise a try for a few weeks.	4	3	2	1
10. I am willing to set aside time at least three times a week for exercise.	4	3	2	1
11. I can find a place to exercise (the streets, a park, a YMCA, a health club).	4	3	2	1
12. I can find other people who would like to exercise with me.	4	3	2	1
13. I will exercise when I am moody, fatigued, and even when the weather is bad.	4	3	2	1
14. I am willing to spend a small amount of money for adequate exercise clothing (shoes, shorts, leotards, swimsuit).	4	3	2	1
15. If I have any doubts about my present state of health, I will see a physician before beginning an exercise program.	4	3	2	1
16. Exercise will make me feel better and improve my quality of life.	4	3	2	1

Scoring Your Test:

This questionnaire allows you to examine your readiness for exercise. You have been evaluated in four categories: mastery (self-control), attitude, health, and commitment. Mastery indicates that you can be in control of your exercise program. Attitude examines your mental disposition toward exercise. Health measures the strength of your convictions about the wellness benefits of exercise. Commitment shows dedication and resolution to carry out the exercise program. Write the number you circled after each statement in the corresponding spaces below. Add the scores on each line to get your totals. Scores can vary from 4 to 16. A score of 12 and above is a strong indicator that that factor is important to you, and 8 and below is low. If you score 12 or more points in each category, your chances of initiating and adhering to an exercise program are good. If you fail to score at least 12 points in three categories, your chances of succeeding at exercise may be slim. You need to be better informed about the benefits of exercise, and a retraining process may be required.

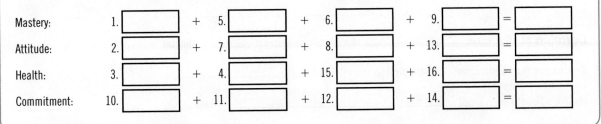

Mastery: 1. ☐ + 5. ☐ + 6. ☐ + 9. ☐ = ☐

Attitude: 2. ☐ + 7. ☐ + 8. ☐ + 13. ☐ = ☐

Health: 3. ☐ + 4. ☐ + 15. ☐ + 16. ☐ = ☐

Commitment: 10. ☐ + 11. ☐ + 12. ☐ + 14. ☐ = ☐

Activity 3.3 Exercise Prescription Forms

Name _____ **Date** _____

Course _____ **Section** _____

I. Cardiorespiratory Exercise Prescription

Intensity of Exercise

1. Estimate your own maximal heart rate (MHR)

   MHR $= 207 - (.70 \times$ age)

   MHR $= 207 - (.70 \times$ [_____] $) =$ [_____] bpm

2. Resting heart rate (RHR) = [_____] bpm

3. Heart rate reserve (HRR) = MHR − RHR

   HRR = [_____] − [_____] = [_____] beats

4. Training intensity (TI) = HRR × % TI + RHR

   30% TI = [_____] × .30 + [_____] = [_____] bpm

   40% TI = [_____] × .40 + [_____] = [_____] bpm

   60% TI = [_____] × .60 + [_____] = [_____] bpm

   90% TI = [_____] × .90 + [_____] = [_____] bpm

5. Cardiorespiratory training zone: Unconditioned individuals, persons in the poor cardiorespiratory fitness category, and older adults starting an exercise program should use a 30 to 40 percent TI. Individuals in fair and average fitness are encouraged to exercise between 40 and 60 percent TI. Active individuals in the good or excellent categories should exercise between 60 and 90 percent TI.

   Light-intensity cardiorespiratory training zone (30% to 40% TI): [_____] to [_____] bpm

   Moderate-intensity cardiorespiratory training zone (40% to 60% TI): [_____] to [_____] bpm

   Vigorous-intensity cardiorespiratory training zone (60% to 90% TI): [_____] to [_____] bpm

Mode of Exercise: List any activity or combination of aerobic activities that you will use in your cardiorespiratory training program:

_____

Duration of Exercise: Indicate the length of your exercise sessions: _____ minutes

Frequency of Exercise: Indicate the days you will exercise: _____

Student's Signature: _____ Date: _____

Activity 3.3 **Exercise Prescription Forms** *(continued)*

II. Strength-Training Prescription

Design your own strength-training program using a minimum of eight exercises. Indicate the number of sets, repetitions, and approximate resistance that you will use. Also, state the days of the week, time, and facility that will be used for this program.

Strength-training days: M ☐   T ☐   W ☐   Th ☐   F ☐   Sa ☐   Su ☐

Time of day: ☐☐☐☐☐☐   Facility: ☐☐☐☐☐☐☐☐☐☐☐

Exercise	**Sets / Reps / Resistance**
1.	
2.	
3.	
4.	
5.	
6.	
7.	
8.	
9.	
10.	
11.	
12.	
13.	
14.	
15.	
16.	

© Fitness & Wellness, Inc.

Activity 3.3 Exercise Prescription Forms *(continued)*

III. Muscular Flexibility Prescription

Perform all of the recommended flexibility exercises given in Appendix B, pages 281–283. Use a combination of slow-sustained and proprioceptive neuromuscular facilitation stretching techniques. Indicate the technique(s) used for each exercise and, where applicable, the number of repetitions performed and the length of time that the final degree of stretch was held.

Stretching Schedule (Indicate days, time, and place where you will stretch):

Flexibility-training days: M ☐ T ☐ W ☐ Th ☐ F ☐ Sa ☐ Su ☐   Time of day: ☐

Place: ☐

Stretching Exercises

Exercise	Stretching Technique	Repetitions	Length of Final Stretch
Lateral head tilt			NA*
Arm circles			NA
Side stretch			
Body rotation			
Chest stretch			
Shoulder hyperextension stretch			
Shoulder rotation stretch			NA
Quad stretch			
Heel cord stretch			
Adductor stretch			
Sitting adductor stretch			
Sit-and-reach stretch			
Triceps stretch			

*Not Applicable

Activity 3.3 **Exercise Prescription Forms** *(continued)*

IV. Low Back Conditioning Program

Perform all of the recommended exercises for the prevention and rehabilitation of low back pain given in Appendix C, pages 284–286. Indicate the number of repetitions performed for each exercise.

Exercise	Repetitions
Hip flexors stretch	
Single-knee-to-chest stretch	
Double-knee-to-chest stretch	
Upper and lower back stretch	
Sit-and-reach stretch	
Gluteal stretch	
Back extension stretch	
Trunk rotation and lower back stretch	
Hip flexors stretch	
Pelvic clock	
Pelvic tilt	
Cat stretch	
Abdominal crunch or abdominal curl-up	

Proper Body Mechanics

Perform the following tasks using the proper body mechanics given in Figure 3.6 (page 84). Check off each item as you perform the task:

- ☐ Standing (carriage) position
- ☐ Sitting position
- ☐ Bed posture
- ☐ Resting position for tired and painful back
- ☐ Lifting an object

Behavior Modification

Using Figure 3.6 on page 84, indicate what changes you need to make in daily activities to improve posture and body mechanics and prevent low back pain.

_____

_____

_____

_____

_____

Activity 3.4 Goal-Setting Form and Exercise Logs

Name _____ **Date** _____

Course _____ **Section** _____

I. Instructions

Indicate your general goal for the four health-related components of fitness and write the specific actions you will use to accomplish these goals in the next few weeks.

Cardiorespiratory endurance goal: _____

Specific actions:

1. _____
2. _____
3. _____

Muscular strength/endurance goal: _____

Specific actions:

1. _____
2. _____
3. _____

Muscular flexibility goal: _____

Specific actions:

1. _____
2. _____
3. _____

Body composition goal: _____

Specific actions:

1. _____
2. _____
3. _____

My signature _____ Witness signature _____

Today's date _____ Date of completion _____

Activity 3.4 **Goal-Setting Form and Exercise Logs** *(continued)*

II. Aerobic Exercise Log

Date	Body Weight	Exercise Heart Rate	Type of Exercise	Distance in Miles	Time Hrs./Min.	Daily Steps*
1						
2						
3						
4						
5						
6						
7						
8						
9						
10						
11						
12						
13						
14						
15						
16						
17						
18						
19						
20						
21						
22						
23						
24						
25						
26						
27						
28						
29						
30						
31						
			Total			

*Daily steps can be determined using a pedometer.

© Fitness & Wellness, Inc.

Activity 3.4 **Goal-Setting Form and Exercise Logs** *(continued)*

Name		Course		Section		

III. Strength-Training Log

Date Exercise	St/Reps/Res*	St/Reps/Res*	St/Reps/Res*	St/Reps/Res*	St/Reps/Res*	St/Reps/Res*	St/Reps/Res*

*St/Reps/Res = Sets, Repetitions, and Resistance (e.g., 1/10/125 = 1 set of 10 repetitions with 125 pounds)

Activity 3.4 **Goal-Setting Form and Exercise Logs** *(continued)*

| Name | | | Course | | | Section | |

III. Strength-Training Log

Date Exercise	St/Reps/Res*	St/Reps/Res*	St/Reps/Res*	St/Reps/Res*	St/Reps/Res*	St/Reps/Res*	St/Reps/Res*

*St/Reps/Res = Sets, Repetitions, and Resistance (e.g., 1/10/125 = 1 set of 10 repetitions with 125 pounds)

© Fitness & Wellness, Inc.

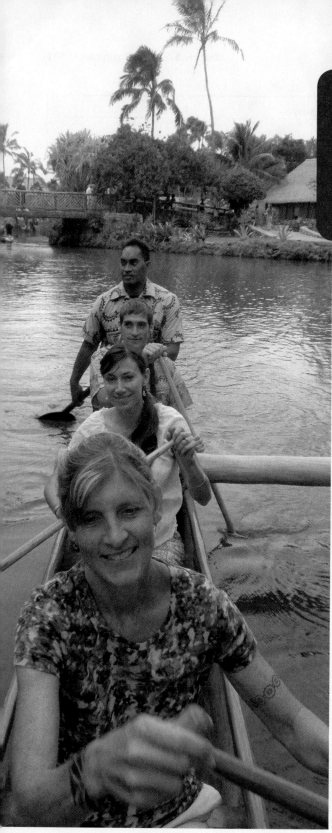

Evaluating Fitness Activities

"To give anything less than your best is to sacrifice the Gift."
—*Steve Prefontaine*

Objectives

> Learn the benefits and advantages of selected aerobic activities.

> Learn to rate the fitness benefits of aerobic activities.

> Evaluate the contributions of skill-related fitness activities.

> Understand the sequence of a standard aerobic workout.

> Learn ways to enhance your aerobic workouts.

REAL LIFE STORY | Sunitha's Exercise Routine

The extent of my exercise program was all jogging. I like to jog because I ran track my first year in high school. Always running, however, was sometimes boring, and I wasn't enjoying it as much as when I ran track with friends. Sometimes I dreaded going out because I wasn't motivated to go by myself or it was either too cold or too hot to exercise. After enrolling in a college fitness and wellness course, we were required to try a minimum of five aerobic activities. I quickly learned that there was more to "exercise life" than running all the time. I really enjoyed spinning, swimming, and elliptical training. Doing different activities took away the monotony of my exercise routine and I found out that exercise is much more fun

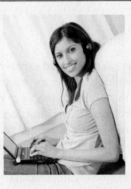

Michaeljung/Shutterstock.com

this way. I also discovered that I am exercising longer and more often than before. I really do feel that cross-training is the way to go if one feels stale or bored of the same exercise routine all the time.

O ne of the fun and alluring aspects of exercise is the sheer variety of activities promoting fitness that are available to you. You can select one or a combination of activities for your program. Your choice should be based on personal enjoyment, convenience, and availability. Exercise that meets these three criteria is likely to be a success. People who choose a form of exercise they view as personal enjoyment are more likely to keep their willpower intact for the remainder of the day and are less inclined to reward themselves in detrimental ways like overeating. A summary of the most popular adult physical activities in the United States is presented in Figure 4.1.

Figure 4.1 Most popular adult physical activities in the United States.

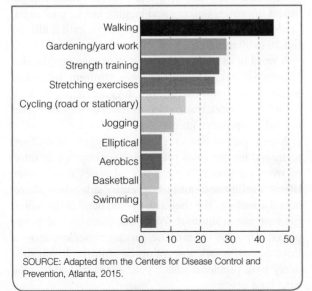

SOURCE: Adapted from the Centers for Disease Control and Prevention, Atlanta, 2015.

A discussion of traditional exercise modalities and new trends in fitness activities follows next in this chapter. In Activity 4.1 at the end of the chapter you will be able to review your participation in various fitness activities during the last 6 months and rate their contribution to the different health-related and motor skill-related components of fitness.

4.1 *Traditional Fitness Activities*

Most people who exercise pick and adhere to a single mode, such as walking, swimming, or jogging. Yet no single activity develops total fitness. Many activities contribute to cardiorespiratory development, but the extent of contribution to other fitness components is limited and varies among the activities. For total fitness, aerobic activities should be supplemented with strength and flexibility exercises. Cross-training can add enjoyment to the program, decrease the risk of incurring injuries from overuse, and keep exercise from becoming monotonous. Cross-training also helps you avoid seeing a plateau in your fitness progress, which can happen in as few as six to eight weeks of a workout as your body becomes efficient at a repeated movement.

Exercise sessions should be convenient. To enjoy exercise, you should select a time when you will not be rushed and a location that is nearby. People do not enjoy driving across town to get to the gym, health club, track, or pool. If parking is a problem, you may get discouraged quickly and quit. Also consider whether you prefer working out alone and enjoying time to yourself, exercising with a partner and looking forward to the social time, or working out under the instruction of a teacher or group that makes you feel motivated. All of these factors, if chosen poorly, can supply excuses to not stick to an exercise program.

Walking

The most natural, easiest, safest, and least expensive form of aerobic exercise is walking. For years, many fitness practitioners believed that walking was not vigorous enough to improve cardiorespiratory functioning, but brisk walking at speeds of 4 miles per hour or faster does improve cardiorespiratory fitness. From a health fitness viewpoint, a regular walking program can prolong life significantly (see the discussion of cardiovascular diseases in Chapter 8). Although walking obviously takes longer than jogging, the caloric cost of brisk walking is only about 10 percent lower than jogging the same distance.

Walking is perhaps the best activity to start a conditioning program for the cardiorespiratory system. Inactive people should start with one-mile walks four or five times per week. Walk times can be increased gradually by five minutes each week. Following three to four weeks of conditioning, a person should be able to walk two miles at a

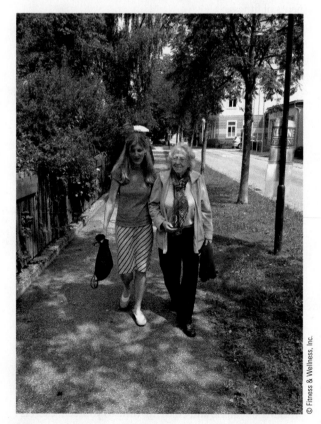

Walking is the most natural aerobic physical activity.

© Fitness & Wellness, Inc.

four-mile-per-hour pace, five times per week. Greater aerobic benefits accrue from walking longer and swinging the arms faster than normal. Light hand weights, a backpack (four to six pounds), or tension belts that add load to the upper body (arms) also add to the intensity of walking. Because of the additional load on the cardiorespiratory system, extra weights or loads are not recommended for people who have or are at risk for cardiovascular disease.

Walking in chest-deep water is an excellent form of aerobic activity, particularly for people who have leg and back problems. Because of the buoyancy of water, individuals submerged in water to armpit level weigh only about 10 percent to 20 percent of their weight outside the water. The resistance the water creates as a person walks in the pool adds to the intensity of the activity and provides a good cardiorespiratory workout.

Jogging

Next to walking, jogging is one of the most accessible forms of exercise. A person can find places to jog almost everywhere. The lone requirement to prevent injuries is a good pair of jogging shoes.

The popularity of jogging in the United States started shortly after publication of Dr. Kenneth Cooper's first *Aerobics* book in 1968. Jim Fixx's *Complete Book of Running*, listed for 11 weeks in 1977 as No. 1 on the NY Times Best-Sellers list, further contributed to the phenomenal growth of jogging as a fitness activity in the United States.

Jogging three to five times a week is one of the fastest ways to improve cardiorespiratory fitness. The risk of injury, however—especially in beginners—is higher with jogging than walking. For proper conditioning, jogging programs should start with 1 to 2 weeks of walking. As fitness improves, walking and jogging can be combined, gradually increasing the jogging segment until it fills the full 20 to 30 minutes.

A word of caution when it comes to jogging: The risk of injury increases greatly as speed (running instead of jogging) and mileage go up. Jogging approximately 15 miles per week is sufficient to reach an excellent level of cardiorespiratory fitness.

A good pair of shoes is a must for joggers. Many foot, knee, and leg problems originate from improperly fitted or worn-out shoes. A good pair of shoes should offer lateral stability and not lean to either side when placed on a flat surface. The shoe also should bend at the ball of the foot, not at midfoot. Worn-out shoes should be replaced. After 500 miles of use, jogging shoes lose about a third of their shock absorption capabilities. If you suddenly have problems, check your shoes first. It may be time for a new pair.

For safety reasons, joggers (and walkers) should follow these precautions:

1. Stay away from high-speed roads.
2. Do not wear headphones so that you can be aware of your surroundings. Using headphones may keep you from hearing a car horn, a voice, or a potential attacker.
3. Go against the traffic so that you can spot and avoid all oncoming traffic.
4. Do not wear dark clothes. Reflective clothing or fluorescent material worn on different parts of the body is highly recommended. A flashlight, particularly an LED light, not only alerts drivers of your presence but also helps illuminate the street. Motorists can see a light from a greater distance than they can spot the reflective material.
5. Wear a billed cap and clear glasses in the dark. The billed cap will hit a branch or other object before such hits your head. Clear glasses can protect your eyes from unseen objects or insects.
6. Cross behind vehicles at intersections, never in front. Drivers often look only in the direction of oncoming traffic and do not look in the opposite direction before proceeding onto the street.
7. Select different routes. A potential attacker may lie in wait if you are predictable in your running route. Running with a partner is also preferable because there is always strength in numbers. And do not wear your hair in a ponytail because it provides an easy grip for a potential attacker.
8. Avoid walking or jogging in unfamiliar areas. When visiting a new area, always inquire as to safe areas to walk or jog.

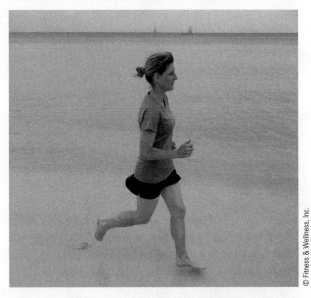

Jogging is one of the most popular forms of aerobic exercise.

© Fitness & Wellness, Inc.

Deep-Water Jogging

An alternative form of jogging, especially for injured people, those with chronic back problems, and overweight individuals, is deep-water jogging—jogging in place while treading water. Deep-water jogging is almost as strenuous as jogging on land. In deep-water jogging, the jogging motions used on land are accentuated by pumping the arms and legs hard through a full range of motion. The participant usually wears a flotation vest to help maintain the body in an upright position. Many elite athletes train frequently in water to lessen the wear and tear on the body caused by long-distance running. These athletes have been able to maintain high oxygen uptake values through rigorous water jogging programs.

Strength Training

Strength training is one of the strongest trends in worldwide fitness. More adults are embracing strength training to enhance muscular fitness, health, and functional capacity, and use it to either complement their aerobic conditioning or in some instances as their primary mode of exercise. Worldwide, fitness participants strength train to further develop or maintain muscular strength and endurance in midlife and throughout the aging process.

Aerobics and Group Cardio Classes

Aerobics is a very popular fitness activity for women in the United States. All cardio classes have in common a group setting where students follow an instructor to complete routines that consist of a combination of stepping, walking, jogging, skipping, kicking, and arm swinging movements performed to music. The music and energy of the group setting, along with a motivational instructor, make this a fun and upbeat option for promoting cardiorespiratory fitness.

High-impact aerobics (HIA) is the traditional form of aerobics. The movements exert a great amount of vertical force on the feet as they contact the floor. Proper leg conditioning through other forms of weight-bearing aerobic exercises (brisk walking and jogging), as well as strength training, is recommended prior to participating in HIA.

GLOSSARY

Aerobics A series of exercise routines that include a combination of stepping, walking, jogging, skipping, kicking, and arm swinging movements performed to music.

High-impact aerobics (HIA) Exercises incorporating movements in which both feet are off the ground at the same time momentarily.

HIA is an intense activity, and it produces the highest rate of aerobics injuries. Shin splints, stress fractures, low back pain, and tendinitis are all too common in HIA enthusiasts. These injuries are caused by the constant impact of the feet on firm surfaces. As a result, several alternative forms of aerobics have been developed.

In **low-impact aerobics (LIA)**, the impact is reduced because each foot contacts the surface separately, but the recommended intensity of exercise is more difficult to maintain than with HIA. To help elevate the exercise heart rate, all arm movements and weight-bearing actions that lower the center of gravity should be accentuated. Sustained movement throughout the program is also crucial to keep the heart rate in the target cardiorespiratory zone.

Step aerobics (SA) is an activity in which participants step up and down from a bench. Benches range in height from 2 to 10 inches. SA adds another dimension to the aerobics program. As noted previously, variety adds enjoyment to aerobic workouts. SA is considered a high-intensity but low-impact activity. The intensity of the activity can be controlled easily by the height of the bench. Aerobic benches or plates can be stacked together safely to adjust the height of the steps. Beginners are encouraged to use the lowest stepping height and then advance gradually to a higher bench. This will decrease the risk for injury. Even though one foot is always in contact with the floor or bench during step aerobics, this activity is not recommended for individuals with ankle, knee, or hip problems.

Other forms of aerobics include a combination of HIA and LIA, as well as **moderate-impact aerobics (MIA)**. MIA incorporates **plyometric training**. This type of training is used frequently by jumpers (high, long, and triple jumpers) and athletes in sports that require quick jumping ability, such as basketball and gymnastics. With MIA, one foot is in contact with the ground most of the time. Participants, however, continuously try to recover from all lower-body flexion actions. This is done by extending the hip, knee, and ankle joints quickly without allowing the foot (or feet) to leave the ground. These quick movements make the exercise intensity of MIA quite high.

Swimming

Swimming, another excellent form of aerobic exercise, uses many of the major muscle groups in the body. This provides a good training stimulus for the heart and lungs. Swimming is a great exercise option for individuals who cannot jog or walk for extended periods.

Compared to other activities, the risk of injuries from swimming is low. The aquatic medium helps to support the body, taking pressure off bones and joints in the lower extremities and the back.

Maximal heart rates during swimming are approximately 10 to 13 beats per minute (bpm) lower than during running. The horizontal position of the body is thought to aid blood flow distribution throughout the body, decreasing the demand on the cardiorespiratory system. Cool water temperatures and direct contact with the water seem to help dissipate body heat more efficiently, further decreasing the strain on the heart.

Some exercise specialists recommend that this difference in maximal heart rate (10 to 13 bpm) be subtracted prior to determining cardiorespiratory training intensities. For example, the estimated maximal swimming heart rate for a 20-year-old would be approximately 180 bpm [207 − (.7 × 20) − 13]. Studies are inconclusive as to whether this decrease in heart rate in water also occurs at submaximal intensities below 70 percent of maximal heart rate.[1]

To produce better training benefits during swimming, swimmers should minimize gliding periods such as those in the breaststroke and sidestroke. Achieving proper training intensities with these strokes is difficult. The forward crawl is recommended for better aerobic results.

Overweight individuals have to swim fast enough to achieve an adequate training intensity. Excessive body fat makes the body more buoyant, and often the tendency is to float along. This may be good for reducing stress and relaxing, but it does not greatly increase caloric expenditure to aid with weight loss. Walking or jogging in waist- or armpit-deep water is a better choice for overweight individuals who cannot walk or jog on land for an extended period of time.

With reference to the principle of specificity of training, cardiorespiratory improvements from swimming cannot be measured adequately with a land-based walk/jog test. This is because most of the work with swimming is done by the upper body musculature.

Although the heart's ability to pump more blood improves significantly with any type of aerobic activity, the primary increase in the ability of cells to utilize oxygen (VO_2, or oxygen uptake) with swimming occurs in the upper body and not the lower extremities. Therefore, fitness improvements with swimming are best assessed by comparing changes in distance a person swims in a given time, say, 12 minutes.

! Critical Thinking

Participation in sports is a good predictor of adherence to exercise later in life. • What previous experiences have you had with participation in sports? • Were these experiences positive, and what effect do they have on your current physical activity patterns?

Water Aerobics

Water aerobics is fun and safe for people of all ages. Besides developing fitness, it provides an opportunity for socialization and fun in a comfortable, refreshing setting.

Water aerobics incorporates a combination of rhythmic arm and leg actions performed in a vertical position while submerged in waist- to armpit-deep water. The vigorous limb movements against the water's resistance during water aerobics provide the training stimuli for cardiorespiratory development.

The popularity of water aerobics as an exercise modality to develop the cardiorespiratory system can be attributed to several factors:

1. Water buoyancy reduces weight-bearing stress on joints and thereby lessens the risk for injuries.
2. Water aerobics is a more feasible type of exercise for overweight individuals and those with arthritic conditions who may not be able to participate in weight-bearing activities such as walking, jogging, and aerobics.
3. Water aerobics is an excellent exercise modality to improve functional fitness in older adults (see Chapter 9, pages 260–262).
4. Heat dissipation in water is beneficial to obese participants who seem to undergo a higher heat strain than average-weight individuals.
5. Water aerobics is available to swimmers and nonswimmers alike.

The exercises used during water aerobics are designed to elevate the heart rate, which contributes to cardiorespiratory development. In addition, the aquatic medium provides increased resistance for strength improvement with virtually no impact. Because of this resistance to movement, strength gains with water aerobics seem to be better than with land-based aerobic activities.

Another benefit is the reduction of pain and fear of injuries common to many people who initiate exercise programs. Water aerobics provides a relatively safe environment for injury-free participation in exercise. The cushioned environment of the water allows patients recovering from leg and back injuries, individuals with joint problems, injured athletes, pregnant women, and obese people to benefit from water aerobics.

As in swimming, maximal heart rates achieved during water aerobics are lower than during running. The difference between water aerobics and running is about 10 bpm.[2] Further, research comparing physiologic differences between self-paced treadmill running and self-paced water aerobics exercise showed that even though individuals work at a lower heart rate intensity in water, the oxygen

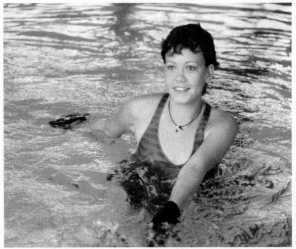

Water aerobics offers fitness and fun in an environment relatively low in risk for injury.

uptake level was the same for both treadmill and water exercise modalities.[3] Apparently healthy people, therefore, can sustain land-based exercise intensities during a water aerobics workout and experience fitness benefits similar to or greater than those acquired during land aerobics.[4]

Cycling

Most people learn cycling in their youth. Because it is a non-weight-bearing activity, cycling is a good exercise modality for people with lower-body or lower back injuries. Cycling helps to develop the cardiorespiratory system, as well as muscular strength and endurance in the lower extremities.

Because cycling is a non-weight-bearing activity, raising the heart rate to the proper training intensity is more difficult. As the amount of muscle mass involved during aerobic exercise decreases, so does the demand placed on the cardiorespiratory system. The thigh muscles do most of the work in cycling, making it harder to achieve and maintain a high cardiorespiratory training intensity.

GLOSSARY

Low-impact aerobics (LIA) Exercises in which at least one foot is in contact with the ground or floor at all times.

Step aerobics (SA) A form of exercise that combines stepping up onto and down from a bench with arm movements.

Moderate-impact aerobics (MIA) Aerobics that include plyometric training.

Plyometric training A form of exercise that requires forceful jumps or springing off the ground immediately after landing from a previous jump.

Maintaining a continuous pedaling motion and eliminating coasting periods helps the participant achieve a faster heart rate. Exercising for longer periods also helps to compensate for the lower heart rate intensity during cycling. Comparing cycling to jogging, similar aerobic benefits take roughly three times the distance at twice the speed of jogging. Cycling, however, puts less stress on muscles and joints than jogging does, making the former a good exercise modality for people who cannot walk or jog.

The height of the bike seat should be adjusted so the knee is flexed at about 30 degrees when the foot is at the bottom of the pedaling cycle. The body should not sway from side to side as the person rides. The cycling cadence also is important for maximal efficiency. Bike tension or gears should be set at a moderate level so the rider can achieve about 60 to 100 revolutions per minute.

Safety is a key issue in road cycling. According to the CDC, each year about 500,000 emergency room visits in the United States are the result of bicycle-related injuries. These occur most often among children, teens, and males in their early 20s. Of these accidents, 800 result in death. Three quarters of deaths are a result of head trauma, with one quarter being related to alcohol consumption. Proper equipment and common sense are necessary. A well-designed and well-maintained bike is easier to maneuver. Toe clips are recommended to keep feet from sliding and to maintain equal upward and downward force on the pedals.

Skill is important in both road and mountain cycling. Cyclists must be in control of the bicycle at all times. They have to be able to maneuver the bike in traffic, maintain balance at slow speeds, switch gears, apply the brakes, watch for pedestrians and stoplights, ride through congested areas, and overcome a variety of obstacles. Stationary cycling, in contrast, does not require special skills. Nearly everyone can do it.

Bike riders must follow the same rules as motorists. Many accidents happen because cyclists run traffic lights and stop signs. Some further suggestions are as follows:

1. Select the right bike. Frame size is important. The size is determined by standing flatfooted while straddling the bike. Regular bikes (road bikes) should have a 1- to 2-inch clearance between the groin and the top tube of the frame. On mountain bikes, the clearance should be about 3 inches. The recommended height of the handlebars is about 1 inch below the top of the seat. Upright handlebars are available for individuals with neck or back problems. Hard, narrow seats on road or racing bikes tend to be especially uncomfortable for women. To avoid saddle soreness, use wider and more cushioned seats such as gel-filled saddles.

2. Use bike hand signals to let the traffic around you know of your intended actions.

3. Don't ride side by side with another rider; single file is safer.

4. Do ride in pairs or groups whenever possible. Drivers are more likely to notice and take caution around a group of cyclists than a solo cyclist.

5. Be aware of turning vehicles and cars backing out of alleys and parking lots; always yield to motorists in these situations; take special care to stay out of the blind spot of drivers.

6. Be on the lookout for storm drains, railroad tracks, and cattle guards, which can cause unpleasant surprises. Front wheels can get caught and riders may be thrown from the bike if these hazards are not crossed at the proper angle (preferably 90 degrees).

7. Wear a good helmet, certified by the Snell Memorial Foundation or the American National Standards Institute. Many serious accidents and even deaths have been prevented by the use of helmets. Fashion, aesthetics, comfort, or price should not be a factor when selecting and using a helmet for road cycling. Health and life are too precious to give up because of vanity and thriftiness.

8. Wear appropriate clothes and shoes. Clothing should be bright, very visible, lightweight, and not restrict movement. Cycling shorts are recommended to prevent skin irritation. For greater comfort, the shorts have extra padding sewn into the seat and crotch areas. They do not tend to wrinkle, and they wick away perspiration from the skin. Shorts should be long enough to keep the skin from rubbing against the seat. Experienced cyclists also wear special shoes with a cleat that snaps directly onto the pedal.

9. Take extra warm clothing in a backpack during the winter months in case you have a breakdown and have to walk a long distance for assistance.

10. Watch out for ice in cold weather. If you see ice on car windows, expect ice on the road. Be especially careful on and under bridges because they tend to have ice even when the roads elsewhere are dry.

11. Use the brightest bicycle lights you can when riding in the dark, and always keep the batteries well charged. For additional safety, wear reflectors on the upper torso, arms, and legs so passing motorists are alerted to you. Stay on streets that have good lighting and plenty of room on the side of the road, even if that means riding an extra few minutes to get to your destination.

12. Take a cell phone if you have one, and let someone else know where you are going and when to expect you back.

Behavior Modification Planning

Tips for People Who Have Been Inactive for a While

- Take the sensible approach by starting slowly.
- Begin by choosing moderate-intensity activities you enjoy the most. By choosing activities you enjoy, you'll be more likely to stick with them.
- Gradually build up the time spent exercising by adding a few minutes every few days or so until you can comfortably perform a minimum recommended amount of exercise (20 minutes per day).
- As the minimum amount becomes easier, gradually increase either the length of time exercising or the intensity of the activity, or both.

- Vary your activities, both for interest and to broaden the range of benefits.
- Explore new physical activities.
- Reward and acknowledge your efforts.

Try It

Fill out the cardiorespiratory exercise prescription in Activity 3.3. In your Online Journal or class notebook, describe how well you implement the above suggestions.

SOURCE: Adapted from Centers for Disease Control and Prevention, Atlanta.

Before buying a stationary bike, though, be sure to try the activity for a few days. If you enjoy it, you may want to purchase one. Invest with caution. If you opt to buy a lower-priced model, you may be disappointed. Good stationary bikes have comfortable seats, are stable, and provide a smooth and uniform pedaling motion. A sticky bike that is hard to pedal leads to discouragement and ends up being stored in the corner of a basement.

Cross-Training

Cross-training combines two or more activities. This type of training is designed to enhance fitness, provide needed rest for tired muscles, decrease injuries, and eliminate the monotony and burnout of single-activity programs. Cross-training may combine aerobic and nonaerobic activities such as moderate jogging, speed training, and strength training.

Cross-training can produce better workouts than a single activity. For example, jogging develops the lower body and swimming builds the upper body. Rowing contributes to upper-body development and cycling builds the legs. Combining activities such as these provides good overall conditioning and at the same time helps to improve or maintain fitness. As exercisers have become more savvy about achieving results and avoiding injury, cross-training is popping up more often in health-club programs and fitness classes. Combined activity classes, such as a spin class where participants do pushups off the handlebars and other strength exercises, are now available and more popular. Cross-training also offers an opportunity to develop skill and have fun with differing activities.

Speed training often is coupled with cross-training. Faster performance times in aerobic activities (running and cycling) are generated with speed or **interval training**. People who want to improve their running times often run shorter intervals at faster speeds than the actual racing pace. For example, a person wanting to run a 6-minute mile may run four 440-yard intervals at a speed of 1 minute and 20 seconds per interval. A 440-yard walk/jog can become a recovery interval between fast runs.

Strength training is used commonly with cross-training. It helps to condition muscles, tendons, and ligaments. Improved strength enhances overall performance in many activities and sports. For example, although road cyclists in one study who trained with weights showed no improvement in aerobic capacity, the cyclists' riding time to exhaustion improved 33 percent when exercising at 75 percent of their maximal capacity.[5]

Cross-Country Skiing

Many people consider cross-country skiing the ultimate aerobic exercise because it requires vigorous lower- and upper-body movements. The large amount of muscle mass involved in cross-country skiing makes the intensity of the activity high, yet it places little strain on muscles and joints. One of the highest maximal oxygen

GLOSSARY

Interval training A repeated series of exercise work bouts (intervals) interspersed with low-intensity or rest intervals.

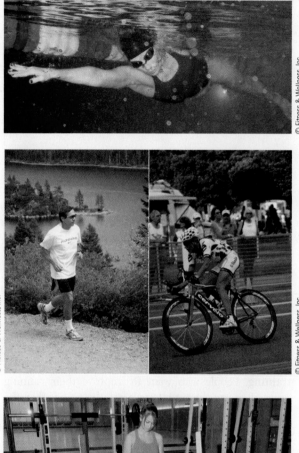

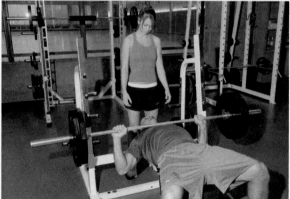

Cross-training enhances fitness, decreases the rate of injuries, and eliminates the monotony of single-activity programs.

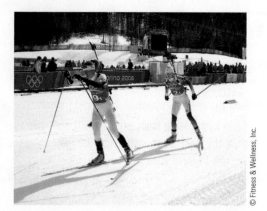

Cross-country skiing requires more oxygen and energy than most other aerobic activities.

uptakes ever measured (85 mL/kg/min) was found in an elite cross-country skier.

In addition to being an excellent aerobic activity, cross-country skiing is soothing. Skiing through the beauty of the snow-covered countryside can be highly enjoyable. Although the need for snow is an obvious limitation, simulation equipment for year-round cross-country training is available at many sporting goods stores.

Some skill is necessary to be proficient at cross-country skiing. Poorly skilled individuals are not able to elevate the heart rate enough to cause adequate aerobic development. Individuals contemplating this activity should seek instruction to be able to fully enjoy and reap the rewards of cross-country skiing.

Rowing

Rowing is a low-impact activity that provides a complete body workout. It mobilizes most major muscle groups, including those in the arms, legs, hips, abdomen, trunk, and shoulders. Rowing is a good form of aerobic exercise, and because of the nature of the activity (constant pushing and pulling against resistance), it also promotes strength development.

To accommodate different fitness levels, workloads can be regulated on most rowing machines. Stationary rowing, however, is not among the most popular forms of aerobic exercise. As with stationary bicycles, people should try the activity for a few weeks before purchasing a unit.

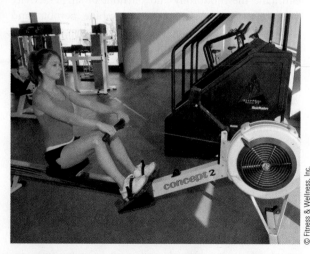

In addition to aerobic development, rowing also contributes to good strength development.

Elliptical Training/Stair Climbing

If sustained for at least 20 minutes, elliptical training and stair climbing are very efficient forms of aerobic exercise. Precisely because of the high intensity of stair climbing, many people stay away from stairs and instead take escalators and elevators. Many people dislike living in two-story homes because they have to climb the stairs frequently.

Elliptical training and stair climbing are relatively safe exercise modalities. Because the feet never leave the climbing surface, they are considered low-impact activities. Joints and ligaments are not strained while climbing. The intensity of exercise is controlled easily because the equipment can be programmed to regulate the workload, making them suitable for participants at all fitness levels, as well as a great option for performing high intensity interval training.

Racquet Sports

In racquet sports such as tennis, racquetball, squash, and badminton, the aerobic benefits are dictated by players' skill, the intensity of the game, and the length of time spent playing. Skill is necessary to participate effectively in these sports and also is crucial to sustain continuous play. Frequent pauses during play do not allow people to maintain the heart rate in the appropriate target zone to stimulate cardiorespiratory development.

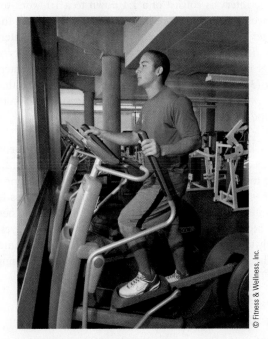

Elliptical training provides a rigorous aerobic workout.

Many people who participate in racquet sports do so for enjoyment, social fulfillment, and relaxation. For cardiorespiratory fitness development, these people supplement the sport with other forms of aerobic exercise such as jogging, cycling, or swimming.

If a racquet sport is the main form of aerobic exercise, participants need to try to run hard, fast, and as constantly as possible during play. They should not have to spend much time retrieving balls (or, in badminton, the bird or shuttlecock). Similar to low-impact aerobics, all movements should be accentuated by reaching out and bending more than usual, for better cardiorespiratory development.

Yoga

Yoga consists of a system of exercises designed to help align the musculoskeletal system and develop flexibility, muscular fitness, and balance. Yoga is also used as a relaxation technique for stress management. The exercises involve a combination of postures (known as "asanas") along with diaphragmatic breathing, relaxation, and meditation techniques. Different forms of yoga exist, including Anuara, Ashtanga, Bikram, Integral, Iyengar, Kripalu, Kundalini, and Sivananda, Viniyoga, Yogalates, and Yogaerobics yoga. Most recently, yoga has become popular as a compliment to other training modalities to aid in recovery and in preparation for upcoming workouts.

Critical Thinking

In your own experience with personal fitness programs throughout the years, what factors have motivated you and helped you the most to stay with a program? • What factors have kept you from being physically active, and what can you do to change these factors?

4.2 New Fitness Trends

Life in the 21st century requires that we participate in physical activities that promote and maintain fitness, health, and wellness. As people search for proven programs, fitness trends emerge to achieve these goals. Some of the activity trends have been with us and continue to evolve to gain popularity among participants, whereas others have been recently developed and gained approval among fitness enthusiasts. According to the American College of Sports Medicine's Worldwide Survey of Fitness Trends in 2013, among the newest fitness activities the following trends have emerged:

High-Intensity Interval Training

A type of training that has become very popular among exercisers and the subject of much research lately is **high-intensity interval training (HIIT)**. This aerobic/anaerobic training modality (80 percent to 90 percent of maximal capacity) had primarily been used by athletes, but it is now used by fitness participants seeking better, faster, and more effective development.

Many people think that high-intensity exercise is only for athletes and unsafe for the average fitness enthusiast. On the contrary, HIIT has been examined as part of short and long workouts using people of all ages and with different exercise modalities. High-risk patients facing a variety of chronic illnesses—including chronic obstructive pulmonary disease, Parkinson's disease, and disability from stroke—have successfully carried out and benefitted from HIIT under close supervision by a physician. For some individuals, a short HIIT workout has been reported to be not only more effective, but also more manageable than a comparable workout of steady exertion. Any individual who is considered medium to high risk, nonetheless, should seek medical clearance and direction from their physician prior to attempting a HIIT program.

Following an appropriate warm-up, HIIT includes high- to very high-intensity intervals that are interspersed with a low- to moderate-intensity recovery phase. Typically, a 1:3, 1:2, or 1:1 work-to-recovery ratio is used; the more intense the interval, the longer the recovery period. HIIT can be performed with a variety of activities, including running, cycling, elliptical training, stair climbing, and swimming. You may use the same activity for your entire HIIT, or you may use a combination of activities.

Research indicates that additional health and fitness benefits are reaped as the intensity of exercise increases. HIIT produces the greatest improvements in aerobic capacity (VO_{2max}) and increases the capability to exercise at a higher percentage of that capacity (anaerobic threshold), thus allowing the participant to burn more calories during the exercise session. HIIT also improves vital aspects of health, including elasticity of arteries and blood glucose control.

The data also show that HIIT increases the capacity for fat oxidation during exercise. Although the fuel used during high-intensity intervals is primarily glucose (carbohydrates), molecular changes occur in the muscles that increase the body's capability for fatty acid oxidation (fat burning).

Furthermore, following light- to moderate-intensity aerobic activity, resting metabolism returns to normal in about 90 minutes. Depending on the volume of training (intensity and number of intervals performed), with HIIT it takes 24 to 72 hours for the body to return to its "normal" resting metabolic rate. Thus, a greater amount of calories (primarily from fat) are burned up to three days following HIIT. While the extra calories burned during recovery can make a difference in the long run, keep in mind that the most significant factor is the number of calories burned during the actual HIIT session. The extra calories burned during recovery are minimal compared to those used during training.

Performing a HIIT program for the first time can be challenging. Exercising near full capacity may certainly seem an unpleasant prospect, and participants may need a few tricks to get through those first workouts. To begin, avoid an all-or-nothing approach. Remember to work within your own personal functional capacity, a pace that will allow you to get through the workout. If your intensity is not as high as you would like it to be, it will come. You may also consider listening to your favorite music as you exercise.

Four training variables impact HIIT. The acronym *DIRT* is frequently used to denote these variables:

D = Distance of each speed interval
I = Interval or length of recovery between speed intervals
R = Repetitions or number of speed intervals to be performed
T = Time of each speed interval

Using these four variables, a person can practically design an unlimited number of HIIT sessions.

The intervals consist of a 1:4 down to a 1:1 work-to-recovery ratio. The more intense the speed interval, the longer the required recovery interval. For aerobic intervals (lasting longer than 3 minutes), 1:2, 1:1, or even lower ratios are used. For intense anaerobic speed intervals (30 seconds to 3 minutes), recovery intervals that last two to four times as long (1:2 to 1:4) as the work period are required.

A 1:3 ratio, for example, indicates that you'll work at a fairly high intensity for, say, 30 seconds and then spend 90 seconds on light- to moderate-intensity recovery. Be sure to keep moving during the recovery phase. Perform four or five intervals at first, then gradually progress to 10 intervals. As your fitness improves, you can lengthen the high-intensity proportion of the intervals progressively to 1 minute and/or decrease the total recovery time.

The following are sample programs performed using HIIT.

Five-Minute Very Hard-Intensity Aerobic Intervals

Exercise at a "very hard" rate (about 90 percent of maximal capacity) for 5 minutes, followed by 5 to 10 minutes of recovery at a "light" to "moderate" intensity. Start with one interval and work up to three by the third to fifth training session. Initially, use a 1:2 work-to-recovery ratio. Gradually decrease the recovery to a 1:1 ratio.

Step-Wise Intensity Interval Training

Using 3- to 5-minute intervals, start at a "light" intensity rate and progressively step up to the "very hard" intensity level (light, moderate, somewhat hard, vigorous, hard, and very hard). Start with 3-minute intervals and as you become more fit, increase to 5 minutes each. As time allows and you develop greater fitness, you can add a step-down approach by stepping down to hard, vigorous, somewhat hard, moderate, and light.

Fartlek Training

The word fartlek means "speed play" in Swedish. It is an unstructured form of interval training where intensity (speed) and distance of each interval are varied as the participant wishes. There is no set structure, and the individual alternates intensity (from "somewhat hard" to "very hard") and the length of each speed interval, along with the recovery intervals ("light" to "moderate") and length thereof. Total duration of fartlek training is between 20 and 60 minutes.

Tempo Training

Although no formal intervals are conducted with tempo training, the intensity of training qualifies it as an HIIT program. Tempo runs involve continuous training between "vigorous" (70 percent) and "hard" (80 percent) for 20 to 60 minutes at a time.

All-Out or Supramaximal Interval Training

All-out interval training involves 10 to 20 supramaximal or "sprint" intervals lasting 30 to 60 seconds each. Depending on the level of conditioning and the length of the speed interval, 2 to 5 minutes of recovery at a "light" to "moderate" level are allowed.

Cardio/Resistance Training Program

You may use a combination of aerobic and resistance training for HIIT. Following a brief aerobic and strength training warm-up, select about eight resistance training exercises that you can alternate with treadmill running, cycling, elliptical training, or rowing. Perform one set of 8 to 20 RM (based on personal preference) on each exercise followed by 90 seconds of aerobic work after each set. You can pace the aerobic intensity according to the preceding strength-training set. For example, you may choose a "light" intensity aerobic interval following a 10 RM for the leg press exercise and a "vigorous" aerobic interval after a 10 RM arm curl set. Allow no greater recovery time (2 to 5 seconds) between exercise modes than what it takes to walk from the strength-training exercise to the aerobic station (and vice versa).

Stability Exercise Balls

A stability exercise ball is a large, flexible, and inflatable ball used for exercises that are specifically designed to develop abdominal, hip, chest, and spinal muscles by addressing core stabilization while the exerciser maintains a balanced position over the ball. Particular emphasis is placed on correct movement and maintenance of proper body alignment to involve as much of the core as possible. Although the primary objective is core strength and stability, many stability exercises can be performed to strengthen other body areas as well.

Stability exercises are thought to be more effective than similar exercises on the ground. For instance, just sitting on the ball requires the use of stabilizing core muscles (including the rectus abdominis, and the external and internal obliques) to keep the body from falling off the ball. Traditional strength-training exercises are primarily for strength and power development and do not contribute as much to body balance.

When performing stability exercises, choose a ball size based on your height. Your thighs should be parallel to the floor when you sit on the ball. A slightly larger ball may be used if you suffer from back problems. For best results, a trained specialist should teach you proper technique and watch your form while you learn the exercises. Individuals who have a weak muscular system or poor balance or who are over the age of 65 should perform stability exercises under the supervision of a qualified trainer.

Core Training

The "core" of the body consists of the muscles that stabilize the trunk (spine) and pelvis. Core training emphasizes strength-conditioning exercises of all the muscles around the abdomen, pelvis, lower back, and hips. These muscles enhance body stability, activities of daily living, and sport performance and support the lower back. Core conditioning can be done without equipment, as in exercises like "the plank." Core training, however, often incorporates the use of stability balls, foam rollers, and

---

GLOSSARY

High-intensity interval training (HIIT) A training program consisting of high- to very high-intensity intervals (80 percent to 90 percent of maximal capacity) that are interspersed with low- to moderate-intensity recovery intervals.

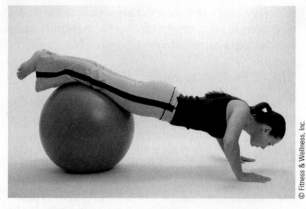

Stability ball exercises can be used to enhance stability, balance, and muscular strength.

wobble boards, among other pieces of equipment. Suspension training is also popular and requires a system of hanging ropes or webs that allow participants to juxtapose their body weight while completing the exercises.

Group Personal Training

Personal trainers are increasingly working with small groups of two to three exercisers to continue providing individualized instruction while keeping costs reasonable. Participants appreciate the accountability they have to the trainer and the group, as well as the sense of belonging that comes from small-group settings. A trainer who understands and can make the most of a group dynamic also enhances the experience.

Outdoor Training

Spurred especially by the growing popularity of adventure races, sports including trail running, cycling, cross country skiing, fast packing, and rowing are growing in popularity. The outdoor setting itself seems to boost mood during exercise, which may explain why even bodyweight training, HIIT, and group sessions with personal trainers are increasingly taking to the open air.

Fitness Boot Camp

A primarily vigorous-intensity outdoor/indoor group exercise program, **fitness boot camp** combines traditional calisthenics, running, interval training, strength training (using body weight exercises such as push-ups, lunges, pull-ups, burpees, and squats), plyometrics, and competitive games to develop cardiorespiratory fitness, muscular strength, and muscular flexibility and to lose body fat. This program is based on military-style training and also

aims at developing camaraderie and team effort. The program (camp) typically lasts four to eight weeks. Fitness boot camps are challenging, and the group dynamic truly helps to motivate participants.

Circuit Training

Circuit training has also been around for decades. It was often used to condition elite athletes and military personnel in the middle of the 20th century. Circuit training involves a combination of 6 to 12 aerobic and body-weight-training (strength) exercises performed in rapid sequence one after the other, with very limited rest between exercise stations. Each exercise is performed for a given period of time (10 to 30 seconds) or by a specified number of repetitions (10 to 20 repetitions), typically interspaced by short rest periods of 10 to 30 seconds between exercises. Early on, you may use a moderate intensity (less time or repetitions per exercise) and allow longer rest (30 seconds) between exercises. Over the course of several weeks, you can gradually increase the intensity (time and/or repetitions) and decrease the rest interval between exercises. The exercise-sequence is set in an order that allows for opposing muscle groups to alternate between exercise stations. For instance, push-ups can be followed by step-ups and abdominal crunches. For best results, all major muscle groups of the body should be used in each circuit.

Because of the high intensity and limited rest intervals used with this type of training, the exercise modality is often referred to as **high-intensity circuit training or HICT**.[6] The combination of high-intensity aerobic and body-weight-strength training, with limited rest between exercises, can elicit similar or greater health and fitness benefits in a much shorter period of time than the traditional 20 to 60 minute sessions. An HICT session involving 12 different exercises can be performed in less than 10 minutes per circuit. One to three circuits with 2 to 3 minutes rest between circuits can be performed per training session. When time is of the essence and a traditional training session is not realistic, an HICT session is recommended.

Functional Fitness

Functional fitness involves primarily weight-bearing exercises to develop balance, coordination, good posture, muscular fitness, and muscular flexibility to enhance the person's ability to perform activities of daily living (walking, climbing stairs, lifting, bending) with ease and with minimal risk for injuries. With its roots in physical therapy, functional fitness often maintains a focus on movements that correct misalignment and simultaneously use muscles that specialize in stabilization and mobility. The

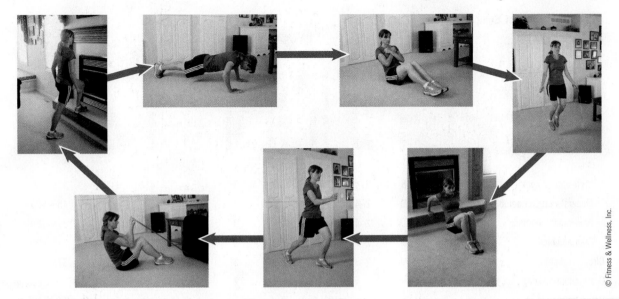

Several modalities of circuit training can be used to enhance overall fitness.

program goal is to "train people for real life," rather than a specific fitness component or a given event. Fitness trainers may plan classes to target specific everyday activities, even focusing movement around a theme. One class for seniors, for example, targets all the movements used for an evening out to the theater; from side stepping down the isle, to sitting in and rising from the seat. Functional fitness training often requires use of fitness equipment such as stability balls, foam blocks, and balancing cushions.

The trend has also gained new meaning for the younger crowd. Many health clubs are setting aside traditional weight machines that isolate one movement at a time in favor of sandbags, hefty ropes, climbing nets, and other equipment that offers members challenging workouts. The goal is to engage major and minor muscle groups along with the body's core in every movement.

Dance Fitness

Gym-goers are embracing a range of dance-inspired group classes that hone in on different fitness goals. A sustained and upbeat cardio workout is the common feature in Zumba classes, which incorporate Latin and international music (cumbia, salsa, merengue, reggaeton, tango, and rock and roll among others) with dance to develop fitness and make exercise fun. The Zumba motto has become, "Ditch the workout; join the party!" More recently, gaining popularity are Barre workouts, based on ballet-inspired movements that offer progressions through flexibility exercises to isometric postures and strength exercises. Barre classes also include exercises not based on traditional dance but that make use of the waist-height barre by having participants hold on and juxtapose their body weight for strength exercises. Other classes are taking their cues from popular hip-hop dance trends, tribal dance, and India-inspired routines, among others.

Rating the Fitness Benefits of Aerobic Activities

The fitness contributions of the aerobic activities discussed in this chapter vary according to the specific activity and the individual. As noted previously, the health-related components of physical fitness are cardiorespiratory endurance, muscular fitness, muscular flexibility, and body composition. Although accurately assessing the contributions to each fitness component is difficult, a summary of likely benefits of these activities is provided in Table 4.1. Instead of a single rating or number, ranges are given for some of the categories because the benefits derived are based on the person's effort while participating in the activity.

GLOSSARY

Fitness boot camp A military-style vigorous-intensity group exercise training program that combines calisthenics, running, interval training, strength training, plyometrics, and competitive games.

High-intensity circuit training (HICT) An exercise modality that combines high-intensity aerobic and bodyweight-strength training exercises with limited rest between exercises.

© Fitness & Wellness, Inc.

Table 4.1 Ratings of Selected Activities

Activity	Recommended Starting Fitness Level[1]	Injury Risk[2]	Potential Cardiorespiratory Endurance Development (VO$_{2MAX}$)[3,4]	Upper Body Strength Development[3]	Lower Body Strength Development[3]	Upper Body Flexibility Development[3]	Lower Body Flexibility Development[3]	Weight Management[3]	MET Level[4,5,6]	Caloric Expenditure (cal/hour)[4,6]
Aerobics										
High-impact aerobics	A	H	3–4	2	4	3	2	4	6–12	450–900
Moderate-impact aerobics	I	M	2–4	2	3	3	2	3	6–12	450–900
Low-impact aerobics	B	L	2–4	2	3	3	2	3	5–10	375–750
Step aerobics	I	M	2–4	2	3–4	3	2	3–4	5–12	375–900
Circuit training	B	M	2–3	3–4	3–4	2	2–3	3–4	5–12	375–900
Cross-country skiing	B	M	4–5	4	4	2	2	4–5	8–16	600–1,200
Cross-training	I	M	3–5	2–3	3–4	2–3	1–2	3–5	6–15	450–1,125
Cycling										
Road	I	M	2–5	1	4	1	1	3	6–12	450–900
Stationary	B	L	2–4	1	4	1	1	3	6–10	450–750
Functional fitness	B	L	2–3	2–3	2–3	2–3	2–3	2–3	5–10	375–750
High-intensity interval training	I	M	4–5	2	3–4	1	1	4–5	8–16	600–1,200
Jogging	I	M	3–5	1	3	1	1	5	6–15	450–1,125
Jogging, deep water	I	L	3–5	2	2	1	1	5	5–12	375–900
Racquet sports	I	M	2–4	3	3	3	2	3	6–10	450–750
Rowing	B	L	3–5	4	2	3	1	4	8–14	600–1,050
Elliptical training/stair climbing	B	L	3–5	1	4	1	1	4–5	8–15	600–1,125
Strength training	B	L	1	4–5	4–5	2–3	2–3	3–4	4–8	300–600
Swimming (front crawl)	B	L	3–5	4	2	3	1	3	6–12	450–900
Walking	B	L	1–2	1	2	1	1	3	4–6	300–450
Walking, water, chest-deep	I	L	2–4	2	3	1	1	3	5–10	375–750
Water aerobics	B	L	2–4	3	3	3	2	3	6–10	450–750
Yoga	B	L	1	1–2	1–2	3–5	3–5	1–3	4–8	300–600
Zumba	B	M	3–4	2	3	3	2	3–4	6–12	450–900

[1]B= Beginner, I= Intermediate, A= Advanced

[2]L= Low, M= Moderate, H= High

[3]1= Low, 2= Fair, 3= Average, 4= Good, 5= Excellent

[4]Varies according to the person's effort (intensity) during exercise.

[5]1 MET represents the rate of energy expenditure at rest (3.5 mL/kg/min). Each additional MET is a multiple of the resting value. For example, 5 METs represents an energy expenditure equivalent to five times the resting value, or about 17.5 L/kg/min.

[6]Varies according to body weight.

© Cengage Learning 2015.

Regular participation in aerobic activities provides notable health benefits, including an increase in cardiorespiratory endurance, quality of life, and longevity. The extent of cardiorespiratory development (improvement in VO_{2max}) depends on the intensity, duration, and frequency of the activity. The nature of the activity often dictates potential aerobic development. For example, jogging is much more strenuous than walking.

The effort during exercise also influences the amount of physiological development. The training benefits of just going through the motions of a low-impact aerobics routine are less than those of accentuating all motions (see earlier discussion of low-impact aerobics). Table 4.1 includes a starting fitness level for each aerobic activity. Beginners should start with low-intensity activities that have a minimum risk for injuries. In some cases, such as in high-impact aerobics and rope skipping, the risk of injuries remains high despite adequate conditioning. These activities should be used only to supplement training and are not recommended for beginners or as the sole mode of exercise.

Physicians who work with cardiac patients frequently use METs to measure activity levels. One **MET** represents the body's energy requirement at rest, or the equivalent of a VO_2 of 3.5 mL/kg/min. A 10-MET activity requires a 10-fold increase in the resting energy requirement, or approximately 35 mL/kg/min. MET levels for a given activity vary according to the individual's effort. The harder a person exercises, the higher the MET level. The MET ranges for the various activities are included in Table 4.1.

The various aerobic activities' effectiveness in aiding weight management also is indicated in Table 4.1. As a rule, the greater the muscle mass involved during exercise, the better the results. Rhythmic and continuous activities that involve considerable muscle mass are most effective in burning calories.

Higher-intensity activities burn more calories as well. Increasing exercise time will compensate for lower intensities. If carried out long enough (60 to 90 minutes, 5 to 6 times per week), even brisk walking can be a good exercise mode to lose weight. Additional information on a comprehensive weight management program is given in Chapter 6.

4.3 *Skill-Related Fitness*

Skill-related fitness is needed for success in athletics and effective performance of lifetime sports and activities. The components of skill-related fitness, defined in Chapter 1, are agility, balance, coordination, power, speed, and reaction time. All of these are important, to varying degrees, in sports and athletics.

For example, outstanding gymnasts must achieve good skill-related fitness in all components. Significant agility is necessary to perform a double back somersault with a full twist—a skill in which the athlete must rotate simultaneously around one axis and twist around a different one. Static balance is essential for maintaining a handstand or a scale. Dynamic balance is needed to perform many of the gymnastics routines (for example, balance beam, parallel bars, and pommel horse).

Coordination is important to successfully integrate into one routine various skills requiring varying degrees of difficulty. Power and speed are needed to propel the body into the air, such as when tumbling or vaulting. Quick reaction time is necessary in determining when to end rotation upon a visual clue, such as spotting the floor on a dismount.

As with the health-related fitness components, the principle of specificity of training applies to skill-related components. According to this principle, the training program must be specific to the type of skill the individual is trying to achieve.

Development of agility, balance, coordination, and reaction time is highly task-specific. To attain a certain skill, the individual must practice the same task many times. There is little crossover learning effect from one skill to another.

For instance, proper practice of a hand-stand (balance) eventually will lead to successful performance of that skill, but complete mastery of the skill does not ensure that the person will immediately be able to transfer this mastery to other static balance positions in gymnastics. Power and speed may be improved with a specific strength-training program or frequent repetition of the specific task to be improved, or both.

The rate of learning in skill-related fitness varies from person to person, mainly because these components seem to be determined to a large extent by hereditary factors. Individuals with good skill-related fitness tend to do better and learn faster when performing a wide variety of skills. Nevertheless, few individuals enjoy complete success in all skill-related components. Furthermore, though skill-related fitness can be enhanced with practice, improvements in reaction time and speed are

---

GLOSSARY

MET One "MET," short for metabolic equivalent, represents the rate of energy expenditure while sitting quietly at rest. This energy expenditure is approximately 3.5 milliliters of oxygen per kilogram of body weight per minute (mL/kg/min) or 1.2 calories per minute for a 70-kilogram person. A 3-MET activity requires three times the energy expenditure of sitting quietly at rest.

limited and seem to be related primarily to genetic endowment.

Although we do not know how much skill-related fitness is desirable, everyone should attempt to develop and maintain a better-than-average level. This type of fitness is crucial for athletes and also is important in leading a better and happier life. Improving skill-related fitness affords an individual more enjoyment and success in a wider variety of lifetime sports (for instance, basketball, tennis, and racquetball) and also can help a person cope more effectively in emergency situations. For example:

1. Good reaction time, balance, coordination, and agility can help you avoid a fall or break a fall and thereby minimize injury.
2. The ability to generate maximum force in a short time (power) may be crucial to ameliorate injury or even preserve life in a situation in which you may be called upon to move a person out of danger or lift a heavy object that has fallen.
3. In our society, with an expanding average lifespan, maintaining speed can be especially important for older adults. Many of them and, for that matter, many unfit and overweight young people no longer have the speed they need to cross an intersection safely before the light changes for oncoming traffic.

Regular participation in a health-related fitness program can heighten performance of skill-related components, and vice versa. For example, significantly overweight people do not have good agility or speed. Because participating in aerobic and strength-training programs helps take off body fat, an overweight individual who loses weight through an exercise program may also improve agility and speed. A sound flexibility program decreases resistance to motion around body joints, which may increase agility, balance, and overall coordination. Improvements in strength definitely help develop power.

Similar to the fitness benefits of the aerobic activities discussed previously in this chapter and given in Table 4.1, the contributions of skill-related activities also vary among activities and individuals. The extent to which an activity helps develop each skill-related component varies by the effort the individual makes and, most important, by proper execution (technique) of the skill (correct coaching is highly recommended) and the individual's potential based on genetic endowment. A summary of potential contributions to skill-related fitness for selected activities is provided in Table 4.2.

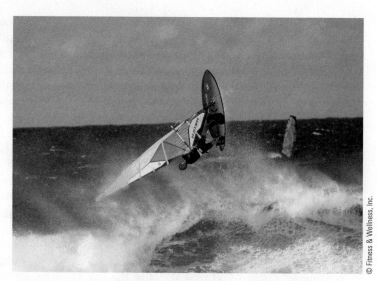

A high degree of skill-related fitness is required to participate in elite level windsurfing.

© Fitness & Wellness, Inc.

Table 4.2 Contributions of Selected Activities to Skill-Related Components

Activity	Agility	Balance	Coordination	Power	Reaction Time	Speed
Alpine Skiing	4	5	4	2	3	2
Archery	1	2	4	2	3	1
Badminton	4	3	4	2	4	3
Baseball	3	2	4	4	5	4
Basketball	4	3	4	3	4	3
Bowling	2	2	4	1	1	1
Cross-country Skiing	3	4	3	2	2	1
Football	4	4	4	4	4	3
Golf	1	2	5	3	1	3
Gymnastics	5	5	5	4	3	3
Ice skating	5	5	5	3	3	3
In-line skating	4	4	4	3	2	4
Judo/karate	5	5	5	4	5	4
Racquetball	5	4	4	4	5	4
Soccer	5	3	5	5	3	4
Table tennis	5	3	5	3	5	3
Tennis	4	3	5	3	5	3
Volleyball	4	3	5	4	5	3
Water skiing	3	4	3	2	2	1
Wrestling	5	5	5	4	5	4

1 = Low, 2 = Fair, 3 = Average, 4 = Good, 5 = Excellent

© Cengage Learning

4.4 *Team Sports*

Choosing activities that you enjoy will greatly enhance your adherence to exercise. People tend to repeat things they enjoy doing. Enjoyment by itself is a reward. Therefore, combining individual activities (such as jogging or swimming) with team sports can deepen your commitment to fitness.

People with good skill-related fitness usually participate in lifetime sports and games, which in turn helps develop health-related fitness. Individuals who enjoyed basketball or soccer in their youth tend to stick to those activities later in life. The availability of teams and community leagues may be all that is needed to stop contemplating and start participating. The social element of team sports provides added incentive to participate. Team sports offer an opportunity to interact with people who share a common interest. Being a member of a team creates responsibility—another incentive to exercise because you are expected to be there. Furthermore, team sports foster lifetime friendships, strengthening the social and emotional dimensions of wellness.

For those who were not able to participate in youth sports, it's never too late to start (see the discussion of behavior modification and motivation in Chapter 1). Don't be afraid to select a new activity, even if that means learning new skills. The fitness and social rewards will be ample.

4.5 *Tips to Enhance Your Aerobic Workout*

A typical aerobic workout is divided into three parts (see Figure 4.2):

1. A 5- to 10-minute warm-up phase during which the heart rate is increased gradually to the target zone
2. The actual aerobic workout, during which the heart rate is maintained in the target zone for 20 to 60 minutes
3. A 10- to 15-minute aerobic/stretching cooldown phase when the heart rate is lowered gradually toward the resting level

To monitor the target training zone, you will have to check your exercise heart rate. As described in Chapter 2, the pulse can be checked on the radial or the carotid artery. When you check the heart rate, begin with zero and count the number of beats in a 10-second period, then multiply by 6 to get the per-minute pulse rate. You should take your exercise heart rate for 10 seconds rather than a full minute because the heart rate begins to slow down 15 seconds after you stop exercising.

Feeling the pulse while exercising is difficult. Therefore, participants should stop during exercise to check the pulse. If the heart rate is too low, increase the intensity of the exercise. If the rate is too high, slow down. You

Figure 4.2 Typical aerobic workout pattern.

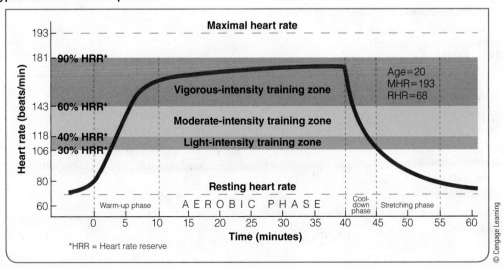

may want to practice taking your pulse several times during the day to become familiar with the technique. Inexpensive heart rate monitors can also be obtained at sporting goods stores or through the Internet. These monitors increase the accuracy of monitoring the heart rate during exercise.

For the first few weeks of your program, you should monitor your heart rate several times during the exercise session. As you become familiar with your body's response to exercise, you may have to monitor the heart rate only twice—once at five to seven minutes into the exercise session and a second time near the end of the workout.

Another technique sometimes used to determine your exercise intensity is simply to talk during exercise and then take your pulse immediately after that. Learning to associate the amount of difficulty when talking with the actual exercise heart rate will allow you to develop a sense of how hard you are working. Generally, if you can talk easily, you are not working hard enough. If you can talk but are slightly breathless, you should be close to the target range. If you cannot talk at all, you are working too hard.

In its latest guidelines, the American College of Sports Medicine (ACSM) recommends at least 10 minutes of stretching exercises performed immediately following the warm-up phase (prior to exercising in the appropriate target zone) or after the cool-down phase.[7] The purpose of stretching following either the warm-up or the cool-down phase is because warm muscles achieve a greater range of motion, thus helping enhance the flexibility program. While two to three stretching sessions per week are recommended, near daily stretching is most effective.

If you have difficulty keeping up with your exercise program, you may need to reconsider your goals and start much more slowly. Behavior modification is a process. From a physiological and psychological point of view, initially, you may not be able to carry out an exercise session for a full 20 to 30 minutes. For the first 2 to 3 weeks, therefore, you may just want to take a few 10-minute daily walks. As your body adapts physically and mentally, you may increase the length and intensity of the exercise sessions gradually.

Most important, learn to listen to your body. At times you will feel unusually fatigued or have much discomfort. Pain is the body's way of letting you know that something is wrong. If you have pain or undue discomfort during or after exercise, you need to slow down or discontinue your exercise program and notify the course instructor. The instructor may be able to pinpoint the reason for the discomfort or recommend that you consult your physician. You also will be able to prevent potential injuries by paying attention to pain signals and making adjustments accordingly.

Assess Your Behavior

1. Are you able to incorporate a variety of activities into your exercise program?

2. Do you participate in recreational sports as a means to further enhance fitness and add enjoyment to your exercise program?

3. Do you have an alternate plan in case of inclement weather (rain/cold) or injury that would keep you from your regular training program (jogging or cycling)?

Assess Your Knowledge

1. Using a combination of aerobic activities to develop overall fitness is known as
   a. health-related fitness.
   b. circuit training.
   c. plyometric exercises.
   d. cross-training.
   e. skill-related fitness.

2. The best aerobic activity choice for individuals with leg or back injuries is
   a. walking in chest-deep water.
   b. jogging.
   c. step aerobics.
   d. rope skipping.
   e. cross-country skiing.

3. The approximate jogging mileage to reach the excellent cardiorespiratory fitness classification is
   a. 5 miles.
   b. 10 miles.
   c. 15 miles.
   d. 25 miles.
   e. 50 miles.

4. To help elevate the exercise heart rate during low-impact aerobics, a person should
   a. accentuate arm movements.
   b. sustain movement throughout the program.
   c. accentuate weight-bearing actions.
   d. All of the above are correct choices.
   e. None of the above choices is correct.

5. Achieved maximal heart rates during swimming are approximately what beats per minute (bpm) lower than during running?
   a. 2–4
   b. 5–9
   c. 10–13
   d. 14–20
   e. 20–25

6. Fitness boot camp is primarily a(n) ___ activity?
   a. body weight strength-training
   b. interval training
   c. running
   d. competitive games
   e. All of the above are exercise movements in spinning.

7. HIIT programs
   a. include high to very high-intensity intervals.
   b. require an all-out effort during the entire training program.
   c. were developed primarily for body-building athletes.
   d. are low-intensity activity programs.
   e. All are incorrect choices.

8. An MET represents
   a. the symbol used to indicate that the exercise goal has been met.
   b. a unit of measure that is used to express the value achieved during the Metabolic Exercise Test.
   c. the Maximal Exercise Time achieved.
   d. the rate of energy expenditure at rest.
   e. All choices are incorrect.

9. Which of the following is not a component of skill-related fitness?
   a. mobility
   b. coordination
   c. reaction time
   d. agility
   e. All are skill-related components.

10. When checking exercise heart rate, one should
    a. continue to exercise at the prescribed rate while checking the heart rate.
    b. stop exercising and take the pulse for no longer than 15 seconds.
    c. exercise at a low-to-moderate intensity.
    d. stop exercise and take the heart rate for a full minute.
    e. All choices are valid ways to check exercise heart rate.

Correct answers can be found on page 307.

Activity 4.1   My Personal Fitness Program

Name _____ **Date** _____

Course _____ **Section** _____

I. In the spaces below, provide a list of five activities in which you have participated during the last 6 months. In addition to fitness activities (jogging, aerobics, swimming, strength training), you may list other activities in which you frequently participate that require physical effort (for example, walking, cycling, sweeping, vacuuming, gardening).

According to your own effort of participation, rate each activity for its health-related and motor skill-related benefits (1 = low, 2 = fair, 3 = average, 4 = good, 5 = excellent). Also indicate the frequency and duration of participation (list times per week, month, or 6 months) and add comments regarding your personal feelings related to your participation in the respective activity (liked it, was fun, too hard, got hurt, need more skill, could do it forever, etc.).

	Cardiorespiratory Endurance	Muscular Fitness	Muscular Flexibility	Weight Management	Agility	Balance	Coordination	Power	Reaction Time	Speed
1.										
Comments										
2.										
Comments										
3.										
Comments										
4.										
Comments										

Activity 4.1 **My Personal Fitness Program** (continued)

	Cardiorespiratory Endurance	Muscular Fitness	Muscular Flexibility	Weight Management	Agility	Balance	Coordination	Power	Reaction Time	Speed
5.										

Comments

II. On a separate sheet of paper, keep a 7-day log of all physical activities that you perform. On a daily basis, keep a record of the exact minutes throughout the day that you are active and rate each activity according to its intensity (moderate- or vigorous-intensity). Total your minutes for each day and compute a daily average for all activities. Attach the log to this activity and then answer the following questions:

A. Did you exercise aerobically at least 3 times per week for 20 to 30 minutes each session?

_____ Yes   _____ No

B. Did you accumulate an average of 60 minutes of daily physical activity?

_____ Yes   _____ No

C. What percentage of your total physical activity was moderate intensity,

_____ %

and what percentage was vigorous intensity?

_____ %

III. According to items I and II above, evaluate your current level of physical activity. State how you feel about your results and indicate if your program is primarily conducive to health fitness or physical fitness (or neither). Do you deem any changes necessary to meet previously stated goals (see Activity 3.4, page 98)?

_____

_____

_____

_____

_____

_____

_____

_____

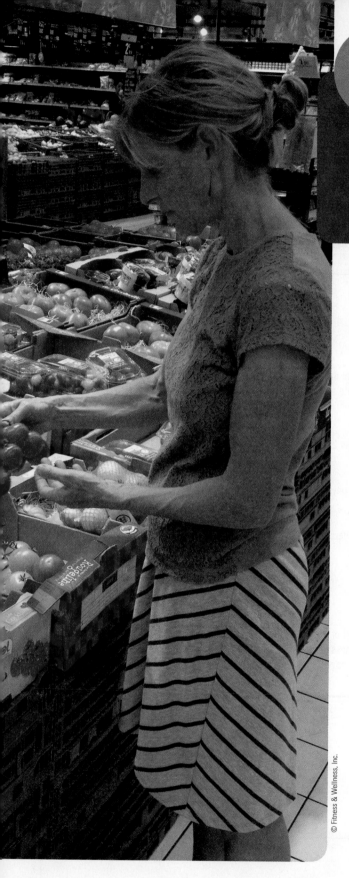

5

Nutrition for Wellness

Healthy nutrition significantly enhances health and quality of life: Preparing most meals at home is one of the surest ways to eat healthier and enjoy a longer, more productive, and better life. If you feel that you don't have time to cook, or don't care to cook, sooner or later you will have to make time to treat and care for illness and disease.

Objectives

> Define nutrition and describe its relationship to health and well-being.

> Learn the functions of nutrients in the human body.

> Become familiar with nutrients, food groups, and nutrient standards, and learn how to achieve a balanced diet through the use of the USDA MyPlate guidelines.

> Become familiar with eating disorders and with their associated medical problems and behavior patterns.

> Identify myths and fallacies regarding nutrition.

> Learn dietary guidelines for Americans.

REAL LIFE STORY | Brandon's Diet

My parents didn't like to cook. They both worked, and the last thing on their minds was to fix an evening meal. We ate a lot of prepackaged meals at home, or fast foods were brought in for the evening meal. I didn't mind it that much as I enjoyed fast foods a whole lot. In our family, we all struggle with weight. My parents, now in their early 50s, are pre-diabetic and my dad has high blood pressure. I have been working for several years, but I am now back part time in school. I never really knew much about nutrition until I took my lifetime fitness course. My instructor was very dynamic and enthusiastic. You could tell that he believed and practiced what he was teaching.

As a course requirement, we had to do a three-day nutrient analysis. Was that a shock to me! I was con-

suming 42 percent of my calories in the form of fat, about a third of them in the form of saturated fat and about 4 grams of daily trans fat. My sodium intake was over 5,000 milligrams per day, fiber intake was only 10 grams per day, and I exceeded my caloric allowance by an approximate 300 daily calories. I knew that my diet was partially responsible for my weight problem, but I had no clue that the way I was eating was also seriously increasing my own risk for high blood pressure, heart disease, and even cancer. Although I can still make improvements—and I do crave fast foods—I make it a point to plan my meals and shop wisely. I eat many fruits, vegetables, and whole grains

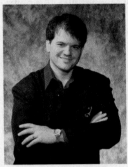
Tony Wear/Shutterstock.com

on most days of the week. I limit my consumption of red meat and whole milk products, and I get my protein mostly from skinless chicken and fish. As much as I crave them, I avoid processed and prepackaged foods and I no longer eat out often. I have lost 15 pounds this last year, I have more energy, and I am sure that health wise I am doing much better. I have learned that eating healthy takes planning and preparation and lots of discipline if you are not used to it. I am very happy that I took that fitness course—and as far as I am concerned, it has made a difference in my life.

Good **nutrition** is clearly linked by scientific studies to overall health and well-being. Proper nutrition means that one's diet supplies all the essential **nutrients** to carry out normal tissue growth, repair, and maintenance. It also implies that the diet will provide enough **substrates** to produce the energy necessary for work, physical activity, and relaxation.

Too much or too little of any nutrient can precipitate serious health problems. The typical U.S. diet is too high in calories, sugar, saturated fat, trans fat, and sodium, and not high enough in whole grains, fruits, and vegetables—factors that undermine good health. Food availability is not the problem. The problem is overconsumption.

According to the office of the U.S. Surgeon General, diseases of dietary excess and imbalance are among the leading causes of death in the United States. Similar trends are observed in developed countries throughout the world. In the report, based on more than 2,000 scientific studies, the Surgeon General said that dietary changes can bring better health to all Americans. Other surveys reveal that, on a given day, nearly half of the

people in the United States eat no fruit and almost a fourth eat no vegetables.

Diet and nutrition often play a crucial role in the development and progression of chronic diseases. A diet high in saturated fat and trans fat increases the risk for atherosclerosis and coronary heart disease. In sodium-sensitive individuals, high salt intake has been linked to high blood pressure. As many as 30 percent to 50 percent of all cancers may be diet-related. Obesity, diabetes, and osteoporosis also have been associated with faulty nutrition.

GLOSSARY

Nutrition The science that studies the relationship of foods to optimal health and performance.

Nutrients Substances found in food that provide energy,

regulate metabolism, and help with growth and repair of body tissues.

Substrates Foods that are used as energy sources (carbohydrates, fat, protein).

5.1 *The Essential Nutrients*

The **essential nutrients** the human body requires are carbohydrates, fats, protein, vitamins, minerals, and water. Carbohydrates, fats, proteins, and water are termed **macronutrients** because people need to take in proportionately large amounts daily. Nutritionists refer to vitamins and minerals as **micronutrients,** because the body requires them in relatively small amounts.

Depending on the amount of nutrients and calories they contain, foods can be classified as high-nutrient density or low-nutrient density. Foods with high-nutrient density contain a low or moderate amount of **calories** but are packed with nutrients. Foods that are high in calories but contain few nutrients are of low-nutrient density and commonly are called "junk food."

Carbohydrates

Carbohydrates are the major source of calories the body uses to provide energy for work, cell maintenance, and heat. They also help regulate fat and metabolize protein. Each gram of carbohydrates provides the human body with four calories. The major sources of carbohydrates are breads, cereals, fruits, vegetables, and milk and other dairy products. Carbohydrates are classified as simple carbohydrates and complex carbohydrates.

Simple Carbohydrates

Simple carbohydrates (such as candy, soda, and cakes), commonly denoted as sugars, have little nutritive value. These carbohydrates are divided into two groups:

- Monosaccharides (glucose, fructose, and galactose)
- Disaccharides (sucrose, lactose, and maltose)

Simple carbohydrates often take the place of more nutritive foods in the diet. Until recently, the most significant health concerns regarding excessive sugar intake included increased caloric intake, weight gain, obesity, tooth decay, and lower nutrient intake. Research indicates, however, that regular soft drink consumers increase coronary heart disease risk by more than 25 percent and have about an 80-percent greater risk for developing type 2 diabetes. Soda consumption in the United States has increased by 500 percent over the past 50 years. Excessive body weight also increases the risk for metabolic complications and heart disease. Most 12-ounce soft drinks contain about 140 calories. An excess of 140 daily calories represents a weight gain of almost 15 pounds per year (140 × 365 ÷ 3,500).

Excessive added sugar in the diet also raises blood fats known as triglycerides, which, along with cholesterol, clog up the arteries. Additionally, people who consume a sugar-heavy diet run a greater risk for pancreatic cancer. Other data indicate that individuals who drink more than five sugary soft drinks per week have reduced bone density in the hips and more than double joint-cushioning cartilage loss in the knees.

Other drinks that are loaded with sugar include fruit drinks, iced teas, sports drinks, and energy drinks. Currently, energy drinks are a major health concern in the United States. Besides sugar, the caffeine content in these drinks can be five times (250 to 500 mg) what's in a cup of coffee (40 to 90 mg). Five deaths have been attributed to these energy drinks, most likely due to an irregular heartbeat caused by the excess caffeine.

Processed and packaged foods are often low in fat but high in refined carbohydrates, sugar, and sodium, all three of which, when consumed in large amounts, are worse for the person than moderate consumption of saturated fat. High refined-carbohydrate diets increase palmitoleic acid, a monounsaturated fatty acid that behaves like a saturated fatty acid and causes an increase in LDL ("bad") cholesterol.

Complex Carbohydrates

Complex carbohydrates are formed when simple carbohydrate molecules are linked together. Three types of complex carbohydrates are

- starches, found commonly in seeds, corn, nuts, grains, roots, potatoes, and legumes.
- dextrins, formed from the breakdown of large starch molecules exposed to dry heat, such as when bread is baked or cold cereals are manufactured.
- glycogen, the animal polysaccharide synthesized from glucose and found in only small amounts in meats. Glycogen constitutes the body's reservoir of glucose. Many hundreds to thousands of glucose molecules are linked to be stored as glycogen in the liver and muscles. When a surge of energy is needed, enzymes in the muscle and the liver break down glycogen and thus make glucose readily available for energy transformation.

Complex carbohydrates provide many valuable nutrients and also are an excellent source of fiber (also called roughage).

Fiber

Fiber is a complex non-digestible carbohydrate. A high-fiber diet gives a person a feeling of fullness without added calories. Dietary fiber is present mainly in plant leaves, skins, roots, and seeds. Processing and refining foods removes almost all of the natural fiber.

Table 5.1 Fiber Content of Selected Foods

Food (gm)	Serving Size	Dietary Fiber
Almonds, shelled	¼ cup	3.9
Apple	1 medium	3.7
Banana	1 small	1.2
Beans (red, kidney)	½ cup	8.2
Blackberries	½ cup	4.9
Beets, red, canned (cooked)	½ cup	1.4
Brazil nuts	1 oz	2.5
Broccoli (cooked)	½ cup	3.3
Brown rice (cooked)	½ cup	1.7
Carrots (cooked)	½ cup	3.3
Cauliflower (cooked)	½ cup	5.0
Cereal		
All Bran	1 oz	8.5
Cheerios	1 oz	1.1
Cornflakes	1 oz	0.5
Fruit and Fiber	1 oz	4.0
Fruit Wheats	1 oz	2.0
Just Right	1 oz	2.0
Wheaties	1 oz	2.0
Corn (cooked)	½ cup	2.2
Eggplant (cooked)	½ cup	3.0
Lettuce (chopped)	½ cup	0.5
Orange	1 medium	4.3
Parsnips (cooked)	½ cup	2.1
Pear	1 medium	4.5
Peas (cooked)	½ cup	4.4
Popcorn (plain)	1 cup	1.2
Potato (baked)	1 medium	4.9
Strawberries	½ cup	1.6
Summer squash (cooked)	½ cup	1.6
Watermelon	1 cup	0.1

© Cengage Learning

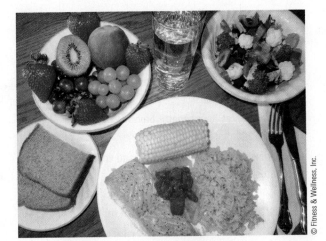
High-fiber foods are essential in a healthy diet.

In the American diet, the main sources of fiber are whole-grain cereals and breads, fruits, vegetables, and legumes. Fiber is important in the diet because it decreases the risk of inflammation, obesity, diabetes, and cardiovascular disease. Increased fiber intake lowers the risk for coronary heart disease and stroke because saturated fats often take the place of fiber in the diet, thus increasing the absorption and formation of cholesterol. Other health disorders that have been tied to low intake of fiber are constipation, diverticulitis, hemorrhoids, and gallbladder disease. Data also shows that increased fiber intake enhances gastrointestinal health and immune function, and promotes the growth of beneficial gut bacteria

The daily recommended amount of fiber intake for adults 50 years and younger is 25 grams for women and 38 grams for men. Most people in the United States eat only 15 grams of fiber per day, putting them at increased risk for disease. A person can increase fiber intake by eating more fruits, vegetables, legumes, grains, and cereals. Research provides evidence that increasing fiber intake by 30 grams per day leads to a significant reduction in heart attacks, cancer of the colon, breast cancer, diabetes, and diverticulitis. Table 5.1 provides the fiber content of selected foods.

Fibers are typically classified according to their solubility in water. Soluble fiber dissolves in water and forms a gel-like substance that encloses food particles. This property allows soluble fiber to bind and excrete fats from the body. Soluble fiber has been shown to decrease blood cholesterol and blood sugar levels. Soluble fibers are found primarily in oats, fruits, barley, legumes, and psyllium.

Insoluble fiber is not easily dissolved in water, and the body cannot digest it. This fiber is important because it binds water, resulting in a softer and bulkier stool that increases peristalsis (involuntary muscle contractions of intestinal walls), forcing the stool onward, and allows food

---GLOSSARY---

Essential nutrients Carbohydrates, fats, protein, vitamins, minerals, and water— the nutrients the human body requires for survival.

Macronutrients The nutrients the body needs in proportionately large amounts; carbohydrates, fats, proteins, and water are examples.

Micronutrients The nutrients the body needs in small quantities— vitamins and minerals—that serve specific roles in transformation of energy and body tissue synthesis.

Calorie The amount of heat necessary to raise the temperature of 1 gram of water 1°C; used to measure the energy value of food and the cost of physical activity.

Carbohydrates Compounds composed of carbon, hydrogen, and oxygen that the body uses as its major source of energy.

Fiber Plant material that human digestive enzymes cannot digest.

Behavior Modification Planning

Tips to Increase Fiber in Your Diet

- Eat more vegetables, either raw or steamed.
- Eat salads daily that include a wide variety of vegetables.
- Eat more fruit, including the skin.
- Choose whole-wheat and whole-grain products.
- Choose breakfast cereals with more than 3 grams of fiber per serving.
- Sprinkle a teaspoon or two of unprocessed bran or 100% bran cereal on your favorite breakfast cereal.
- Add high-fiber cereals to casseroles and desserts.
- Add beans to soups, salads, and stews.

- Add vegetables to sandwiches: sprouts, green and red pepper strips, diced carrots, sliced cucumbers, red cabbage, and onions.
- Add vegetables to spaghetti: broccoli, cauliflower, sliced carrots, and mushrooms.
- Experiment with unfamiliar fruits and vegetables: collards, kale, broccoflower, asparagus, papaya, mango, kiwi, and starfruit.
- Blend fruit juice with small pieces of fruit and crushed ice.
- When increasing fiber in your diet, drink plenty of fluids.

© Cengage Learning

residues to pass through the intestinal tract more quickly. Speeding the passage of food residues through the intestines seems to lower the risk for colon cancer, mainly because cancer-causing agents are not in contact as long with the intestinal wall. Insoluble fiber also is thought to bind with carcinogens (cancer-producing substances), and more water in the stool may dilute the cancer-causing agents, lessening their potency. Sources of insoluble fiber include wheat, cereals, vegetables, and skins of fruits.

A practical guideline to obtain your fiber intake is to eat at least five daily servings of fruits and vegetables and three servings of whole-grain foods (whole-grain bread, cereal, and rice).

Fats

Fats, or **lipids**, are the most concentrated source of energy. Each gram of fat supplies 9 calories to the body. Fats, also part of the cell structure, are used as stored energy and as an insulator to preserve body heat. They absorb shock, supply essential fatty acids, and carry the fat-soluble vitamins A, D, E, and K. The main sources of dietary fat are whole milk and other dairy products, meats, and meat alternatives. Fats are classified into simple, compound, and derived fats.

Simple Fats

Simple fats consist of a glyceride molecule linked to one, two, or three units of fatty acids. According to the number of fatty acids attached, simple fats are divided into monoglycerides (one fatty acid), diglycerides (two fatty acids), and triglycerides (three fatty acids). More than 90 percent of the weight of fat in foods and more than 95 percent of the stored fat in the human body is in the form of triglycerides.

The length of the carbon atom chain and the amount of hydrogen saturation in fatty acids vary. Based on the extent of saturation, fatty acids are said to be saturated or unsaturated. Unsaturated fatty acids, also known as 'healthy fats,' are classified further into monounsaturated and polyunsaturated fats. Saturated fatty acids are mainly of animal origin. Unsaturated fats are found mostly in plant products.

In saturated fatty acids, the carbon atoms are fully saturated with hydrogens; only single bonds link the carbon atoms on the chain. These saturated fatty acids are more commonly known as saturated fats. Examples of foods high in saturated fatty acids are meats, meat fat, lard, whole milk, cream, butter, cheese, ice cream, hydrogenated oils (a process that makes oils saturated), coconut oil, and palm oils. They are also concealed in foods such as cakes, cookies, muffins, biscuits, fried chicken with skin, creamy pasta sauces, mayonnaise, salad dressings, and processed meats.

Saturated fats tend to be solids that typically do not melt at room temperature. Coconut and palm oils are exceptions. In general, saturated fats raise the blood cholesterol level. The data on coconut and palm oils are controversial, as some research indicates that these oils may be neutral in terms of their effects on cholesterol.

In unsaturated fatty acids (unsaturated fats), double bonds form between the unsaturated carbons. Unsaturated fat is usually liquid at room temperature. It is mostly in oils from plants. Try to eat mostly unsaturated fats instead of saturated fat. Unsaturated fats are healthy fats.

Monounsaturated fat and polyunsaturated fat are types of unsaturated fat. Monounsaturated fatty acids (MUFA) have only one double bond along the chain. Examples are olive, canola, rapeseed, peanut, and sesame oils. Polyunsaturated fatty acids (PUFA) contain two or more double bonds between unsaturated carbon atoms along the chain. Corn, cottonseed, safflower, walnut, sunflower, and soybean oils are high in polyunsaturated fatty acids. Polyunsaturated fat is also found in seafood, almonds and pecans.

Omega-3, omega-6, and omega-9 are polyunsaturated fats. Omega-3 fatty acids and omega-6 fatty acids have gained considerable attention in recent years because they are essential to human health and cannot be manufactured by the body. They have to be consumed in the diet. Omega-9 fatty acids are defined as nonessential because the body can synthesize them from other foods we eat, and we don't have to depend on direct dietary sources to obtain them.

Most critical in the diet are omega-3 fatty acids, which provide substantial health benefits. Omega-3 fatty acids tend to decrease cholesterol, triglycerides, inflammation, blood clots, abnormal heart rhythms, and high blood pressure and slow growth of plaque in the arteries. They also decrease the risk for heart attack, abnormal heart rhythms, stroke, Alzheimer's disease, dementia, macular degeneration, and joint degeneration. Fish—especially fresh or frozen salmon, mackerel, herring, tuna, and rainbow trout—are high in omega-3. Other sources include flaxseeds, canola oil, walnuts, wheat germ, and green leafy vegetables.

Body inflammation can be of two types. Normal body inflammation that develops suddenly is a protective response to injury, infection, or the presence of inflammatory stimulants. Typically it lasts a few days or weeks to help kill or encapsulate microbes, form protective scar tissue, and regenerate damaged tissue.

Chronic or low-grade inflammation, however, is a persistent condition with tissue destruction and repair taking place at the same time and can last years or decades before damage is apparent. It occurs as a result of the continuous presence of pro-inflammatory stimulants and the body's inability to provide sufficient anti-inflammatory compounds. Chronic inflammation is a major risk factor for disease development and it is primarily related to unhealthy lifestyle choices. Most people are unaware of its existence until age-related chronic disease occurs. It is triggered by eating an unhealthy diet, being physically inactive and obese, not getting enough sleep, smoking, drinking too much alcohol, or having an internal injury or infection that produces no outward signs or symptoms (see Figure 5.1).

Figure 5.1 Low-grade inflammation leads to an array of chronic diseases.

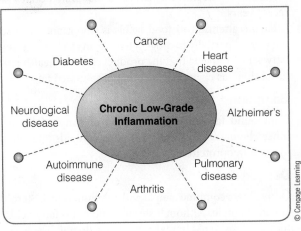

© Cengage Learning

Omega-6 fatty acids include linoleic acid (LA), gamma-linolenic acid (GLA), and arachidonic acid (AA). Unfortunately, most of the polyunsaturated fatty acid consumption in the United States comes from omega-6; about 10 to 20 times more omega-6 than omega-3. Most omega-6 fatty acids come in the form of LA from vegetable oils, the primary oil ingredient added to most processed foods, including salad dressing. LA-rich oils include corn, soybean, sunflower, safflower, and cottonseed oils.

Trans fat (trans fatty acids) has been receiving a lot of attention in recent years. Hydrogen often is added to monounsaturated and polyunsaturated fats to increase shelf life and to solidify them so they are more spreadable. During this process, called "partial hydrogenation," the position of hydrogen atoms may be changed along the carbon chain, transforming the fat into a trans fat. Some margarines, spreads, shortening, creamy pasta sauces, pastries, nut butters, crackers, cookies, frozen breakfast foods, dairy products, snacks and chips, cake mixes, meats, processed foods, fried chicken, and fast foods contain trans fatty acids.

Trans fats are not essential and provide no known health benefit. In truth, health-conscious people minimize their intake of these types of fats because diets high in trans fat increase rigidity of the coronary arteries, elevate cholesterol, and contribute to the formation of blood clots that may lead to heart attacks and strokes. Trans-fat consumption has been associated with an

-GLOSSARY-

Fats (lipids) A class of nutrients that the body uses as a source of energy.

increased risk of all-cause mortality, accounting for an estimated 7 percent of all death in the United States in recent years.

Paying attention to food labels is important because the words "partially hydrogenated," "trans fat," and "trans fatty acids" indicate that the product carries a health risk just as high as or higher than that of saturated fat.

Compound Fats

Compound fats are a combination of simple fats and other chemicals. Examples are phospholipids, glucolipids, and lipoproteins.

Derived Fats

Derived fats combine simple and compound fats. Sterols are an example. Although sterols contain no fatty acids, they are considered lipids because they do not dissolve in water. The most often mentioned sterol is cholesterol, which is found in many foods and is manufactured from saturated fats in the body.

Proteins

Proteins are used to build and repair tissues including muscles, blood, internal organs, skin, hair, nails, and bones. They are a part of hormones, enzymes, and antibodies, and they help maintain a normal balance of body fluids. Proteins can also be used as a source of energy, but only if not enough carbohydrates are available. The primary sources are meats, meat alternatives, milk, and other dairy products.

Proteins are composed of **amino acids**, containing nitrogen, carbon, hydrogen, and oxygen. Because the body cannot produce them, 9 of the 20 amino acids are called essential amino acids. The other 11, termed nonessential amino acids, can be manufactured in the body if food proteins in the diet provide enough nitrogen. For normal body function, all amino acids must be present in the diet.

Proteins that contain all the essential amino acids, known as "complete" or "higher-quality" proteins, are usually of animal origin. If one or more of the essential amino acids are missing, the proteins are termed incomplete or lower-quality proteins. The essential amino acid that is missing in an incomplete protein is called the limiting amino acid. All plant products, including grains, fruits, vegetables, grains, beans, nuts, and seeds, are incomplete proteins. The only exceptions of complete proteins found in plant products are soy and quinoa (a grain-like crop grown for its edible seed).

Individuals have to take in enough protein to ensure nitrogen for adequate production of all amino acids. On a vegetarian diet, consumption of a variety of food sources is required so that the diet supplies all the essential amino acids within a meal or a given day. When different foods are consumed, the limiting amino acid in one food can be obtained from another food source. This principle is referred to as complementing proteins. For example, grains and legumes complement each other. Legumes and nuts also complement each other. Nuts and grains, however, are not complementary proteins. Soy and quinoa can also be used to complement the limiting amino acids in grains, legumes, nuts, and seeds.

A word of caution is in order as to your dietary protein sources. Several recent research studies provide strong evidence that excessive red meat consumption increases the risk of premature death, primarily from heart disease, stroke, some cancers, and type 2 diabetes. Consumption of both unprocessed red meat (beef, pork, and lamb) and processed red meat (cold cuts, ham, bacon, bologna, sausage, hot dogs) leads to this outcome.

The most compelling evidence comes from a 2012 study of more than 120,000 people showing a 30 percent increased risk of premature death among people who eat the most red meat as compared to those who eat the least (about a half a serving per day).[1] In the study, three ounces of unprocessed red meat were considered as one serving, but only one ounce of processed red meat was viewed as a serving. The mortality rate was highest among processed red-meat eaters. Eating just one serving per day increased the risk between 13 percent (unprocessed) and 20 percent (processed).

The data also indicated that replacing one serving a day of red meat with fish, poultry, nuts, beans, low-fat dairy, or whole grains decreased the chances of premature death in the range of 7 percent to 19 percent. The researchers concluded that, "*The message we want to communicate is it would be great if you could reduce your intake of red meat consumption to half a serving a day or two to three servings a week, and severely limit processed red meat intake.*"

The role of protein in the American diet is gaining relevance as *adequate protein intake with each meal* is crucial for satiety and weight management and to help build, repair, and maintain lean tissue. The latter has even greater relevance for people who are physically active. Loss of lean tissue with sedentary living, aging, exhaustive exercise training, and while dieting (negative caloric balance) without proper energy and protein intake is inevitable. Loss of lean tissue is never desirable because of the decrease in functional physical capacity (the ability to perform ordinary and unusual tasks of daily living), as well as in the resting metabolic rate.

Protein is also important for bone health. About 50 percent of bone volume and 30 percent of bone mass

Table 5.2 Recommended Daily Protein Intake

Category	Grams/kg of Body Weight
Sedentary	0.8 g/kg
Healthy older adults (65+)	1.0–1.2 g/kg
Physically active	1.0–1.2 g/kg
Athlete	1.2–2.0 g/kg
Weight gain/loss	1.5–2.0 g/kg

© Cengage Learning 2017

is protein. Data indicate that when consumed during the same meal, protein and calcium interact and help improve bone health. An intake above the recommended RDA of 0.8 g/day can improve health by helping prevent obesity, osteoporosis, and metabolic syndrome. The current RDA, nonetheless, is the same for people of all ages. During growth in youth, body hormones help the body use proteins quite efficiently. Such is not the case as people age. In fact, adults have greater protein needs to maintain lean tissue (muscles and bones) necessary for a healthy metabolic rate, blood sugar regulation, and bone health. Protein requirement is actually higher in older adults because caloric intake typically decreases as people age, yet the protein need does not.

As an individual, you can prevent or even completely reverse muscle tissue loss. The recommendation is that we distribute our protein intake in equal parts throughout the day. To do so, determine your daily intake in grams (see Table 5.2) and divide by three (meals per day). For example, if you weigh 141 pounds (64 kg) and you are physically active, your total protein intake should be between 64 and 77 grams per day (64 × 1.0 and 64 × 1.2 or the equivalent of 256 to 308 calories derived from protein each day—each gram of protein supplies the body with 4 calories) or 21 to 26 grams of protein per meal.

Vitamins

Vitamins function as **antioxidants** and as coenzymes (primarily the B complex), which regulate the work of enzymes, and vitamin D even functions as a hormone.

Based on their solubility, vitamins are classified into two types: fat-soluble vitamins (A, D, E, and K) and water-soluble vitamins (B complex and C). With the exception of vitamins A, D, and K, the body cannot manufacture vitamins; they can be obtained only through a well-balanced diet. Vitamin A is produced from beta-carotene, found mainly in yellow/orange foods such as carrots, pumpkin, and sweet potatoes. Vitamin D is found in certain foods and is created when ultraviolet light from the sun transforms 7-dehydrocholesterol, a compound in human skin. Vitamin K is created in the body by intestinal bacteria. Additional information on the importance of vitamins is presented later in this chapter.

Minerals

Minerals serve several important functions. They are constituents of all cells, especially those in hard parts of the body (bones, nails, teeth). They are crucial in maintaining water balance and the acid–base balance. They are essential components of respiratory pigments, enzymes, and enzyme systems, and they regulate muscular and nervous tissue excitability.

Water

Water, the most important nutrient, is involved in almost every vital body process: in digesting and absorbing food, in producing energy, in the circulatory process, in regulating body heat and electrolyte balance, in removing waste products, in building and rebuilding cells, in transporting essential nutrients, and in cushioning joints and organs.

Water is contained in almost all foods, but primarily in liquid foods, fruits, and vegetables. Although for decades the recommendation was to consume at least 8 cups of water per day, a panel of scientists of the Institute of Medicine of the National Academy of Sciences indicated that people are getting enough water from liquids (milk, juices, sodas, coffee) and the moisture content of solid foods. Caffeine-containing drinks are also acceptable as a water source because data indicate that people who regularly consume such beverages do not have a greater 24-hour urine output than those who don't.

Most Americans and Canadians remain well hydrated simply by using thirst as their guide. An exception to this practice, however, is when an individual exercises in the heat or does so for an extended time. Water lost under these conditions must be replenished regularly, without waiting for the onset of thirst.

GLOSSARY

Proteins A class of nutrients that the body uses to build and repair body tissues.

Amino acids The basic building blocks of protein.

Vitamins Organic substances essential for normal bodily metabolism, growth, and development.

Antioxidants Compounds that prevent oxygen from combining with other substances it might damage.

Minerals Inorganic elements needed by the body.

5.2 *Nutrition Standards*

Nutritionists use a variety of nutrient standards. The most widely known is the Recommended Dietary Allowances (RDA). This is not the only standard, though. Nutrition standards include the Dietary Reference Intakes and the Daily Values on food labels. Each standard has a different purpose and utilization in dietary planning and assessment.

Dietary Reference Intakes

To help people meet dietary guidelines, the National Academy of Sciences has developed a set of dietary nutrient intakes for healthy people in the United States and Canada, the **Dietary Reference Intakes (DRIs)**. The DRIs are based on a review of the most current research on adequate amounts and maximum safe nutrient intakes of healthy people. The DRI reports are written by the Food and Nutrition Board of the Institute of Medicine in cooperation with scientists from Canada.

Within the umbrella of DRI are four types of reference values for planning and assessing diets:

1. Estimated Average Requirements (EAR)
2. Recommended Dietary Allowances (RDA)
3. Adequate Intakes (AI)
4. Tolerable Upper Intake Levels (UL)

The type of reference value used for a given nutrient and a specific age/gender group is determined according to available scientific information and the intended use of the dietary standard.

The **Estimated Average Requirements (EAR)** is the amount of nutrient that is estimated to meet the nutrient requirement of half the healthy people in specific age and gender groups. At this nutrient intake level, the nutritional requirements of the upper 50 percent of the people are not met.

The **Recommended Dietary Allowances (RDA)** set forth the daily amount of a nutrient considered adequate to meet the known nutrient needs of nearly all healthy people in the United States. The RDAs for selected nutrients are presented in Table 5.3. Because

Table 5.3 Recommended Dietary Allowances and Adequate Intakes for Selected Nutrients

	Thiamin (mg)	Riboflavin (mg)	Niacin (mg NE)	Vitamin B₆ (mg)	Folate (mg)	Vitamin B₁₂ (mg)	Phosphorus (mg)	Magnesium (mg)	Vitamin A (mg)	Vitamin C (mg)	Vitamin D (mg)	Vitamin E (mg)	Selenium (mcg)	Iron (mg)	Calcium (mg)	Fluoride (mg)	Panthothenic acid (mg)	Biotin (mg)	Choline (mg)
	Recommended Dietary Allowances (RDA)															Adequate Intakes (AI)			
Males																			
14–18	1.2	1.3	16	1.3	400	2.4	1,250	410	900	75	15	15	55	11	1,300	3	5	25	550
19–30	1.2	1.3	16	1.3	400	2.4	700	400	900	90	15	15	55	8	1,000	4	5	30	550
31–50	1.2	1.3	16	1.3	400	2.4	700	420	900	90	15	15	55	8	1,000	4	5	30	550
51–70	1.2	1.3	16	1.7	400	2.4	700	420	900	90	15	15	55	8	1,000	4	5	30	550
>70	1.2	1.3	16	1.7	400	2.4	700	420	900	90	20	15	55	8	1,200	4	5	30	550
Females																			
14–18	1	1	14	1.2	400	2.4	1,250	360	700	65	15	15	55	15	1,300	3	5	25	400
19–30	1.1	1.1	14	1.3	400	2.4	700	310	700	75	15	15	55	18	1,000	3	5	30	425
31–50	1.1	1.1	14	1.3	400	2.4	700	320	700	75	15	15	55	8	1,000	3	5	30	425
51–70	1.1	1.1	14	1.5	400	2.4	700	320	700	75	15	15	55	8	1,200	3	5	30	425
>70	1.1	1.1	14	1.5	400	2.4	700	320	700	75	20	15	55	27	1,200	3	5	30	425
Pregnant (19–30)	1.4	1.4	18	1.9	600	*	140	350	770	85	15	15	60		1,000	3	6	30	450
Lactating (19–30)	1.4	1.6	17	2	500	*	*	310	1,300	120	15	19	70	9	1,000	3	7	35	550

*Values for these nutrients do not change with pregnancy or lactation. Use the value listed for women of comparable age.

SOURCE: Adapted from "Dietary Reference Intakes: Recommended Dietary Allowances and Adequate Intakes, Vitamins," "Dietary Reference Intakes: Recommended Dietary Allowances and Adequate Intakes, Elements," and "Dietary Reference Intakes for Calcium and Vitamin D," 2011 by the National Academy of Sciences. Courtesy of the National Academies Press, Washington, DC.

the committee must decide what level of intake to recommend for everybody, the RDA is set well above the EAR and covers about 98 percent of the population. Stated another way, the RDA recommendation for any nutrient is well above almost everyone's actual requirement.

The RDA could be considered a goal for adequate intake. The process for determining the RDA depends on being able to set an EAR. RDAs are statistically determined from the EAR values. If an EAR cannot be set, no RDA can be established.

When data are insufficient or inadequate to set an EAR, an **Adequate Intakes (AI)** value is determined instead of the RDA. The AI value is derived from approximations of observed nutrient intakes by a group or groups of healthy people. The AI value for children and adults is expected to meet or exceed the nutritional requirements of a specific healthy population.

The **Tolerable Upper Intake Levels (UL)**, which eventually will be available for all nutrients, establish the highest level of nutrient intake that seems to be safe for most healthy people and beyond which there is an increased risk of adverse effects. As intakes increase above the UL, so does the risk for adverse effects. Generally speaking, the optimum nutrient range for healthy eating is between the RDA and the UL. The established ULs for selected nutrients are presented in Table 5.4.

Daily Values

The **Daily Values (DVs)** are reference values for nutrients and food components for use on commercial food labels. The DVs are based on a 2,000-calorie diet and may therefore require adjustments depending on an individual's daily **estimated energy requirement (EER)** in calories.

For example, on a 2,000-calorie diet (EER), recommended carbohydrate intake is about 300 grams (about 60 percent of EER), and fat is less than 65 grams (about 30 percent of EER) (see Figure 5.2). The vitamin, mineral, and protein DVs were adapted from the RDAs. The DVs are also not as specific for age and gender groups as are the DRIs.

The food label is a good guide for planning a daily diet. For example, if the DV for carbohydrates in a given meal adds up to only 35 percent, you know that several additional high-carbohydrate food items are required throughout that day to reach the 100 percent DV. Further, if the DV for fat from another food item is 60 percent or

Table 5.4 Tolerable Upper Intake Levels (UL) of Selected Nutrients for Adults (19–70 years)

Nutrient	UL per Day
Calcium	2.5 gr
Phosphorus	4.0 gr*
Magnesium	350 mg
Vitamin D	50 mcg
Fluoride	10 mg
Niacin	35 mg
Iron	45 mg
Vitamin B$_6$	100 mg
Folate	1,000 mcg
Choline	3.5 gr
Vitamin A	3,000 mcg
Vitamin C	2,000 mg
Vitamin E	1,000 mg
Selenium	400 mcg

*3.5 gr per day for pregnant women.

SOURCE: Adapted from the National Academy of Sciences, Institute of Medicine. Dietary Reference Intakes for Tolerable Upper Intake Levels, Vitamins. Washington D.C.: National Academy Press, 2011.

GLOSSARY

Dietary Reference Intakes (DRIs) Four types of nutrient standards that are used to establish adequate amounts and maximum safe nutrient intakes in the diet: Estimated Average Requirements (EAR), Recommended Dietary Allowances (RDA), Adequate Intakes (AI), and Tolerable Upper Intake Levels (UL).

Estimated Average Requirements (EAR) The amount of a nutrient that meets the dietary needs of half the people.

Recommended Dietary Allowances (RDA) The daily amount of a nutrient (statistically determined from the EARs) considered adequate to meet the known nutrient needs of almost 98 percent of all healthy people in the United States.

Adequate Intakes (AI) The recommended amount of a nutrient intake when sufficient evidence is not available to calculate the EAR and subsequent RDA.

Tolerable Upper Intake Levels (UL) The highest level of nutrient intake that appears to be safe for most healthy people without an increased risk of adverse effects.

Daily Values (DVs) Reference values for nutrients and food components used in food labels.

Estimated energy requirement (EER) The average dietary energy (caloric) intake that is predicted to maintain energy balance in a healthy adult of defined age, gender, weight, height, and level of physical activity, consistent with good health.

Figure 5.2 Food label using Daily Values.

1 Design
Nutrition Facts
The food label provides information on the macronutrients and other food components important to decrease the risk of developing chronic diseases.

2 Serving size
Check here first
Serving sizes typically are unrealistic. Most people consume more than the small portion sizes listed. If you eat more, you need to adjust all nutrients, including the increase in calories consumed.

3 Percent Daily Value (% DV)
How much are you really getting?
The % DV are based on a 2,000 calories/day diet. You will need to adjust your values based on how much you eat in a serving. This listing can help you choose foods rich in nutrients deficient in your diet (choose items with at least 20% DV) or decrease food items you need to limit for health reasons.

4 Limit these nutrients
Know what you want to minimize
These are nutrients that most people need to limit on a daily basis: Trans fat, saturated fat, sodium, and cholesterol. Be on the lookout for hydrogenated and partially-hydrogenated oils. For poly-unsaturated and monounsaturated fats, you may consume up to 10 percent and 20 percent, respectively, of your total daily calories. For better health, make sure to choose items with less than 5% DV for foods you wish to avoid. Note also that if there is less than .5 g trans fat per serving, manufacturers do not have to list it here and it may simply state 0%. 20% DV is high in sodium.

5 Know your nutrients
Know the nutrients to increase
For good health, consume sufficient beneficial nutrients like dietary fiber, protein, calcium, vitamins, and nutrients needed every day. Be sure, however, to consume primarily complex carbohydrates and limit the intake of food items with a close ratio of total carbohydrates to sugars. Limit foods with more than 5 g of sugar per serving. Check the protein content to make sure you meet the recommended daily requirement, particularly if you are highly active, on a weight loss program, or if you are an older adult.

6 Ingredient list
Always read the list
The ingredients are listed in descending order of predominance (the ingredient that weighs the most is listed first and the ingredient that weighs the least is listed last). Choose whole, minimally processed foods with ingredients that you are familiar with in your kitchen. Foods with a shorter ingredient list indicates that the foods are less processed. A good guideline is to choose items with 5 or fewer ingredients. In particular pay attention to and minimize the use of foods with the following ingredients on the list: trans fats, saturated fat, hydrogenated and partially-hydrogenated oils, grains that are not 100 percent whole grain, added sugars, high fructose corn syrup (and other sugars), artificial ingredients, nitrates, and nitrites.

7 Other facts
Descriptors, health claims, and allergies
Certain terms such as "good source of fiber," "low-fat," and "fat-free," as well as selected health claims are allowed on food labels. Laws require that such descriptors and claims meet legal definitions. Food labels must also list major food allergens (milk, eggs, fish, crustacean shellfish, tree nuts, wheat, peanuts, and soybeans).

Nutrition Facts

Serving Size 1 cup (240g)

Servings Per Container about 2

Amount Per Serving

Calories 200	
Calories from Fat	70

% Daily Value*

Total Fat 10g	**12%**
Saturated Fat 3g	**9%**
Trans Fat 0g	
Polyunsaturated Fat 3g	
Monounsaturated Fat 4g	
Cholesterol 15mg	**5%**
Sodium 860mg	**36%**
Potassium 620mg	**18%**
Total Carbohydrate 21g	**7%**
Dietary Fiber 2g	**8%**
Sugars 2g	
Protein 6g	

Vitamin A	0%	Vitamin C	0%
Calcium	2%	Iron	4%

* Percent Daily Values are based on a 2,000 calorie diet.

Ingredients: Clam Broth, Potatoes*, Clams, Soybean Oil, Water, Onions, Modified Food Starch, Contains less than 2% of: Butter, Artificial Color, Cream, Sugar, DATEM, Brandy, Sodium Phosphate, Celery*, Potassium Chloride, Yeast Extract, Parsley*, Chablis Wine, Salt, Natural Flavor. Soy Protein Concentrate,   *Dried

CONTAINS CLAM, MILK AND SOY INGREDIENTS.

Gluten Free

70 percent, you should limit your fat intake during the rest of that day.

Both the DRIs and the DVs apply only to healthy adults. They are not intended for people who are ill and may require additional nutrients or dietary adjustments.

> **! Critical Thinking**
>
> What do the nutrition standards mean to you? • How much of a challenge would it be to apply those standards in your daily life?

5.3 *Macronutrient Composition Guidelines*

Most people would like to live life to its fullest, have good health, and lead a productive life. One of the ways to do this is through a well-balanced diet. As illustrated in Table 5.5, the recommended guidelines by the National Academy of Sciences (NAS) state that daily caloric intake should be distributed so that 45 percent to 65 percent of the total calories come from carbohydrates (mostly complex carbohydrates and less than 25 percent from sugar), 20 to 35 percent from fat, and 10 to 35 percent from protein.[2] These ranges offer greater flexibility in planning diets according to individual health and physical activity needs. The fat percentage is up to 35 percent to accommodate individuals with metabolic syndrome (see Chapter 8, page 218), who have an abnormal insulin response to carbohydrates and may need additional fat in the diet. For all other individuals, daily fat intake should not exceed 30 percent of total caloric intake.

In addition to macronutrients, the diet must include all of the essential vitamins and minerals. The source of fat calories is also critical. In late 2013 the American Heart Association (AHA) and the American College of Cardiology released a new recommendation that saturated fat should constitute less than 5 to 6 percent, whereas polyunsaturated fat can be up to 10 percent, and monounsaturated fat up to 20 percent of total daily calories. Rating a given diet accurately is difficult without a complete nutrient analysis. You have an opportunity to perform this analysis in Activity 5.1, page 152.

The NAS recommendations will be effective only if people consistently replace saturated and trans fatty acids with unsaturated fatty acids. Such a dietary change will require dramatic changes in the typical "unhealthy" American diet, which is generally high in red meats, whole dairy products, and fast foods—all of which are high in saturated and/or trans fatty acids.

5.4 *Caloric Content of Food*

As illustrated in Figure 5.3, each gram of carbohydrates and protein supplies the body with four calories, and fat provides nine calories per gram consumed (alcohol yields seven calories per gram). In this regard, just looking at the total amount of grams consumed for each type of food can be misleading.

For example, a person who consumes 160 grams of carbohydrates, 100 grams of fat, and 70 grams of protein has a total intake of 330 grams of food. This indicates that 30 percent of the total grams of food is in the form of fat (100 grams of fat ÷ 330 grams of total food × 100).

Table 5.5 Current and Recommended Intake of Carbohydrate, Fat, and Protein Expressed as a Percentage of Total Calories

	Current	Recommended*
Carbohydrates	50%	45–65%
Simple	26%	Less than 25%
Complex	24%	20–40%
Fat	34%	20–35%**
Monounsaturated	11%	Up to 20%
Polyunsaturated	10%	Up to 10%
Saturated	13%	Less than 6%
Protein	16%	10–35%

*Adapted from the 2002 recommended guidelines by the National Academy of Sciences.
© Cengage Learning

Figure 5.3 Calories per gram of food.

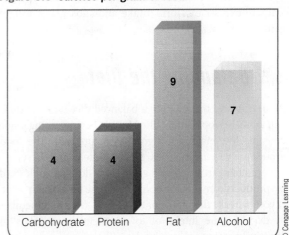

© Cengage Learning

Figure 5.4 Determining percent calories from fat in food.

Serving = 120 calories   Fat = 5 g

Percent fat calories = (g of fat × 9)
÷ calories per serving × 100

5 g of fat × 9 calories per g of fat =
45 calories from fat

45 calories from fat ÷ 120 calories per
serving × 100 = 38% fat

© Cengage Learning

Figure 5.5 MyPlate food guide.

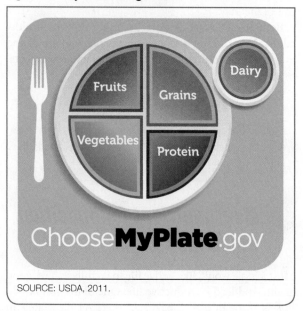

SOURCE: USDA, 2011.

Almost half of this diet, however, consists of fat calories. In the diet, 640 calories are derived from carbohydrates (160 grams × 4 calories/gram), 280 calories from protein (70 grams 3 × calories/gram), and 900 calories from fat (100 grams × 9 calories/gram), for a total of 1,820 calories. If 900 calories are derived from fat, you can see that almost half of the total caloric intake is in the form of fat (900 ÷ 1,820 × 100 = 49.5 percent).

Most people need to be careful with their caloric intake. Realizing that each gram of fat provides 9 calories is a useful guideline to monitor total daily caloric consumption. To determine fat content in food, all you have to do is multiply the grams of fat by 9 and divide by the total calories in that specific food. Multiply that number by 100 to get the percentage (see Figure 5.4). For example, if a food label lists a total of 120 calories and 7 grams of fat, the fat content is 53 percent of total calories (7 × 9 ÷ 120 × 100). For proper weight-management, however, keep in mind that fat is very calorie dense—it contains more than twice the amount of calories per gram of food than carbohydrates or protein. Some healthy fat is recommended in the diet to increase satiety and for heart health, but consumption of too much fat typically leads to excessive caloric intake and subsequent weight gain.

5.5 *Balancing the Diet*

Achieving and maintaining a balanced diet is not as difficult as most people think. The MyPlate healthy eating guide contains five major food groups (Figure 5.5). The food groups are vegetables, fruits, grains, protein, and dairy.

Vegetables, fruits, whole grains, and low-fat milk (and by-products) provide the nutritional base for a healthy diet. If you increase the intake of these food groups, remember to decrease the intake of low-nutrient-dense foods to effectively balance caloric intake with energy needs.

In addition to providing nutrients crucial to health, vegetables and fruits are the sole source of **phytonutrients** ("phyto" comes from the Greek word for plant). The main function of phytonutrients in plants is to protect them from sunlight. In humans, phytonutrients seem to have a powerful ability to block the formation of cancerous tumors. Their actions are so diverse that, at almost every stage of cancer, phytonutrients have the ability to block, disrupt, slow down, or even reverse the process (also see Chapter 8).

These compounds are not found in pills. The message here is to eat a diet with ample fruits and vegetables. The daily recommended amount of vegetables and fruits has absolutely no substitute. People can't expect to eat a poor diet, pop a few pills, and derive the same benefits.

Whole grains are a major source of fiber as well as other nutrients. Whole grains contain the entire grain seed (the bran, germ, and endosperm). Examples include whole-wheat flour, whole cornmeal, oatmeal, cracked wheat (bulgur), and brown rice.

Refined grains have been milled, a process that removes the bran and germ. The process also removes fiber, iron, and many B vitamins. Refined grains include white flour, white bread, white rice, and degermed cornmeal. Refined grains are often enriched to add back B vitamins and iron. Fiber, however, is not added back.

The amount of flavorful whole grain products in supermarkets today has substantially increased. Ten to 20 years ago, most whole grain products were not very flavorful. Nowadays, excellent choices of whole grain breads, flour, rice, pasta, crackers, and pancake and waffle mixes are available. Many of these products, such as brown, multi-grain, and wild rices can now also be cooked in microwaves in less than two minutes. Available also are many products made with whole-wheat white flour (derived from a different strain of wheat) that is lighter in color and flavor, but still provides the nutrient benefits of whole grains.

Dairy (milk and milk products—select low-fat or non-fat) can decrease the risk of low bone mass (osteoporosis) throughout life. Besides providing calcium, milk is also a good source of potassium, vitamin D, and protein.

The recommendation for poultry, fish, or meat is to eat three ounces—and no more than six ounces—daily. All visible fat and skin should be trimmed off meats and poultry before cooking.

The difficult part for most people is retraining themselves to adopt a lifetime healthy nutrition plan. You can achieve a balanced diet if you (a) avoid excessive fats, oils, sweets, sodium (salt), and alcohol; (b) increase your fiber intake; and (c) eat the minimum number of servings recommended for each of the major groups in MyPlate.

Nutrient Analysis

To aid you in balancing your diet, Activity 5.1, page 152, provides a form for you to record your daily food intake. First, make as many copies as the number of days you wish to analyze. Whenever you eat something, record the food and the amount eaten. Doing this immediately after each meal enables you to keep track of your actual food intake more easily.

At the end of each day, consult the list of foods in Appendix E and record the number of calories for all foods consumed. Referring to Activity 5.1, record the amount and calories under the respective food groups. If you eat twice the amount of a standard serving, double the calories and the amount.

You can evaluate the diet by comparing your food intake recorded in Activity 5.1 against MyPlate guidelines (Figure 5.6). To start the activity, go to http://www.choosemyplate.gov/ and establish your personal Daily Food Plan based on your age, gender, height, weight, and physical activity level. To do so, select the 'Super-Tracker' tab and choose 'Create Your Profile.' Whenever you have something to eat, record the food and the amount eaten according to the MyPlate standard amounts (ounce, cup, or teaspoon—Figure 5.6). Do this immediately after each meal so you will be able to keep track of your actual food intake more easily. At the end of the day, evaluate your diet by checking whether you ate the minimum required amounts for each food group.

If you meet the minimum required servings at the end of each day and your caloric intake is in balance with the recommended amount, you are taking good steps to a healthier you.

In addition to meeting the daily amount guidelines, a complete nutrient analysis is recommended to rate your diet accurately. A nutrient analysis can pinpoint potential problem areas in your diet, such as too much fat, saturated fat, cholesterol, sodium, and the like. A complete nutrient analysis can be an educational experience because most people do not realize how detrimental and non-nutritious many common foods are.

You can also do the analysis by logging on to http://www.cengagebrain.com and using the information you have recorded already on the form provided in Activity 5.1. Up to seven days may be analyzed when using the software. Before running the software, fill out the information at the top of the form (age, weight, height, gender, and activity rating), and make sure the foods are recorded by the standard amounts given in the list of selected foods in Appendix E. The analysis also accommodates vegetarianism.

Vegetarianism

More than 7 million people in the United States are vegetarians and another 23 million people follow a vegetarian-inclined diet. **Vegetarians** rely primarily on foods from the grains and fruit and vegetable groups and avoid foods from animal sources including the milk, yogurt, and cheese and meat groups.

Following are five basic types of vegetarians:

1. Vegans: those who eat no animal products at all
2. Ovovegetarians: those who allow eggs in the diet
3. Lactovegetarians: those who allow foods from the milk group
4. Ovolactovegetarians: those who include egg and milk products in the diet
5. Semivegetarians: those who do not eat red meat but include fish (pescovegetarian) and poultry in addition to milk products and eggs in their diets

Well-planned vegetarian diets are healthful, are consistent with the Dietary Guidelines for Americans, and can meet the DRIs for nutrients. Vegetarians who do not

---

GLOSSARY

Phytonutrients Compounds found in vegetables and fruits with cancer-fighting properties.

Vegetarians Individuals whose diet is of vegetable or plant origin.

Figure 5.6 **MyPlate food guide.**

VEGETABLES	FRUITS	GRAINS	PROTEIN	DAIRY
Any vegetable or 100% vegetable juice counts as a member of the Vegetable Group. Vegetables may be raw or cooked; fresh, frozen, canned, or dried/dehydrated; and may be whole, cut-up, or mashed. Vegetables are organized into 5 subgroups, based on their nutrient content: Dark green vegetables, red and orange vegetables, beans and peas, starchy vegetables, and other vegetables.	Any fruit or 100% fruit juice counts as part of the Fruit Group. Fruits may be fresh, canned, frozen, or dried, and may be whole, cut-up, or pureed.	Any food made from wheat, rice, oats, cornmeal, barley, or another cereal grain is a grain product. Bread, pasta, oatmeal, breakfast cereals, tortillas, and grits are examples of grain products. Grains are divided into 2 subgroups: whole grains and refined grains.	All foods made from meat, poultry, seafood, beans and peas, eggs, processed soy products, nuts, and seeds are considered part of the Protein Foods Group (beans and peas are also part of the Vegetable Group). Select at least 8 ounces of cooked seafood per week. Meat and poultry choices should be lean or low-fat. Young children need less, depending on their age and calorie needs. The advice to consume seafood does not apply to vegetarians. Vegetarian options in the Protein Foods Group include beans and peas, processed soy products, and nuts and seeds.	All fluid milk products and many foods made from milk are considered part of this food group. Most Dairy Group choices should be fat-free or low-fat. Foods made from milk that retain their calcium content are part of the group. Foods made from milk that have little to no calcium, such as cream cheese, cream, and butter, are not. Calcium-fortified soymilk (soy beverage) is also part of the Dairy Group.
Make half your plate fruit and vegetables.	Make half your plate fruit and vegetables.	Make at least half your grains whole grains.	Choose fish and lean or low-fat meat and poultry.	Switch to fat-free or low-fat (1%) milk.

Recommended Daily Amounts

Women	Vegetables	Fruits	Grains	Protein	Dairy
19–30 years old	2½ cups	2 cups	6 oz. equivalents	5½ oz. equivalents	3 cups
31–50 years old	2½ cups	1½ cups	6 oz. equivalents	5 oz. equivalents	3 cups
51+ years old	2 cups	1½ cups	5 oz. equivalents	5 oz. equivalents	3 cups
Men					
19–30 years old	3 cups	2 cups	8 oz. equivalents	6½ oz. equivalents	3 cups
31–50 years old	3 cups	2 cups	7 oz. equivalents	6 oz. equivalents	3 cups
51+ years old	2½ cups	2 cups	6 oz. equivalents	6½ oz. equivalents	3 cups

SOURCE: USDA, 2011.

© Cengage Learning

select their food combinations properly, however, can develop nutritional deficiencies of protein, vitamins, minerals, and even calories. Even more attention should be paid when planning vegetarian diets for infants and children. Without careful planning, a strictly plant-based diet will prevent proper growth and development.

Protein deficiency is a concern in some vegetarian diets. Vegans in particular must be careful to eat foods that provide a balanced distribution of essential amino acids, such as grain products and legumes. Strict vegans also need a supplement of vitamin B_{12}. This vitamin is not found in plant foods; its only source is animal foods.

A deficiency of this vitamin can lead to anemia and nerve damage.

The key to a healthful vegetarian diet is to eat foods with complementary proteins. Most plant-based products lack one or more essential amino acids in adequate amounts. For example, both grains and legumes are good protein sources, but neither provides all the essential amino acids. Grains and cereals are low in the amino acid lysine, and legumes lack methionine. As noted under *Proteins* on pages 130–131, grains and legumes complement each other and legumes and nuts complement each other, but nuts and grains are not complementary proteins. For example, tortillas and beans, rice and beans, rice and soybeans, or wheat bread and peanuts, will complement each other. These complementary proteins may be consumed over the course of the day, but it is best if they are consumed during the same meal.

MyPlate can also be used as a guide for vegetarians. The key is food variety. Most vegetarians today consume dairy products and eggs. Meat can be replaced with legumes, nuts, seeds, eggs, and meat substitutes (tofu, tempeh, soy milk, and commercial meat replacers such as veggie burgers and soy hot dogs). For additional MyPlate healthy eating tips for vegetarians and ways to get enough of the previously mentioned nutrients, go to http://www.choosemyplate.gov/.

Consumption of nuts and soy foods, commonly used in vegetarian diets, has received considerable attention in recent years. Although nuts are 70 percent to 90 percent fat, most of it is unsaturated fat. And research indicates that people who eat nuts several times a week have a lower incidence of heart disease. Eating 2 to 3 ounces (about one-half cup) of almonds, walnuts, or macadamia nuts a day may decrease high blood cholesterol by about 10 percent.

Heart-health benefits are attributed to the unsaturated fats and also to other nutrients found in nuts, such as vitamin E and folic acid. Nuts are also packed with additional B vitamins, calcium, copper, potassium, magnesium, fiber, and phytonutrients. Many of these nutrients are cancer- and cardio-protective.

Nuts do have a drawback: They are high in calories. A handful of nuts provides as many calories as a piece of cake. Therefore, you should avoid using nuts as a snack. Nuts are recommended for use in place of high-protein foods such as meats, bacon, and eggs, or as part of a meal in fruit or vegetable salads, homemade bread, pancakes, casseroles, yogurt, and oatmeal. Peanut butter is also healthier than cheese or some cold cuts in sandwiches.

The increasing popularity of soy foods is attributed primarily to Asian research that points to less heart disease and fewer hormone-related cancers in people who regularly consume soy foods. The benefits of soy lie in its high protein content and plant chemicals, known as isoflavones, which act as antioxidants and may protect against estrogen-related cancers (breast, ovarian, and endometrial).

The compound genistein, one of many phytonutrients in soy, may reduce the risk for breast cancer, and soy consumption also may lower the risk for prostate cancer. Limited animal studies have suggested an actual increase in breast cancer risk. Human studies are still inconclusive but tend to favor a slight protective effect in premenopausal women.

Those who are interested in vegetarian diets should consult other resources. A thorough discussion of such diets cannot be covered adequately in a few paragraphs.

Nutrient Supplementation

Approximately half of all adults in the United States take daily nutrient **supplements**. The Academy of Nutrition and Dietetics, however, states that consuming a wide variety of nutrient-dense foods is more effective for good health and chronic disease prevention than taking vitamin and mineral supplements. Nutrient requirements for the body normally can be met by consuming as few as 1,500 calories per day, as long as the diet contains the recommended amounts of food from the different food groups.

Most supplements do not seem to provide additional benefits for healthy people who eat a balanced diet. They do not help people run faster, jump higher, relieve stress, improve their sexual prowess, cure a common cold, or boost energy levels. Some of the special cases are discussed below.

A supplement cannot replace the array of nutrients found in whole foods. These nutrients often work in synergy; that is, the interaction of the nutrients when combined is greater than the sum of their individual effects. The synergy between nutrients in one particular food item or between fruits, vegetables, and whole grains explains why people do not derive the same benefits when taking isolated supplements as compared to eating whole foods. Studies published show that there is no clear health benefit to most vitamin and mineral supplements.

People should not take **megadoses** of vitamins and minerals. For some nutrients, a dose of five times the

---

GLOSSARY

Supplements Tablets, pills, capsules, liquids, or powders that contain vitamins, minerals, amino acids, herbs, or fiber that are taken to increase the intake of these substances.

Megadoses For most vitamins, 10 times the RDA or more; for vitamins A and D, 5 and 2 times the RDA, respectively.

RDA taken over several months may create problems. For others, such a dose may not pose any threat to human health. With the possible exception of vitamin D (see discussion on page 141–143), vitamin and mineral intake should not exceed the ULs. For nutrients that do not have an established UL, a person should not take a dosage higher than three times the RDA.

Iron deficiency (determined through blood testing) is more common in women than men. Iron supplementation is frequently recommended for women who have a heavy menstrual flow. Pregnant and lactating women also may require supplements. The average pregnant woman who eats an adequate amount of a variety of foods should take a low dose of iron supplement daily. Women who are pregnant with more than one baby may need additional supplements. Adults older than 60, people with nutrient deficiencies, alcoholics, street-drug users, vegans, individuals on low-calorie diets (fewer than 1,500 calories per day), and people with disease-related disorders or who are taking medications that interfere with proper nutrient absorption can benefit from nutrient supplementation.

Antioxidants

Much research and discussion are taking place regarding the effectiveness of antioxidants in thwarting several chronic diseases. Although foods probably contain more than 4,000 antioxidants, the four more studied antioxidants are vitamins E and C, beta-carotene (a precursor to vitamin A), and the mineral selenium (see Table 5.6).

Table 5.6 Antioxidant Nutrients, Sources, and Functions

Nutrient	Good Sources	Antioxidant Effect
Vitamin C	Citrus fruit, kiwi fruit, cantaloupe, strawberries, broccoli, green or red peppers, cauliflower, and cabbage	Appears to inactivate oxygen free radicals.
Vitamin E	Vegetable oils, yellow and green leafy vegetables, margarine, wheat germ, oatmeal, almonds, whole-grain breads, and cereals	Protects lipids from oxidation.
Beta-carotene	Carrots, squash, pumpkin, sweet potatoes, broccoli, and green leafy vegetables	Soaks up oxygen free radicals.
Selenium	Seafood, Brazil nuts, meat, and whole grains	Helps prevent damage to cell structures.

© Cengage Learning

Oxygen is utilized during metabolism to change carbohydrates and fats into energy. During this process oxygen is transformed into stable forms of water and carbon dioxide. A small amount of oxygen, however, ends up in an unstable form, referred to as oxygen free radicals.

Free radicals attack and damage proteins and lipids, in particular cell membranes and DNA. This damage is thought to contribute to the development of conditions such as cardiovascular disease, cancer, emphysema, cataracts, Parkinson's disease, and premature aging. Environmental factors that seem to encourage the formation of free radicals include solar radiation, cigarette smoke, air pollution, radiation, some drugs, injury or infection, and chemicals (such as pesticides), among others.

The body's own antioxidant defense systems typically neutralize free radicals so they don't cause any damage. When free radicals are produced faster than the body can neutralize them, they can damage the cells, foster inflammation, and interfere with blood glucose control, blood vessel function, and normal cell growth. Research also indicates that the body's antioxidant defense system improves as fitness improves. That is, physically fit people have greater protection against free radicals.

Antioxidants work best in the prevention and progression of disease, but they cannot repair damage that has already occurred or cure people with disease. The benefits are obtained primarily from food sources themselves, and controversy surrounds the benefits of antioxidants taken in supplement form.

For years people believed that taking antioxidant supplements could further prevent free-radical damage, but a report published in the *Journal of the American Medical Association* indicated that antioxidant supplements actually increase the risk of death.[3] Vitamin E, beta-carotene, and vitamin A all have been shown to increase the risk of mortality between 4 and 16 percent. Vitamin C had no effect on mortality, while selenium decreased risk by 9 percent.

Antioxidant nutrients Antioxidants are found abundantly in food, especially in fruits and vegetables. Unfortunately, most Americans do not eat the minimum daily recommended amounts of fruits and vegetables. Plant foods enhance the body's defense system to help combat oxidative stress and its damaging effects.

The RDA for vitamin E is 15 mg or 22 international units (IU). Although no evidence indicates that vitamin E supplementation below the upper limit of 1,000 mg per day is harmful, little or no clinical research supports any health benefits. Vitamin E is found primarily in oil-rich seeds and vegetable oils. Foods high in vitamin E include almonds, hazelnuts, peanuts, canola oil, safflower oil, cottonseed oil, kale, sunflower seeds, shrimp, wheat germ, sweet potato, avocado, and tomato sauce. You should incorporate some of these foods regularly in your diet to obtain the RDA.

Studies have shown that vitamin C may offer benefits against heart disease, cancer, and cataracts. People who consume the recommended amounts of daily fruits and vegetables, nonetheless, need no supplementation because they obtain their daily vitamin C requirements through diet alone.

Vitamin C is water-soluble, and the body eliminates it in about 12 hours. For best results, consume vitamin C-rich foods twice a day. High intake of a vitamin C supplement, above 500 mg per day, is not recommended. The body absorbs very little vitamin C beyond the first 200 mg per serving or dose. Foods high in vitamin C include oranges and other citrus fruit, kiwi fruit, cantaloupe, guava, bell peppers, strawberries, broccoli, kale, cauliflower, and tomatoes.

Obtaining the daily recommended dose of beta-carotene (20,000 IU) from food sources rather than supplements is preferable. Clinical trials have found that beta-carotene supplements do not offer protection against heart disease or cancer or provide any other health benefits. Therefore, the recommendation is to "skip the pill and eat the carrot." One medium raw carrot contains about 20,000 IU of beta-carotene. Other foods high in beta-carotene include sweet potatoes, pumpkin, cantaloupe, squash, kale, broccoli, tomatoes, peaches, apricots, mangoes, papaya, turnip greens, and spinach.

Based on the current body of research, 100 to 200 mcg of selenium per day seems to provide the necessary amount of antioxidant for this nutrient. A person has no reason to take more than 200 mcg daily. In fact, the UL for selenium has been set at 400 mcg. Too much selenium can damage cells rather than protect them. One Brazil nut (unshelled) that you crack yourself provides about 100 mcg of selenium. Shelled nuts found in supermarkets average only about 20 mcg each. Other selenium-containing foods include seafood (salmon, tuna, oysters, and shrimp), whole grains, sunflower seeds, chicken, turkey, eggs, and mushrooms.

Multivitamins

Although much interest has been generated in the previously mentioned individual supplements, the American people still prefer multivitamins as supplements. At present, there is no solid scientific evidence that they decrease the risk of either cardiovascular disease or cancer. The most convincing data came in a study on more than 161,000 postmenopausal women taking multivitamin pills.[4] The results showed no benefits in terms of cardiovascular, cancer, or premature mortality risk reduction

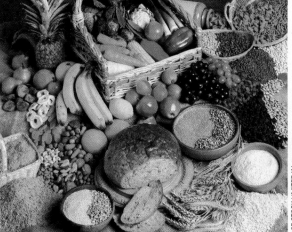

The best sources for disease-prevention nutrients (antioxidants and phytonutrients) are fruits, vegetables, and grains.

in women taking a multivitamin complex for an average of eight years compared to those who did not.

If you take multivitamins for general health reasons, you may help fill in certain deficiencies, but it doesn't grant you a license to eat carelessly. Multivitamins are not magic pills. They don't provide energy, fiber, or phytonutrients. People who eat a healthy diet, with ample amounts of fruits, vegetables, and grains, have a low risk of cardiovascular disease and cancer compared to people with deficient diets who take a multivitamin complex.

Vitamin D

Vitamin D is attracting a lot of attention because research suggests that the vitamin possesses anti-cancer properties, especially against breast, colon, and prostate cancers and possibly lung and digestive cancers. It also decreases inflammation, fighting cardiovascular disease, periodontal disease, and atherosclerosis. Furthermore, vitamin D strengthens the immune system, controls blood pressure, helps maintain muscle strength, decreases the risk for arthritis, prevents birth defects, and may help deter diabetes and fight depression; it is also necessary for the absorption of calcium, a nutrient critical for dental health and for building and maintaining bones to prevent osteoporosis.

The theory that vitamin D protects against cancer is based on studies showing that people who live farther north, who have less sun exposure during the winter months, have a higher incidence of cancer. Additionally, people diagnosed with breast, colon, or prostate cancer during the summer months, when vitamin D production by the body is at its highest, are 30 percent less likely to die from cancer, even 10 years following the initial diagnosis. Researchers believe that the vitamin D level at the time of cancer onset affects survival rates.

The current recommended daily intake ranges between 200 and 600 IU (5 and 15 mcg—based on your age), an amount believed to be too low for most individuals, especially during the winter months. The UL has been set at 2,000 IU (50 mcg). Experts believe that this figure needs revision because there are no data implicating toxic effects up to 10,000 IU (250 mcg) a day.[5]

During the winter months, most people in the United States living north of latitude 35 degrees (above the states of Georgia and Texas) and in Canada are not getting enough vitamin D. The body uses ultraviolet B rays (UVB) to generate vitamin D. UVB rays are shorter than ultraviolet A rays (UVA), so they penetrate the atmosphere at higher angles. During the winter season, the sun is too far south for the UVB rays to get through.

The Institute of Medicine of the National Academy of Sciences recommends a daily intake level of vitamin D of 600 IU for children and adults up to 70 years of age. Older adults should get 800 IU per day. This level is not as high as vitamin D researchers recommend. Preliminary evidence suggests that we should get between 1,000 and 2,000 IU (25 to 50 mcg) per day.[6]

The most accurate test to measure how much vitamin D is in your body is through the 25-hydroxyvitamin D test. Blood levels should remain between 50 and 80 ng/mL all year long. To increase your levels, the Vitamin D Council recommends that all adults supplement with 5,000 IU of vitamin D daily for 3 months and then take a 25-hydroxyvitamin D test.[7] You may then adjust your supplement dosage based on your test results, daily sun exposure, and the season of the year.

Depending on skin tone and sun intensity, about 15 minutes of unprotected sun exposure (without sunscreen) of the face, arms, hands, and lower legs during peak daylight hours (10:00 a.m. and 4:00 p.m.—when your shadow is shorter than your actual height) generates between 2,000 and 5,000 IU of vitamin D. Thus, it makes no sense that the UL is set at 2,000 when the human body manufactures more than that in just 15 minutes of unprotected sun exposure. The UL of 2,000 IU will most likely be revised in the next update of the DRIs.

Good sources of vitamin D in the diet include salmon, mackerel, tuna, and sardines. Fortified milk, yogurt, orange juice, margarines, and cereals are also good sources. To obtain up to 2,000 IU per day from food sources alone, however, is difficult (see Table 5.7). Thus, daily safe sun exposure and/or supplementation (especially during the winter months) is highly recommended.

The best source of vitamin D is sunshine. UVB rays lead to the production on the surface of the skin of inactive

Table 5.7 Good Sources of Vitamin D

Food	Amount	IU*
Multivitamins (most brands)	daily dose	400
Salmon	3.5 oz	360
Mackerel	3.5 oz	345
Sardines (oil/drained)	3.5 oz	250
Shrimp	3.5 oz	200
Orange juice (D-fortified)	8 oz	100
Milk (any type/D-fortified)	8 oz	100
Margarine (D-fortified)	1 tbsp	60
Yogurt (D-fortified)	6–8 oz	60
Cereal (D-fortified)	¾–1 c	40
Egg	1	20

*IU—International units

© Cengage Learning

oil-soluble vitamin D_3. The inactive form is then transformed by the liver, and subsequently the kidneys, into the active form of vitamin D. Sun-generated vitamin D is better than that obtained from foods or supplements.

Vitamin D_3 generated on the surface of the skin, however, doesn't immediately penetrate into the blood. It takes up to 48 hours to absorb most of the vitamin. Because soap is an oil-soluble compound, experts recommend avoiding its use following safe sun exposure, as it would wash off most of the vitamin. You may use soap for your armpits, groin area, and feet, but avoid doing so on the newly sun-exposed skin.

Excessive sun exposure can lead to skin damage and skin cancer. It is best to strive for daily "safe sun" exposure, that is, 10 to 20 minutes (based on skin tone and sun intensity) of unprotected sun exposure during peak hours of the day a few times a week. Generating too much vitamin D from the sun is impossible because the body generates only what it needs. If you have extremely sensitive skin, you may start with five minutes and progressively increase sun exposure by one minute per day. If your skin turns a slight pink following exposure, you have overdone it and need to cut back on the time that you are out in the sun.

People at the highest risk for low vitamin D levels are older adults, those with dark skin, and individuals who spend most of their time indoors and get little sun exposure. On average, a 65-year-old person synthesizes only about 25 percent as much vitamin D as a 20-year-old from similar sun exposure. People with darker skin may need 5 to 10 times the sun exposure of lighter-skinned people to generate the same amount of vitamin D. The skin's dark pigment reduces the ability of the body to synthesize vitamin D from the sun by up to 95 percent.

In the United States and Canada, most of the population does not make vitamin D from the sun during the winter months when UVB rays do not get through, most of the time is spent indoors, and extra clothing is worn to protect against the cold. During periods of limited sun exposure, you should consider a daily vitamin D_3 supplement of up to 2,000 IU per day. Some vitamins contain vitamin D_2, which is a less potent form of the vitamin.

Folate

A folate (a B vitamin) supplement has been recommended for all premenopausal women. In particular, folate supplements are encouraged prior to and during pregnancy. This includes women who might become pregnant. Studies have shown that high folate intake (400 mcg per day) during early pregnancy can prevent serious birth defects. Folate also seems to offer protection against colon and cervical cancers. In all the above instances, supplements should be taken under a physician's supervision.

Increasing evidence indicates that taking 400 mcg of folate along with vitamins B_6 and B_{12} prevents heart attacks by reducing homocysteine levels in the blood (see Chapter 8). High concentrations of homocysteine accelerate the process of plaque formation (atherosclerosis) in the arteries. Five servings of fruits and vegetables per day usually meet the needs for these nutrients. Currently, close to 9 in 10 adults in the United States do not meet the recommended 400 mcg of folate per day. Because of the critical role of folate in preventing heart disease, some experts also recommend a daily vitamin B complex that includes 400 mcg of folate.

In an updated recommendation released in 2014, the U.S. Preventive Services Task Force concludes that "the current evidence is insufficient to assess the balance of benefits and harms of the use of multivitamins for the prevention of cardiovascular disease or cancer." Many nutrition supplements are promoted to prevent disease, yet the scientific evidence does not support this notion.

A further word of caution when taking supplements: the quality and safety of dietary supplements in today's market is questionable. Supplements are exempt from the strict regulatory oversight applied to prescription drugs and often times they do not contain the ingredient(s) or nutrient(s) listed on the label. According to the *American College of Gastroenterology*, some of these supplements taken over a long term or in high doses can be toxic to the human body. There is no shortcut to healthy nutrition: you are better off by eating right and not relying on supplements for health and wellness.

5.6 *Benefits of Foods*

In its latest position statement on nutrient supplements, the American Dietetic Association stated, "The best nutrition-based strategy for promoting optimal health and reducing the risk of chronic disease is to wisely choose a wide variety of foods. Additional nutrients from supplements can help some people meet their nutrient needs as specified by science-based nutrition standards such as the Dietary Reference Intakes."[8]

Fruits and vegetables are the richest sources of antioxidants and phytonutrients. Researchers at the U.S. Department of Agriculture compared the antioxidant effects of vitamins C and E with those of various common fruits and vegetables. The results indicated that three-fourths cup of cooked kale (which contains only 11 IU of vitamin E and 76 mg of vitamin C) neutralized as many free radicals as approximately 800 IU of vitamin E or 600 mg of vitamin C supplements. Other excellent sources of antioxidants found by these researchers include blueberries, strawberries, spinach, Brussels sprouts, plums, broccoli, beets, oranges, and grapes.

Many people who eat unhealthy diets think they need supplementation to balance their diet. This is a fallacy about nutrition. The problem here is not necessarily a lack of vitamins and minerals, but a diet too high in calories, saturated fat, and sodium. Vitamin, mineral, and fiber supplements do not supply all of the nutrients and other beneficial substances present in food and needed for good health.

Wholesome foods contain vitamins, minerals, carbohydrates, fiber, proteins, fats, phytonutrients, and other substances not yet discovered. Researchers do not know if the protective effects are caused by the antioxidants alone, or in combination with other nutrients (such as phytonutrients), or by some other nutrients in food that have not been investigated yet. Many nutrients work in **synergy**, enhancing chemical processes in the body.

Supplementation will not offset poor eating habits. Pills are no substitute for common sense. If you think your diet is not balanced, you first need to conduct a nutrient analysis (see Activity 5.1 on page 152) to determine which nutrients you lack in sufficient amounts. Eat more of them, as well as foods that are high in antioxidants and phytonutrients. After you perform a nutrient

--- GLOSSARY ---

Synergy A reaction in which the result is greater than the sum of its two parts.

Behavior Modification Planning

Guidelines for a Healthy Diet

- Base your diet on a large variety of foods.
- Consume ample amounts of green, yellow, and orange fruits and vegetables.
- Eat foods high in complex carbohydrates, including at least three one-ounce servings of whole-grain foods per day.
- Obtain most of your vitamins and minerals from food sources.
- Eat foods rich in vitamin D.
- Maintain adequate daily calcium intake and consider a vitamin D_3 supplement if you do not get regular safe sun exposure.
- Daily protein consumption should be within the recommended amount for your activity level or age category.
- Limit daily fat, trans fat, and saturated fat intake.
- Limit unprocessed and processed red meat consumption to less than three ounces and one ounce per day

respectively. Consume cold-water fish (salmon, mackerel, herring, tuna, and rainbow trout) at least twice per week

- Limit sodium intake to 2,300 mg per day.
- Limit sugar intake and avoid sweets, soda pop, and foods with added sugars.
- If you drink alcohol, do so in moderation (one daily drink for women and two for men—women with a family or personal history of breast, esophagus, larynx, rectum, and liver cancers are encouraged to abstain from alcohol).

Try It

Carefully analyze the above guidelines and note the areas where you can improve your diet. Work on one guideline each week until you are able to adhere to all of the above guidelines.

© Cengage Learning

---

assessment, a **registered dietitian** can help you decide what supplement(s), if any, might be necessary.

The American Heart Association does not recommend antioxidant supplements until more definite research is available. If you take supplements in pill form, look for products that meet the USP (U.S. Pharmacopoeia) disintegration standards on the bottle. The USP symbol suggests that the supplement should completely dissolve in 45 minutes or less. Supplements that do not dissolve, of course, cannot get into the bloodstream.

! Critical Thinking

Do you take supplements? If so, for what purposes are you taking them—and do you think you could restructure your diet so you could do without them?

Probiotics

Yogurt is rated in the "super foods" category because, in addition to being a good source of calcium, riboflavin, and protein, it contains probiotics. These health-promoting microorganisms live in the intestines and help break down

foods and prevent disease-causing organisms from settling in. Probiotics have been found to offer protection against gastrointestinal infections, boost immune activity, and even help fight certain types of cancer.

Yogurts are cultured with *L. bulgaricus* and *S. thermophilus* probiotics. When selecting yogurt, preferably, look for products that also contain *L-acidophilus*, *Bifidus*, and the prebiotic (substances on which probiotics feed) inulin. The latter, a soluble fiber, appears to enhance calcium absorption. Avoid yogurt with added fruit jam, sugar, and candy.

A fast growing trend in nutrition is the relationship between a healthy diet and *gut microbes*. These microorganisms have a remarkable impact on the immune system and disease prevention. They feed primarily on complex/fiber-rich carbohydrates and introduce additional live bacteria to the gut. Thus, a diet high in whole plant foods, including whole grains, legumes, fruit, vegetables, seeds, nuts, and fermented foods, results in increased microbial diversity and positive health outcomes.

Fish

Potential contaminants in fish, in particular mercury, have created concerns among some people. Mercury, a naturally occurring trace mineral, can be released into the air from industrial pollution. As mercury falls into streams and oceans, it accumulates in the aquatic food chain. Larger fish accumulate larger amounts of mercury because they eat medium and small fish. Of particular concern are shark, swordfish, king mackerel, pike, bass, and tilefish that have higher levels.

The American Heart Association recommends consuming fish twice a week. The risk of adverse effects from eating fish is extremely low and primarily theoretical in nature.[9] For most people, eating two servings (up to 6 ounces) of fish per week poses no health threat. Pregnant and nursing women and young children, however, should avoid mercury in fish. Farm-raised salmon also have slightly higher levels of polychlorinated biphenyls (PCBs), which the U.S. Environmental Protection Agency lists as a "probable human carcinogen."

The best recommendation is to balance the risks against the benefits. If you are concerned, consume no more than 12 ounces per week of a variety of fish and shellfish that are lower in mercury, including canned light tuna, wild salmon, shrimp, pollock, catfish, and scallops. A review of more than 200 studies on the effects of fish consumption on health concluded that the benefits exceed the potential risks, and seafood appears to be the single most important food a person can consume for good health.[10]

Advanced Glycation End Products

A new area of research in nutrition has to do with **advanced glycation end products (AGEs)**, compounds that have been implicated in aging, adverse effects, and chronic diseases by increasing oxidation and inflammation. AGEs are thought to contribute to the development of atherosclerosis, heart disease, diabetes and diabetes-related complications, kidney disease, osteoarthritis, rheumatoid arthritis, and Alzheimer's disease, among others. These compounds are produced when glucose combines with proteins, lipids, and other ingredients in foods.

AGEs are found primarily in foods cooked in dry heat, at high temperatures, in processed foods, and in foods high in fat content. Broiling, grilling, and frying create the highest levels of AGEs, whereas braising, steaming, stewing, roasting, boiling, and poaching decrease the levels. French-fried potatoes have about eight times the amount of AGEs compared with a baked potato. Fast-food restaurants take advantage of the flavor-enhancing effects of AGEs by adding these toxic compounds to their foods to increase the foods' appeal to the consumer. The take-home message to the consumer here is once

again moderation. You do not have to completely eliminate grilling, frying, and fast foods, but common sense is vital to maintain good health.

The following guidelines can help you decrease AGEs in your diet:

1. Limit cooking meats at high temperatures.
2. Avoid high-fat foods (whole milk products and meats).
3. Increase intake of fruits, vegetables, grains, fish, and low-fat milk products.
4. Choose unprocessed over processed foods by cooking fresh foods from scratch.
5. Eat at home most of the time and avoid prepackaged and fast foods as much as possible.
6. Avoid browning because the process of browning sugars and proteins on food surfaces increases the formation of AGEs.

5.7 *Eating Disorders*

Eating disorders are medical illnesses that involve critical disturbances in eating behaviors thought to stem from some combination of environmental pressures. These disorders are characterized by an intense fear of becoming fat, which does not disappear even after the individual has lost extreme amounts of weight. The two most common types of eating disorders are **anorexia nervosa** and **bulimia nervosa**, although **binge eating**, also known as compulsive overeating, is recognized as an eating disorder as well.

Most people who have eating disorders are afflicted by significant family and social problems. They may lack

---

GLOSSARY

Registered dietitian (RD) A person with a college degree in dietetics who meets all certification and continuing education requirements of the American Dietetic Association or Dietitians of Canada.

Advanced glycation end products (AGEs) Derivatives of glucose-protein and glucose-lipid interactions that are linked to aging and chronic diseases.

Anorexia nervosa An eating disorder characterized by self-imposed starvation to lose weight and then maintain very low body weight.

Bulimia nervosa An eating disorder characterized by a pattern of binge eating and purging.

Binge-eating disorder An eating disorder characterized by uncontrollable episodes of eating excessive amounts of food within a relatively short time.

fulfillment in many areas of their lives. The eating disorder then becomes the coping mechanism to avoid dealing with these problems. Taking control over their own body weight helps them feel that they are restoring some sense of control over their lives.

Anorexia nervosa and bulimia nervosa are common in industrialized nations where society encourages low-calorie diets and thinness. Although frequently seen in young women, the majority seeking treatment are between the ages of 25 and 50. Surveys, nonetheless, indicate that as many as 40 percent of college-age women are struggling with an eating disorder.

Eating disorders are not limited to women. Every 1 in 10 cases exists in men. But because the role of men in society and their body image are viewed differently, these cases often go unreported.

Individuals who have clinical depression and obsessive-compulsive behavior are more susceptible. About half of all people with eating disorders have some sort of chemical dependency (alcohol and drugs), and a majority of them come from families with alcohol and drug-related problems. Of reported cases of eating disorders, a large number are individuals who are, or have been, victims of sexual molestation.

Eating disorders develop in stages. Typically, individuals who are already dealing with significant issues in life start a diet. At first they feel in control and are happy about the weight loss even if they are not overweight. Encouraged by the prospect of weight loss and the control they can exert over their own weight, individuals take dieting to an extreme and often combine it with exhaustive exercise and the overuse of laxatives and diuretics.

Although a genetic predisposition may contribute, most cases are environmentally related. The syndrome typically emerges following emotional issues or a stressful life event and the uncertainty about the ability to cope efficiently. Life experiences that can trigger the syndrome might be gaining weight, starting the menstrual period, beginning college, losing a boyfriend, having poor self-esteem, being socially rejected, starting a professional career, or becoming a wife or a mother.

The eating disorder now takes on a life of its own and becomes the primary focus of attention for the individuals afflicted with it. Their self-worth revolves around what the scale reads every day, their relationship with food, and their perception of how they look each day.

Anorexia Nervosa

An estimated 1 percent of the population in the United States is anorexic. Anorexic individuals seem to fear weight gain more than death from starvation. Furthermore, they have a distorted image of their body and think of themselves as being fat, even when they are emaciated.

Anorexics commonly develop obsessive and compulsive behaviors and emphatically deny their condition. They are preoccupied with food, meal planning, and grocery shopping, and they have unusual eating habits. As they lose weight and their health begins to deteriorate, anorexics feel weak and tired. They might realize they have a problem, but they will not stop the starvation and refuse to consider the behavior abnormal.

Once they have lost a lot of weight and malnutrition sets in, physical changes become more visible. Typical changes are **amenorrhea** (stopping menstruation), digestive problems, extreme sensitivity to cold, hair and skin problems, fluid and electrolyte abnormalities (which may lead to an irregular heartbeat and sudden stopping of the heart), injuries to nerves and tendons, abnormalities of immune function, anemia, growth of fine body hair, mental confusion, inability to concentrate, lethargy, depression, dry skin, lower skin and body temperature, and osteoporosis.

Following are diagnostic criteria for anorexia nervosa:[11]

- Refusal to maintain body weight over a minimal normal weight for age and height (weight loss leading to maintenance of body weight less than 85 percent of that expected or failure to make expected weight gain during periods of growth, leading to body weight less than 85 percent of that expected)
- Intense fear of gaining weight or becoming fat, even though underweight
- Disturbance in the way in which one's body weight, size, or shape is perceived; undue influences of body weight or shape on self-evaluation; or denial of the seriousness of the current low body weight
- In postmenarcheal females, amenorrhea (absence of at least three consecutive menstrual cycles; a woman is considered to have amenorrhea if her periods occur only following estrogen therapy)

Many of the changes induced by anorexia nervosa can be reversed. Individuals with this condition can get better with professional therapy, turn to bulimia nervosa, or they may die from the disorder. Twenty percent of anorexics die as a result of their condition. Anorexia nervosa has the highest mortality rate of all psychosomatic illnesses today. The disorder, however, is 100 percent curable, but treatment almost always requires professional help, and the sooner it is started, the better the chances for reversibility and cure.

Therapy consists of a combination of medical and psychological techniques to restore proper nutrition, prevent medical complications, and modify the environment or events that triggered the syndrome.

Seldom can anorexics overcome the problem by themselves. They strongly deny their condition. They are able to hide it and deceive friends and relatives. Based on their behavior, many of them meet all of the characteristics of anorexia nervosa, but it goes undetected because both thinness and dieting are socially acceptable. Only a well-trained clinician is able to diagnose anorexia nervosa.

Bulimia Nervosa

Bulimia nervosa is more prevalent than anorexia nervosa. As many as one in every five women on college campuses may be bulimic, according to some estimates. Bulimia nervosa also is more prevalent than anorexia nervosa in males, although bulimia is still much more prevalent in females.

Bulimics usually are healthy-looking people, well-educated, and near recommended body weight. They seem to enjoy food and often socialize around it. In actuality, they are emotionally insecure, rely on others, and lack self-confidence and self-esteem. Recommended weight and food are important to them.

The binge-purge cycle usually occurs in stages. As a result of stressful life events or the simple compulsion to eat, bulimics engage periodically in binge eating that may last an hour or longer.

With some apprehension, bulimics anticipate and plan the cycle. Next they feel an urgency to begin, followed by large and uncontrollable food consumption, during which they may eat several thousand calories (up to 10,000 calories in extreme cases). After a short period of relief and satisfaction, feelings of deep guilt, shame, and intense fear of gaining weight ensue. Purging seems to be an easy answer, as the binging cycle can continue without fear of gaining weight.

Following are the diagnostic criteria for bulimia nervosa:[12]

- Recurrent episodes of binge eating. An episode of binge eating is characterized by both of the following:
  - Eating in a discrete period of time (for example, within any two-hour period) an amount of food that is definitely more than most people would eat during a similar period and under similar circumstances.
  - A sense of lack of control over eating during the episode (a feeling that one cannot stop eating or control what or how much one is eating).

- Recurring inappropriate compensatory behaviors to prevent weight gain, such as self-induced vomiting; misuse of laxatives, diuretics, enemas, or other medications; fasting; or excessive exercise.
- The binge eating and inappropriate compensatory behaviors both occur, on average, at least twice a week for three months.
- Self-evaluation is unduly influenced by body shape and weight.

The most typical form of purging is self-induced vomiting. Bulimics, too, frequently ingest strong laxatives and emetics. Near-fasting diets and strenuous bouts of exercise are common. Medical problems associated with bulimia nervosa include cardiac arrhythmias, amenorrhea, kidney and bladder damage, ulcers, colitis, tearing of the esophagus or stomach, tooth erosion, gum damage, and general muscular weakness.

Unlike anorexics, bulimics realize their behavior is abnormal and feel great shame about it. Fearing social rejection, they pursue the binge-purge cycle in secrecy and at unusual hours of the day.

Bulimia nervosa can be treated successfully when the person realizes that this destructive behavior is not the solution to life's problems. A change in attitude can prevent permanent damage or death.

Binge-Eating Disorder

Binge-eating disorder is probably the most common of the three eating disorders. About 2 percent of American adults are afflicted with binge-eating disorder in a 6-month period. Although most people think they overeat from time to time, eating more than one should now and then does not mean the individual has a binge-eating disorder. The disorder is slightly more common in women than in men; three women for every two men have the disorder.

Binge-eating disorder is characterized by uncontrollable episodes of eating excessive amounts of food within a relatively short time. The causes of binge-eating disorder are unknown, although depression, anger, sadness, boredom, and worry can trigger an episode. Unlike bulimics, binge eaters do not purge; thus, most people with

---

GLOSSARY

Amenorrhea Absence (primary amenorrhea) or cessation (secondary amenorrhea) of normal menstrual function.

this disorder are either overweight or obese. Following are typical symptoms of binge-eating disorder:

- Eating what most people think is an unusually large amount of food
- Eating until uncomfortably full
- Eating out of control
- Eating much faster than usual during binge episodes
- Eating alone because of embarrassment over how much food is being consumed
- Feeling disgusted, depressed, or guilty after overeating

Emotional Eating

Emotional eating involves the consumption of large quantities of food, mostly "comfort" and junk food, to suppress negative emotions. Such emotions include stress, anxiety, uncertainty, guilt, anger, pain, depression, loneliness, sadness, boredom, and foods that have a nostalgic or sentimental appeal. In such circumstances, people eat for comfort when they are at their weakest point emotionally. Comfort foods often include calorie-dense, sweet, salty, and fatty foods. Excessive emotional eating hinders proper weight management

Eating Disorder Not Otherwise Specified (EDNOS)

The American Psychiatric Association introduced **eating disorder not otherwise specified (EDNOS)**, a diagnostic category for individuals who don't fall into the previously discussed categories.

Orthoxia

An eating disorder characterized by a fixation with healthy or righteous eating. These individuals attempt to eat organic foods only or avoid anything that isn't "pure in quality," often eliminating entire food groups. They are primarily motivated by fear of bad health and not necessarily thinness.

Pregorexia

This disorder relates to women who fear gaining the recommended 25 to 35 pounds of weight during pregnancy and can lead to anemia, hypertension, depression, a miscarriage, or a malnourished baby born with birth defects.

Drunkorexia

Individuals who decrease caloric intake or skip meals to save those calories for alcohol and binge drinking. One

survey found that close to 30 percent of female college students engage in drunkorexic behavior.

Anorexia Athletica

People who engage daily in compulsive lengthy and rigorous exercise routines to reach and maintain low body weight.

Treatment

Treatment for eating disorders is available on most school campuses through the school's counseling center or the health center. Local hospitals also offer treatment for these conditions. Many communities have support groups, frequently led by professional personnel and often free of charge. All information and the identity of the individual are kept confidential so the person need not fear embarrassment or repercussion when seeking professional help.

5.8 *Dietary Guidelines*

National health organizations often issue dietary guidelines for the general population. These guidelines are intended for healthy people who do not require additional nutrient needs. Due to the dramatic increase in obesity, eating, and physical activity patterns that are focused on consuming fewer calories, making informed food choices and being physically active are emphasized to help people attain and maintain a healthy weight, reduce their risk of chronic disease, and promote overall health. Guidelines provide necessary information to make thoughtful choices of healthier foods in the right portions and to complement those choices with physical activity. Key concepts emphasized by health organization guidelines include:

- Balance calories with physical activity to sustain a healthy weight.
- Focus on consuming nutrient-dense foods and beverages, including a greater consumption of fruits, vegetables, whole grains, fat-free and low-fat dairy products, and seafood; and decrease the consumption of foods with sodium (salt), saturated fats, trans fats, added sugars, and refined grains. Avoid soda pop, sugar-filled drinks, and juices with added sugar. Drink water instead.

Balancing Calories to Manage Weight

1. Prevent and/or reduce overweight and obesity through improved eating and physical activity behaviors.

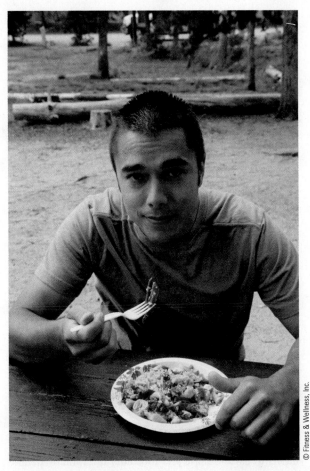

A healthy diet is a critical component of a healthy lifestyle to prevent disease, manage weight, and increase longevity.

2. Control total calorie intake to manage body weight. For people who are overweight or obese, this means consuming fewer calories from foods and beverages.

3. Increase physical activity and reduce time spent sitting and in sedentary behaviors.

4. Maintain appropriate calorie balance during each stage of life—childhood, adolescence, adulthood, pregnancy and breastfeeding, and older age.

5. Reduce daily sodium intake to less than 2,300 milligrams (mg) and further reduce intake to 1,500 mg among persons who are 51 and older and those of any age who are African American or have hypertension, diabetes, or chronic kidney disease. The 1,500-mg recommendation applies to about half of the U.S. population, including children and the majority of adults.

6. Consume less than 6 percent of calories from saturated fatty acids by replacing them with monounsaturated and polyunsaturated fatty acids.

7. Keep trans fatty acid consumption to an absolute minimum.

8. Reduce the intake of calories from solid fats and added sugars.

9. Limit the consumption of unprocessed red meat to less than half a serving (1.5 oz.) per day or two to three servings (3 oz.) per week and severely limit processed red meat intake.

10. Limit the consumption of foods that contain refined grains, especially refined grain foods that contain solid fats, added sugars, and sodium.

11. If alcohol is consumed, it should be consumed in moderation—up to one drink per day for women and two drinks per day for men—and only by adults of legal drinking age.

12. Limit the consumption of highly processed foods. Eat whole foods as close to their natural form as possible.

Foods and Nutrients to Increase

1. Increase vegetable and fruit intake.

2. Eat a variety of vegetables, especially dark-green, red, and orange vegetables, and beans and peas.

3. Consume most grains as whole grains.

4. Increase intake of fat-free or low-fat milk and milk products, such as milk, yogurt, cheese, or fortified soy beverages.

5. Choose a variety of protein foods, including seafood, lean meat and poultry, eggs, beans and peas, soy products, and unsalted nuts and seeds.

6. Increase the amount and variety of seafood consumed by choosing seafood in place of some meat and poultry.

7. Replace protein foods that are higher in solid fats with choices that are lower in solid fats and calories and/or are sources of oils.

8. Use oils to replace solid fats where possible.

9. Choose foods that provide more potassium, dietary fiber, calcium, and vitamin D, which are nutrients of concern in American diets. These foods include vegetables, fruits, whole grains, and low-fat milk and milk products.

GLOSSARY

Emotional eating The consumption of large quantities of food to suppress negative emotions.

Eating Disorder Not Otherwise Specified

(EDNOS) A medical condition used to diagnose individuals who don't fall into the most commonly known eating disorder categories but who have troubled relationships with food or distorted body images.

Recommendations for Specific Population Groups

Women Capable of Becoming Pregnant

1. Choose foods that supply hemeiron, which is more readily absorbed by the body; additional iron sources; and enhancers of iron absorption such as vitamin C-rich foods.
2. Consume 400 micrograms (mcg) per day of synthetic folic acid (from fortified foods and/or supplements) in addition to food forms of folate from a varied diet.

Pregnant or Breastfeeding Women

1. Consume 8 to 12 ounces of seafood per week from a variety of seafood types.
2. Due to their high methyl mercury content, limit white (albacore) tuna to 6 ounces per week and do not eat the following four types of fish: tilefish, shark, swordfish, and king mackerel.
3. If pregnant, take an iron supplement, as recommended by an obstetrician or other health care provider.

For Individuals 50 Years and Older

1. Consume foods fortified with vitamin B_{12}, such as fortified cereals, or dietary supplements.

5.9 *A Lifetime Commitment to Wellness*

Proper nutrition, a sound exercise program, and quitting smoking (for those who smoke) are the three factors that do the most for health, longevity, and quality of life. Achieving and maintaining a balanced diet is not as difficult as most people would think. The difficult part for most people is retraining themselves to follow a lifetime healthy nutrition plan. No single food can provide all the necessary nutrients and other beneficial substances in the amounts the body needs.

A well-balanced diet contains a variety of foods from all food groups, including wise selection of foods from animal sources. Food items vary, and each item provides different combinations of nutrients and other substances needed for good health. A landmark study involving more than 120,000 people, published in the American

Journal of Clinical Nutrition, reported an increase in life expectancy of 15.1 and 8.4 years in women and men respectively who followed a combined healthy lifestyle approach: (1) regular physical activity, (2) eating a Mediterranean diet, (3) not smoking, and (4) maintaining healthy body weight.[13]

A subsequent study published in 2013, the first randomized **clinical study** on the diet, was terminated early because individuals on a Mediterranean diet had an almost 30 percent decreased risk of heart disease.[14] The Mediterranean diet has also been linked to lower risk for metabolic syndrome and stroke, improved brain health and cognitive function, and lower risk for Alzheimer's disease. Although most people in the United States focus on the olive oil component of the diet, olive oil is used mainly as a means to increase consumption of vegetables because vegetables sautéed in oil taste better than steamed vegetables.

> **! Critical Thinking**
>
> What factors in your life and the environment have contributed to your current dietary habits? • Do you need to make changes? • What may prevent you from doing so?

Despite ample scientific evidence linking poor dietary habits to early disease and mortality rates, many people are not willing to change their eating patterns. Even when faced with obesity, elevated blood lipids, hypertension, and other nutrition-related conditions, many people do not change. They remain in the precontemplation stage of change (see the discussion of behavior modification in Chapter 1).

The motivating factor to change one's eating habits seems to be a major health breakdown, such as a heart attack, a stroke, or cancer. An ounce of prevention is worth a pound of cure. The sooner you implement the dietary guidelines presented in this chapter, the better will be your chances of preventing chronic diseases and reaching a higher state of wellness.

GLOSSARY

Clinical study A research study in which the investigator intervenes (makes certain changes or uses certain interventions or programs) to prevent or treat a disease.

Assess Your Behavior

1. Are whole grains, fruits, and vegetables the staple of your diet?

2. Are you meeting your personal MyPlate recommendations for daily fruits, vegetables, grains, meat (or substitutes) and legumes, and milk?

3. Are there dietary changes that you need to implement to meet energy, nutrition, and disease risk-reduction guidelines and to improve health and wellness? If so, list these changes and indicate what you will do to make it happen.

Assess Your Knowledge

1. The science of nutrition studies the relationship of
   a. vitamins and minerals to health.
   b. foods to optimal health and performance.
   c. carbohydrates, fats, and proteins to the development and maintenance of good health.
   d. the macronutrients and micronutrients to physical performance.
   e. kilocalories to calories in food items.

2. Faulty nutrition often plays a crucial role in the development and progression of which disease?
   a. cardiovascular disease
   b. cancer
   c. osteoporosis
   d. diabetes
   e. All are correct choices.

3. According to MyPlate, daily vegetable consumption is measured in
   a. servings.
   b. ounces.
   c. cups.
   d. calories.
   e. All of the above are correct.

4. The daily recommended amount of fiber intake for adults 50 years and younger is
   a. 10 grams per day for women and 12 grams for men.
   b. 21 grams per day for women and 30 grams for men.
   c. 28 grams per day for women and 35 grams for men.
   d. 25 grams per day for women and 38 grams for men.
   e. 45 grams per day for women and 50 grams for men.

5. Unhealthy fats include
   a. unsaturated fatty acids.
   b. monounsaturated fats.
   c. polyunsaturated fatty acids.
   d. saturated fats.
   e. alpha-linolenic acid.

6. The daily recommended carbohydrate intake is
   a. 45 to 65 percent of the total calories.
   b. 10 to 35 percent of the total calories.
   c. 20 to 35 percent of the total calories.
   d. 60 to 75 percent of the total calories.
   e. 35 to 50 percent of the total calories.

7. The amount of a nutrient that is estimated to meet the nutrient requirement of half the healthy people in specific age and gender groups is known as the
   a. Estimated Average Requirement.
   b. Recommended Dietary Allowance.
   c. Daily Value.
   d. Adequate Intake.
   e. Dietary Reference Intake.

8. The percent fat intake for an individual who on a given day consumes 2,385 calories with 106 grams of fat is
   a. 44 percent of total calories.
   b. 17.7 percent of total calories.
   c. 40 percent of total calories.
   d. 31 percent of total calories.
   e. 22.5 percent of total calories.

9. Treatment of anorexia nervosa
   a. almost always requires professional help.
   b. is often accomplished in the home.
   c. is most successful when friends take the initiative to help.
   d. requires that the individual be placed in the environment where the disorder started.
   e. is best done under the supervision of a physician.

10. Which of the following is not a goal of dietary guidelines for healthy people?
    a. Increase daily intake of fruits and vegetables, whole grains, and nonfat or low-fat milk and milk products.
    b. Reduce the intake of calories from solid fats and added sugars.
    c. Increase vegetable and fruit intake.
    d. Increase the amount and variety of seafood consumed by choosing seafood in place of some meat and poultry.
    e. All are correct choices.

Correct answers can be found on page 307.

Activity 5.1 Nutrient Analysis

Name _____ Date _____

Course _____ Section _____

Age _____ Weight _____ Height _____ Gender M F   (Pregnant–P, Nursing–N)

Activity Rating
(check one):

○ Sedentary
○ Lightly active
○ Moderately active
○ Very active
○ Extremely active

Food Groups
Daily Goals
(see Figure 5.6)

No.	Food*	Calories	Fat (gm)	Grains (oz.)	Vegetables (cups)	Fruits (cups)	Dairy (cups)	Protein Foods (oz.)	Oils (tsp.)
1									
2									
3									
4									
5									
6									
7									
8									
9									
10									
11									
12									
13									
14									
15									
16									
17									
18									
19									
20									
21									
22									
23									
24									
25									
26									
27									
28									
29									
30									
Totals									
Recommended Amount: Obtain online at www.choosemyplate.gov based on age, gender, weight, height, and activity level (see page 137 for a complete explanation)		**							
Deficiencies/Excesses									

*See "List of Nutritive Value of Selected Foods" in Appendix E.

**Multiply the recommended amount of calories by .30 (30%) and divide by 9 to obtain the daily recommended amount of grams of fat.

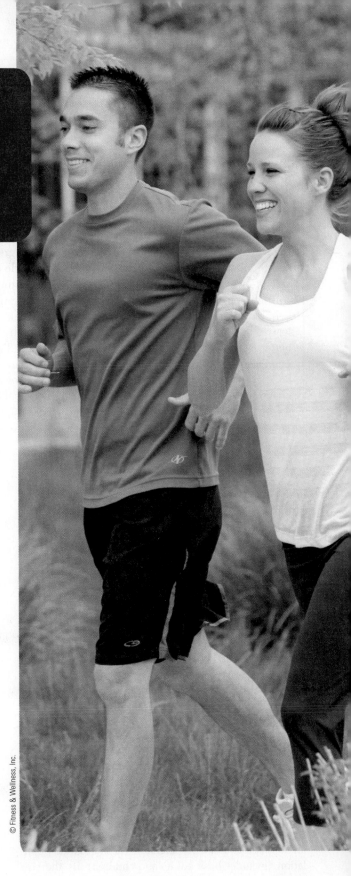

6

Weight Management

Physical activity is the cornerstone of a sound weight management program. If you are unwilling to increase daily physical activity, you might as well not even attempt to lose weight because most likely you won't be able to keep it off.

Objectives

> Recognize myths and fallacies regarding weight management.

> Understand the physiology of weight control.

> Become familiar with the effects of diet and exercise on resting metabolic rate.

> Recognize the role of a lifetime exercise program in a successful weight management program.

> Learn to write and implement weight reduction and weight maintenance programs.

> Identify behavior modification techniques that help a person adhere to a lifetime weight maintenance program.

© Fitness & Wellness, Inc.

REAL LIFE STORY | Megan's Weight Struggles

Similar to most students, I gained several pounds of weight my first year in college. I dieted several times but ended up regaining the weight, and then some more! I put off taking my fitness class because I wanted to lose the weight first and get in shape before I took the class. My roommate, however, took the class the spring semester, and I couldn't help but notice how she had lost weight and looked so much better. After finding out more details about the course, I made an appointment with the course instructor and decided to enroll during the fall semester. That fall, we assessed my body composition and determined that I had 9 pounds to lose to get to 138 pounds and be at 23 percent body fat. With the aid of the instructor, we agreed on a 1,500-calorie diet, along with 45 minutes of walking/jogging 5 times per week and 45 minutes of strength training twice per week. I also had to report every Monday morning to my instructor for a weigh-in and to turn in my weekly food and activity logs. I signed a contract

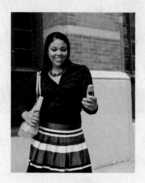

with the instructor that I would adhere to the program as prescribed. I also talked to my roommates so they would understand what my goal was for the next 15 weeks. At the end of the semester, I had lost 10 pounds but actually came in at 22.7 percent body fat at 140 pounds. In essence, because of all my physical activity I had gained about 3 pounds of lean tissue along with 12 pounds of actual fat loss.

Aidon/Jupiter Images

A good physical fitness program will include achieving and maintaining recommended body weight as a major objective. Two terms commonly used in reference to the condition of weighing more than recommended are **overweight** and **obesity**. Obesity levels are established at a point at which excess body fat can lead to significant health problems.

Obesity is a health hazard of epidemic proportions in most developed countries around the world. According to the World Health Organization, an estimated 35 percent of the adult population in industrialized nations is obese. Obesity has been established at a body mass index (BMI) of 30 or higher.

The number of people who are overweight and obese in the United States has increased dramatically in the past three decades, a direct result of physical inactivity and poor dietary habits. About 69 percent of U.S. adults age 20 and older are overweight (have a BMI greater than 25), and 35 percent are obese. More than 120 million people are overweight, and 30 million are obese. The prevalence of obesity is even higher in ethnic groups, especially African Americans and Hispanic Americans.

As illustrated in Figure 6.1, the obesity epidemic continues to escalate. Before 1990, not a single state reported an obesity rate above 15 percent of the state's total population (includes both adults and children). By the year 2013, not a single state had an obesity rate less than 20 percent, more than half had an obesity rate equal to or

greater than 25 percent, including 2 states with a rate above 35 percent.

As of the end of 2012, the average man weighed 196 pounds and the average woman 156 pounds. Unfortunately, the human mind has a tremendous capability to adapt and accept change, even if it is detrimental to one's health. And so it is with body weight. According to a Gallup poll conducted in November 2012, men indicated that their "ideal" body weight was 185 pounds, the highest ever, and 14 pounds greater than the 1990 weight as determined by this same poll. Women indicated their "ideal" weight to be 11 pounds heavier than in 1990, at 140 pounds.

As the nation continues to evolve into a more mechanized and automated society (relying on escalators, elevators, remote controls, computers, electronic mail, cell phones, and automatic-sensor doors), the amount of required daily physical activity continues to decrease. We are being lulled into a high-risk sedentary lifestyle.

More than a third of the population is on a diet at any given moment. People spend about $40 billion yearly attempting to lose weight. More than $10 billion goes to memberships in weight reduction centers and another $30 billion to diet food sales. The total cost attributable to obesity-related disease is approximately $117 billion per year.

Excessive body weight combined with physical inactivity is the second leading cause of preventable death in

Figure 6.1 Incidence of obesity in the United States based on BMI ≥30 or 30 pounds overweight: 1985, 2000, and 2013.

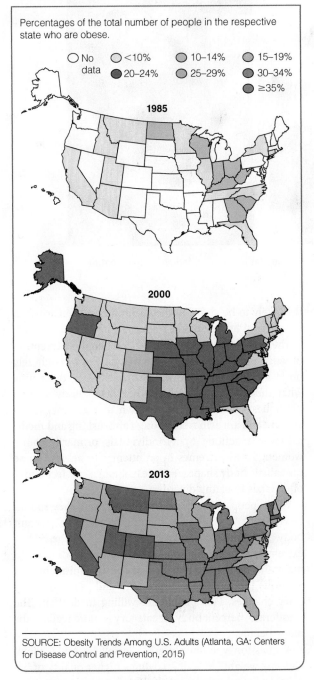

SOURCE: Obesity Trends Among U.S. Adults (Atlanta, GA: Centers for Disease Control and Prevention, 2015)

disease. Estimates by the American Institute for Cancer Research (AICR) also indicate that 122,000 yearly cancer deaths could be prevented if Americans were not overweight or obese. Obesity in itself has been linked to nine different cancers: colorectal, esophageal, post-menopausal breast, endometrial, kidney, pancreatic, ovarian, gallbladder and advanced prostate cancer. Excessive body weight also is implicated in psychological maladjustment and a higher accidental death rate. Extremely obese people have a lower mental health–related quality of life.

Overweight and obese are not the same thing. Many overweight people (people who weigh about 10 to 20 pounds over the recommended weight) are not obese. Although a few pounds of excess weight may not be harmful to most people, this is not always the case. People with excessive body fat who have type 2 diabetes and other cardiovascular risk factors (elevated blood lipids, high blood pressure, physical inactivity, and poor eating habits) benefit from losing weight. People who have a few extra pounds of weight but are otherwise healthy and physically active, exercise regularly, and eat a healthy diet may not be at higher risk for disease and early death. Such is not the case, however, with obese individuals.

Research indicates that individuals who are 30 or more pounds overweight during middle age (30 to 49 years of age) lose about 7 years of life; whereas being 10 to 30 pounds overweight decreases the lifespan by about 3 years.[4] These decreases are similar to those seen with tobacco use. Severe obesity (BMI greater than 45) at a young age, nonetheless, may cut up to 20 years off one's life.[5]

Although the loss of years of life is significant, the decreased life expectancy doesn't even begin to address the loss in quality of life, considerably compromised by obesity, and increased illness and disability throughout the years. Even a modest weight reduction of 2 to 3 percent can reduce the risk for chronic diseases including heart disease, high blood pressure, high cholesterol, and diabetes.[6]

A primary objective of overall physical fitness and enhanced quality of life is to attain recommended body composition. Individuals at recommended body weight

GLOSSARY

Overweight Excess body weight when compared to a given standard such as height or recommended percent body fat.

Obesity A chronic disease characterized by an excessively high amount of body fat (about 20 percent above recommended weight or a BMI at 30 or above).

the United States.[1] Furthermore, obesity is more prevalent than poverty and problem drinking.[2] Obesity and unhealthy lifestyle habits are the most critical public health problems we face in the 21st century.

The American Heart Association has identified obesity as one of the six major risk factors for coronary heart

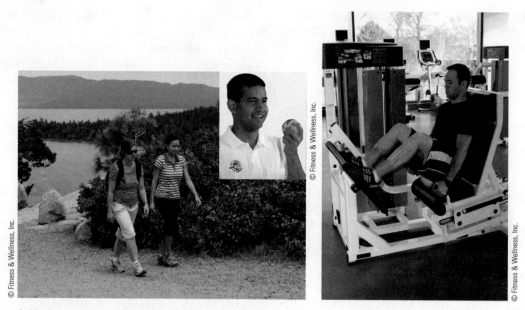

Achieving and maintaining a high physical fitness percent body fat requires a lifetime commitment to regular physical activity, exercise, and proper nutrition.

are able to participate in a wide variety of moderate to vigorous activities without functional limitations. These people have the freedom to enjoy most of life's recreational activities and reach their fullest potential. Excessive body weight does not afford an individual the fitness level to enjoy vigorous lifetime activities such as basketball, soccer, racquetball, surfing, mountain cycling, and mountain climbing. Maintaining high fitness and recommended body weight gives a person a degree of independence throughout life that the majority of people in developed nations no longer enjoy.

> **! Critical Thinking**
>
> Do you consider yourself overweight? • If so, how long have you had a weight problem, what attempts have you made to lose weight, and what has worked best for you?

6.1 *Tolerable Weight*

Many people want to lose weight so they will look better. That's a noteworthy goal. The problem, however, is that they often have a distorted image of what they would really look like if they were to reduce to what they think is their ideal weight. Hereditary factors play a big role, and only a small fraction of the population has the genes for a "perfect body." **Tolerable weight** is a more realistic goal. This is a realistic standard that is not "ideal" but is "acceptable."

It is likely to be closer to the health fitness standard than the physical fitness standard for many people.

The media has a great influence on people's perception of what constitutes ideal body weight. Most people rely on fashion, fitness, and beauty magazines to determine what they should look like. The "ideal" body shapes, physiques, and proportions shown in these magazines are rare and are achieved through airbrushing and medical reconstruction.[7] Many individuals, primarily young women, go to extremes in an attempt to achieve these unrealistic body shapes. Failure to attain a "perfect body" often leads to eating disorders.

When people set their own target weight, they should be realistic. Attaining the "high physical fitness" percent body fat standard shown in Table 2.11 (page 51) is extremely difficult for some. It is even more difficult to maintain, unless the person makes a commitment to a vigorous lifetime exercise program and permanent dietary changes. Few people are willing to do that. The "moderate" percent body fat category is more realistic for many people.

A question you should ask yourself is: Am I happy with my weight? Part of enjoying a higher quality of life is being happy with yourself. If you are not, you either need to do something about it or learn to live with it.

If your percent of body fat is higher than the health fitness standard shown in Table 2.11, page 51 (or a BMI above 25), you should try to reach and stay in this category for health reasons. This is the category that seems to pose no detriment to health.

If you have achieved the health fitness standard but would like to be more fit, ask yourself a second question: How badly do I want it? Enough to implement lifetime exercise and dietary changes? If you are not willing to change, you should stop worrying about your weight and deem the health fitness standard tolerable for you.

6.2 *Fad Dieting*

Few people who begin a traditional weight loss program (without exercise) are able to lose the desired weight. Worse, less than 5 percent of this group is able to keep the weight off for a significant time. Traditional diets have failed in helping people keep the weight off because few diet programs incorporate lifetime changes in food selection and overall increases in daily physical activity and exercise as the keys to successful weight loss and maintenance. Short-term "on and off dieting," are not the solution to lifelong weight management. You need to adopt a sustainable strategy that involves a permanent change in eating behaviors, including healthy food choices, portion control, and regular physical activity.

Fad diets continue to deceive people. Capitalizing on hopes that the latest diet to hit the market will really work this time, fad diets continue to appeal to people of all shapes and sizes. These diets may work for a while, but their success is usually short-lived. Most of these diets are low in calories and deprive the body of certain nutrients, generating a metabolic imbalance that can be detrimental to health. With many of these diets, a large amount of weight loss is in the form of water and protein, not fat.

On a crash diet, close to half of the weight loss is in lean (protein) tissue (see Figure 6.2). When the body uses protein instead of a combination of fats and

Figure 6.2 Effects of three forms of diet on fat loss.

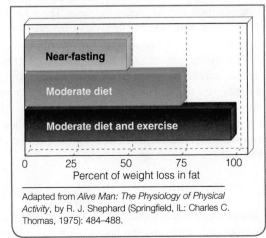

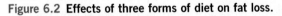

Percent of weight loss in fat

Adapted from *Alive Man: The Physiology of Physical Activity*, by R. J. Shephard (Springfield, IL: Charles C. Thomas, 1975): 484–488.

How to Recognize Fad Diets

Fad diets have characteristics in common. These diets typically

- are nutritionally unbalanced.
- rely primarily on a single food (for example, grapefruit).
- are based on testimonials.
- were developed according to "confidential research."
- are based on a "scientific breakthrough."
- promote rapid and "painless" weight loss.
- promise miraculous results.
- restrict food selection.
- are based on pseudo-claims that excessive weight is related to a specific condition such as insulin resistance, combinations or timing of nutrient intake, food allergies, hormone imbalances, or certain foods (fruits, for example).
- require the use of selected products.
- use liquid formulas instead of foods.
- misrepresent salespeople as individuals qualified to provide nutrition counseling.
- fail to provide information on risks associated with weight loss and of the diet use.
- do not involve physical activity.
- do not encourage healthy behavioral changes.
- are not supported by the scientific community or national health organizations.
- fail to provide information for weight maintenance upon completion of the diet phase.

© Cengage Learning

carbohydrates as a source of energy, the individual loses weight as much as 10 times faster. This is because a gram of protein produces less than half the amount of energy as fat does. In the case of muscle protein, one-fifth of protein is mixed with four-fifths of water. Each pound of muscle yields only one-tenth the amount of energy of a pound of fat. As a result, most of the weight loss is in the form of water, which on the scale, of course, looks good.

Among the popular diets on the market in recent years were the low-carbohydrate/high-protein (LCHP) diet

GLOSSARY

Tolerable weight A realistic body weight that is close to the health fitness percent body fat standard.

plans. Although variations exist among them, in general, "low-carb" diets limit the intake of carbohydrate-rich foods. Examples of these diets are the Atkins Diet, the Zone, Protein Power, the Scarsdale Diet, the Carb Addict's Diet, and Sugar Busters.

Rapid weight loss occurs during LCHP diets because the low carbohydrate intake forces the liver to produce glucose. The source for most of this glucose is body proteins. As mentioned, protein is mostly water; thus, weight is lost rapidly. When a person terminates the diet, the body rebuilds some of the protein tissue and the person quickly regains some weight.

Research studies indicated that individuals on an LCHP (Atkins) diet lose slightly more weight in the first few months than those on a low-fat diet.[8] The effectiveness of the diet, however, seemed to dwindle over time. In one of the studies, at 12 months into the diet, participants in the LCHP diet had regained more weight than those on the low-fat diet plan.

LCHP diets are contrary to the nutrition advice of most national leading health organizations (which recommend a diet low in animal fat and saturated fat and high in complex carbohydrates). Without fruits, vegetables, and whole grains, high-protein diets lack many vitamins, minerals, phytonutrients, and fiber—all dietary factors that protect against an array of ailments and diseases.

The major risk associated with long-term adherence to LCHP diets might be the increased risk of heart disease because high-protein foods are also high in fat content. Low carbohydrate intake also produces loss of vitamin B, calcium, and potassium. Side effects commonly associated with these diets are weakness, nausea, bad breath, constipation, irritability, light-headedness, and fatigue. Potential bone loss can further accentuate the risk for osteoporosis. Long-term adherence to an LCHP diet also can increase the risk for cancer. If you choose to go on an LCHP diet for longer than a few weeks, let your physician know so that he or she may monitor your blood lipids, bone density, and kidney function.

Some diets allow only certain specialized foods. If people would realize that no "magic" foods provide all the necessary nutrients and that a person has to eat a variety of foods to be well nourished, the diet industry would not be as successful. Most of these diets create a nutritional deficiency, which can be detrimental to health. Some people eventually get tired of eating the same thing day in and day out and start eating less—which results in weight loss. If they achieve the lower weight without making permanent dietary changes, however, they gain back the weight quickly if they return to their old eating habits.

A few diets recommend exercise along with caloric restrictions—the best method for weight reduction, of course. People who adhere to these programs will succeed, so the diet has achieved its purpose. Unfortunately, if the people do not change their food selection and activity level permanently, they gain back the weight once they discontinue dieting and exercise.

6.3 Principles of Weight Management

Traditional concepts related to weight control have centered on three assumptions:

1. Balancing food intake against output allows a person to achieve recommended weight.
2. Fat people just eat too much.
3. The human body doesn't care how much (or little) fat is stored.

Although these statements contain some truth, they still are open to much debate and research. We now know that the causes of obesity are complex and combine genetic, behavior, and lifestyle factors.

Energy-Balancing Equation

In keeping with the **energy-balancing equation**, if caloric intake exceeds output, the person gains weight; when caloric output is more than intake, the individual loses weight. Each pound of fat represents 3,500 calories. Therefore, theoretically, to increase body fat (weight) by 1 pound, a person would have to consume an excess of 3,500 calories. Equally, to lose 1 pound, the individual would have to decrease caloric intake by 3,500 calories. This principle seems straightforward, but the human body is not quite that simple.

The rule of thumb is that a person needs a 3,500-calorie deficit to lose a pound of fat. This figure, however, is an oversimplification of what really happens. There are too many individual, behavior, and lifestyle variables that keep weight loss from happening at the same rate among individuals, including gender, body composition, metabolic rate, and activity level. As will be discussed in this chapter, most notable are differences in daily physical activity and the drop in basal metabolic rate as a person loses weight (that is, the body burns fewer calories as weight is lost). The 3,500-calorie rule, nonetheless, is a good guideline to work off when writing weight-loss programs.

Diet and Metabolism

The genetic instinct to survive tells the body that fat storage is vital, and, therefore, the body's weight-regulating mechanism or **setpoint** sets an acceptable fat level for each person. This setpoint remains somewhat constant or may climb gradually because of poor lifestyle habits.

Under strict calorie reduction (fewer than 800 calories per day), the body makes compensatory metabolic adjustments in an effort to maintain its fat storage. The **basal metabolic rate (BMR)** may drop dramatically against a consistent negative caloric balance, and the person may be on a plateau for days or even weeks without losing much weight. When the dieter goes back to the normal or even below-normal caloric intake, at which the weight may have been stable for a long time, he or she quickly regains the fat lost as the body strives to restore a comfortable fat level.

These findings were substantiated by research conducted at Rockefeller University in New York,[9] which showed that the body resists maintaining altered weight. Obese and lifetime nonobese individuals were used in the investigation. Following a 10 percent weight loss, in an attempt to regain the lost weight, the body compensated by burning up to 15 percent fewer calories than expected for the new reduced weight (after accounting for the 10 percent loss). The effects were similar in the obese and nonobese participants. These results imply that after a 10 percent weight loss, a person would have to eat less or exercise more to account for the estimated deficit of about 200 to 300 daily calories.

In this same study, when the participants were allowed to increase their weight to 10 percent above their "normal" body weight (pre–weight loss), the body burned 10 percent to 15 percent more calories than expected. This indicates an attempt by the body to waste energy and return to the preset weight. The study provides another indication that the body is highly resistant to weight changes unless the person incorporates additional lifestyle changes to ensure successful weight management. (Methods to manage weight will be discussed later in this chapter.)

This research shows why most dieters regain the weight they lose through dietary means alone. Let's use a practical illustration: Jim would like to lose some body fat and assumes that he has reached a stable body weight at an average daily caloric intake of 2,500 calories (no weight gain or loss at this daily intake). In an attempt to lose weight rapidly, he now goes on a strict low-calorie diet (or, even worse, a near-fasting diet). Immediately the body activates its survival mechanism and readjusts its metabolism to a lower caloric balance.

After a few weeks of dieting at less than 800 calories per day, the body now can maintain its normal functions at 2,000 calories per day. Having lost the desired weight, Jim terminates the diet but realizes the original intake of

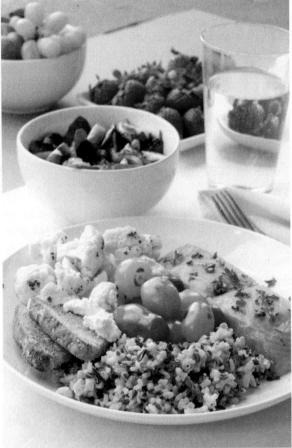

A wide variety of foods is required to maintain a well-nourished body.

2,500 calories per day will have to be lower to maintain the new lower weight. To adjust to the new lower body weight, he restricts his intake to about 2,200 calories per day. Jim is surprised to find that even at this lower daily intake (300 fewer calories), his weight comes back at a rate of about 1 pound every 2 to 3 weeks. After the diet ends, this new lowered metabolic rate may take several months to kick back up to its normal level.

GLOSSARY

Energy-balancing equation A body weight formula stating that when caloric intake equals caloric output, weight remains unchanged.

Setpoint Body weight and body fat percentage unique to each person that are regulated by genetic and environmental factors.

Basal metabolic rate (BMR) Lowest level of caloric intake necessary to sustain life.

From this explanation, individuals clearly should not go on very low calorie diets. Doing so will decrease the resting metabolic rate and also will deprive the body of basic daily nutrients required for normal function. Very low calorie diets should be used only in conjunction with dietary supplements and under proper medical supervision. Furthermore, research indicates that people who go on very low calorie diets are not as effective in keeping the weight off once they terminate the diet.

Recommendation

A daily caloric intake of approximately 1,500 calories provides the necessary nutrients if they are distributed properly over the basic food groups (meeting the daily recommended amounts from each group). Of course, the individual will have to learn to select healthy foods from among 100-percent whole grains, fiber-rich fruits and vegetables, beans, lean proteins, and modest amounts of healthy oils (olive and canola) and nuts while on a calorie-restricted plan. Diets below 1,500 daily calories may require a multivitamin supplement to obtain the daily nutrient requirements.

Under no circumstances should a person go on a diet that calls for a level of 1,200 calories or less for petite women or 1,500 calories or less for most everyone else. Weight (fat) is gained over months and years, not overnight. Likewise, weight loss should be gradual, not abrupt. At 1,200 calories per day, you may require a multivitamin nutrient supplement. Your health care professional should be consulted regarding such a supplement.

Furthermore, when a person tries to lose weight by dietary restrictions alone, **lean body mass** (muscle protein, along with vital organ protein) decreases. The amount of lean body mass lost depends entirely on the caloric limitation. When a person goes on a near-fasting diet, up to half of the weight lost can be lean body mass and the other half, actual fat loss. If the diet is combined with exercise, close to 100 percent of the weight loss is in the form of fat, and lean tissue actually may increase (see Figure 6.2). Loss of lean body mass is not good because it weakens the organs and muscles and slows the metabolism.

Reduction in lean body mass is common in people on severely restricted diets. No diet with caloric intakes below 1,500 calories will prevent loss of lean body mass. Even at this intake level, some loss is inevitable unless the diet is combined with exercise. Although many diets claim they do not alter the lean component, the simple truth is that, regardless of what nutrients may be added to the diet, caloric restrictions always prompt a loss of lean tissue.

Too many people go on low-calorie diets again and again. Every time they do, the metabolic rate slows as more lean tissue is lost. People in their 40s and older who weigh the same as they did when they were 20 often think they are at recommended body weight. During this span of 20 years or more, however, they may have dieted too many times without exercising. Shortly after terminating each diet, they regain the weight, but much of that gain is in fat. Maybe at age 20 they weighed 150 pounds, of which only 15 percent was fat. Now, at age 40, even though they still weigh 150 pounds, they might be 30 percent fat (see Figure 6.3, and also Figure 2.2, page 44). At recommended body weight, they wonder why they are eating so little and still having trouble staying at that weight.

Figure 6.3 Effects of constant dieting without exercise on body weight, percent body fat, and lean body mass.

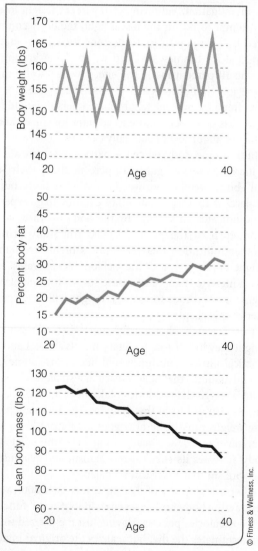

Further, data indicate that diets high in fat and refined carbohydrates, near-fasting diets, and perhaps even artificial sweeteners, keep people from losing weight and, in reality, contribute to fat gain. The only practical and sensible way to lose fat weight is to combine exercise and a sensible diet high in complex carbohydrates and low in fat and sugar.

Because of the effects of proper food management on body weight, most of the successful dieter's effort should be spent in retraining eating habits, increasing the intake of complex carbohydrates and high-fiber foods, and decreasing the consumption of refined carbohydrates (sugars) and fats. This change in eating habits will bring about a decrease in total daily caloric intake. One gram of carbohydrates provides only four calories as contrasted with nine calories per gram of fat. Thus, you could eat twice the volume of food (by weight) when substituting carbohydrates for fat. Some fat, however, is recommended in the diet—preferably polyunsaturated and monounsaturated fats. These so-called good fats do more than help protect the heart; they help delay hunger pangs.

A "diet" cannot be viewed as a temporary tool to aid in weight loss but, instead, as a permanent change in eating behaviors to ensure weight management and better health. The role of increased physical activity also must be considered because successful weight loss and recommended body composition seldom are attainable without a moderate reduction in caloric intake combined with a regular exercise program.

Sleep and Weight Management

Adequate sleep is a key component that enhances health and extends life. New evidence shows that sleep is also important to adequate weight management. Sleep deprivation appears to be conducive to weight gain and may interfere with the body's capability to lose weight.

Current obesity and sleep deprivation data point toward a possible correlation between excessive body weight and sleep deprivation. Sixty-nine percent of the U.S. population is overweight or obese, and according to the National Sleep Foundation, 63 percent of Americans report that they do not get eight hours of sleep per night. The question must be raised: Is there a connection? Let's examine some of the data.

One of the most recent studies examining this issue showed that individuals who get fewer than six hours of sleep per night have a higher average BMI (28.3) compared to those who average eight hours per night (24.5).[10] Another study on more than 68,000 women between the ages of 30 and 55 found that those who got 5 or fewer hours of sleep per night were 30 percent more likely to gain 30 or more pounds compared to women who got 8 hours per night.[11]

Researchers believe that lack of sleep disrupts normal body hormonal balances. Ghrelin and leptin are two hormones that play a critical role in weight gain and weight loss. Ghrelin, produced primarily in the stomach, stimulates appetite; that is, the more ghrelin the body produces, the more you want to eat. Leptin, produced by fat cells, on the other hand, lets the brain know when you are full; the more leptin you produce, the less you want to eat.

Sleep deprivation has now been shown to elevate ghrelin levels and decrease leptin levels, potentially leading to weight gain or keeping you from losing weight.[12] Data comparing these hormone levels in 5-hour versus 8-hour sleepers found that the short sleepers had a 14.9 percent increase in ghrelin levels and a 15.5 percent decrease in leptin levels. The short sleepers also had a 3.6 percent higher BMI than the regular sleepers.[13]

Based on all these studies, the data appear to indicate that sleep deprivation has a negative impact on weight loss or maintenance. Thus, an important component to a well-designed weight management program should be a good night's rest (eight hours of sleep).

Light Exposure and BMI

Although still in early stages, another piece of your weight management program may be the relationship between light exposure, timing of the exposure, and intensity of exposure. Studies are beginning to show that exposure to morning light can influence body weight and the hormones that regulate hunger. Data have shown that people who get more light exposure early in the day have lower BMIs.[19] Light exposure needs to be at least 500 lux (about the brightness of a typical office), but a higher amount could be better. Outside in full daylight exposure, a person gets approximately 10,000 lux. People who had most of their daily exposure to even moderately bright light in the morning had a significantly lower body mass index (BMI) than those who had most of their light exposure later in the day, the study found. The earlier the light exposure takes place in the day, the lower the individuals' BMI. Additional research suggests that sleep deprived individuals with ghrelin and leptin levels out of range showed improvements in their levels following two hours of daylight exposure shortly after waking up.[20] A third study indicated that obese women exposed

GLOSSARY

Lean body mass Nonfat component of the human body.

to bright light for a minimum of 45 minutes of morning light (between 6:00 am and 9:00 am) for three weeks had a slight drop in body fat.[21] Based on these data, weight management researchers indicate that light is a powerful biological signal to the human body and that proper timing (early morning), intensity, and duration of light exposure is important in a sound weight management program.

Monitoring Body Weight

A critical component to lifetime weight management is to regularly monitor your body weight. Get into the habit of weighing yourself, preferably at the same time of day and under the same conditions, for instance, in the morning just as you get out of bed. Depending on your body size, activity patterns, rehydration level, and dietary intake on any given day, your weight will fluctuate by a pound or more from one day to the next. You do not want to be obsessed with body weight, which can potentially lead to an eating disorder, but monitoring your *recommended body weight* (and that is the key: *"healthy" recommended body weight*) on a regular basis allows you to make immediate adjustments in food intake and physical activity if your weight increases and stays there for several days. *Do not adapt and accept* the higher weight as your new stable weight. Understand that it is a lot easier to make sensible short-term dietary and activity changes to lose 1 or 2 pounds of weight rather than having to make drastic long-term changes to lose 10, 20, 50, or more pounds that you allowed yourself to gain over the course of several months or years. Whenever feasible, you also want to do periodic assessments of body composition using experienced technicians and valid techniques.

6.4 Exercise and Weight Management

A more effective way to tilt the energy-balancing equation in your favor is by burning calories through physical activity. Research indicates that exercise accentuates weight loss while on a negative caloric balance (diet) as long as you do not replenish the calories expended during exercise.

Exercise also seems to exert control over how much a person weighs. On average, the typical adult American gains 1 to 2 pounds of weight per year. A 1-pound weight gain per year represents a simple energy surplus of less than 10 calories per day (10 × 365 = 3,650). In many

cases, most of the additional weight accumulated in middle age comes from people becoming less physically active. This simple surplus of less than 10 calories per day is the equivalent of less than 1 teaspoon of sugar. Weight gain is clearly related to a decrease in physical activity and an increase in caloric intake. Physical inactivity, however, might very well be the primary cause leading to excessive weight and obesity. The human body was meant to be physically active and *a minimal level of activity* appears to be necessary to accurately balance caloric intake to caloric expenditure. In sedentary individuals, the body seems to lose control over this fine energy balance.

A few individuals will lose weight by participating in 30 minutes of exercise per day, but most people need 60 to 90 minutes of daily physical activity for proper weight management (the 30 minutes of exercise are included as part of the 60 to 90 minutes of physical activity).

Although 30 minutes of moderate-intensity activity per day provides substantial health benefits, the Institute of Medicine of the National Academy of Sciences recommends that people trying to manage their weight accumulate 60 minutes of moderate-intensity physical activity most days of the week.[14] The evidence shows that people who maintain recommended weight typically accumulate an hour or more of daily physical activity.

As illustrated in Figure 6.4, greater weight loss can be achieved by increasing the amount of weekly physical activity. Of even greater significance, however, only the individuals who remain physically active for more than 60 minutes per day are able to keep the weight off.

Figure 6.4 Approximate decrease in body weight based on total weekly minutes of physical activity (PA) without caloric restrictions.

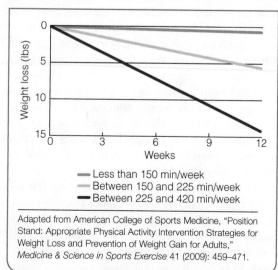

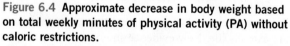

Adapted from American College of Sports Medicine, "Position Stand: Appropriate Physical Activity Intervention Strategies for Weight Loss and Prevention of Weight Gain for Adults," *Medicine & Science in Sports Exercise* 41 (2009): 459–471.

Data from the National Weight Control Registry (http://www.nwcr.ws) on more than 10,000 individuals who have lost an average of 66 pounds and kept it off for 5.5 years, indicate that 90 percent of them exercise on average one hour per day. Furthermore, other data show that individuals who completely stop physical activity regain almost 100 percent of the weight within 18 months of discontinuing the weight loss program. Thus, if weight management is *not* a consideration, 30 minutes of daily activity provides health benefits. *To prevent weight gain, 60 minutes of daily activity are recommended; to maintain substantial weight loss, 90 minutes may be required.* Furthermore, most of the successful "weight maintainers" also show greater dietary restraint and follow a low-fat diet, consuming less than 30 percent of the total daily calories from fat.

A combination of aerobic and strength-training exercises works best in weight loss programs. Aerobic exercise is the best to offset the setpoint, and the continuity and duration of these types of activities cause many calories to be burned in the process. Unfortunately, of those individuals who are attempting to lose weight, only a small percentage decrease caloric intake and exercise the recommended 30 minutes on most days of the week.

Strength training is critical in helping maintain lean body mass. Although the increase in BMR (basal metabolic rate) through increased muscle mass is currently being debated in the literature and merits further research, data indicate that each additional pound of muscle tissue raises the BMR in the range of 6 to 35 calories per day.[15] The latter figure is based on calculations that an increase of 3 to 3.5 pounds of lean tissue through strength training increased basal metabolic rate by about 105 to 120 calories per day.[16]

Most likely, the benefit of strength training goes beyond the new muscle tissue itself. Maybe a pound of muscle tissue requires only 6 calories per day to sustain itself, but as all muscles undergo strength training, they undergo increased protein synthesis to build and repair themselves, resulting in increased energy expenditure of 1 to 1.5 calories per pound in all trained muscle tissue. Such an increase would explain the 105 to 120 calorie-BMR increase in some research studies.

To examine the effects of a small increase in BMR on long-term body weight, let's use a very conservative estimate of an additional 50 calories per day as a result of a regular strength-training program. An increase of 50 calories represents an additional 18,250 calories per year (50 × 365), or the equivalent of 5.2 pounds of fat (18,250 ÷ 3,500). This increase in BMR would more than offset the typical adult weight gain of 1 to 2 pounds per year.

This figure of 18,250 calories per year does not include the actual energy cost of the strength-training workout. If we use an energy expenditure of only 150 calories per strength-training session, done twice per week, over a year's time it would represent 15,600 calories (150 × 2 × 52) or the equivalent of another 4.5 pounds of fat (15,600 ÷ 3,500).

In addition, although the amounts seem small, the previous calculations do not account for the increase in metabolic rate following the strength-training workout (the time it takes the body to return to its pre-workout resting rate—about 2 hours). Depending on the intensity and length of training, this recovery energy expenditure ranges from 20 to 100 calories following each strength-training workout.[17] All these "apparently small" changes make a big difference in the long run.

Another benefit of strength training is a significant decrease in abdominal (visceral) fat. A study on women in their 30s showed that as little as two strength-training sessions per week yielded a 3 percent decrease in abdominal fat over two years as compared to an almost equal increase in inactive women (no strength-training).[18] The strength-trained women also had a 4.3 percent increase in lean body mass.

In men, a study in 2014 on more than 10,000 men over the age of 40 that were followed over 12 years showed that individuals who participated in aerobic exercise lost more weight than those who strength trained for an equal amount of time, but the men who did 20 minutes of daily strength training had a lower increase in age-related abdominal (visceral) fat.[19] With aging, aerobic exercise by itself contributes to both fat and muscle tissue loss. As people age, they also need activities that will help maintain strength and muscle mass.

Although size (inches) and percent body fat both decrease when sedentary individuals begin an exercise program, body weight often remains the same or might even increase during the first couple of weeks after beginning the program. Exercise helps to increase muscle tissue, connective tissue, blood volume (as much as 500 mL, or the equivalent of 1 pound, following the first week of aerobic exercise), enzymes and other structures within the cell, and glycogen (which binds water). All of these changes lead to a higher functional capacity of the human body. With exercise, most of the weight loss becomes apparent after a few weeks of training, when the lean component has stabilized.

One additional benefit of exercise and physical activity is that it attenuates a person's predisposition to obesity. Genetic epidemiological studies have established that genetic factors play a role in obesity development in our 21st century obesogenic environment. Promoting physical

activity, exercise, and an active lifestyle is especially critical for individuals genetically predisposed to obesity.

The Myth of Spot Reducing

Research has revealed the fallacy of
spot reducing or losing cellulite, as
some people call the fat deposits that
bulge out in certain areas of the body.
Cellulite is caused by the herniation
of subcutaneous fat within fibrous
connective tissue, giving it a padded
appearance. Merely doing several sets
of sit-ups daily will not get rid of fat in
the midsection of the body. When fat
comes off, it does so throughout the
entire body, not just in the exercised
area. Although the greatest proportion of fat may come off the biggest fat
deposits, the caloric output of a few
sets of sit-ups has almost no effect on
reducing total body fat. A person has to exercise regularly
for extended periods of time to really see results.

The Role of Exercise Intensity and Duration in Weight Management

A hotly debated and controversial current topic is the
exercise volume required for adequate weight management. Depending on the degree of the initial weight
problem and the person's fitness level, there appears to be

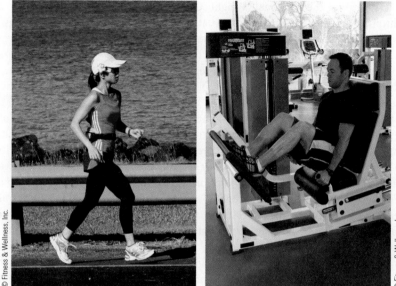

Regular participation in a combined lifetime aerobic and strength-training
exercise program is the key to successful weight management.

a difference in the volume of exercise that is most conducive toward adequate weight loss, weight loss maintenance, and weight management.

We have known for years that compared with vigorous
intensity, a greater proportion of calories burned during
light-intensity exercise are derived from fat. The lower
the intensity of exercise, the higher the percentage of fat
utilization as an energy source. During light-intensity
exercise, up to 50 percent of the calories burned may be
derived from fat (the other 50 percent from glucose [car-
bohydrates]). With vigorous exercise, only 30 percent to

Behavior Modification Planning

**Weight Maintenance
Benefits of Lifetime
Aerobic Exercise**

The authors of this book
have been jogging together a
minimum of 15 miles per week
(3 miles/5 times per week)
for the past 39 years. Without
considering the additional
energy expenditure from their
regular strength-training pro-
gram and their many other sport and recreational activities,
the energy cost of this regular jogging program over

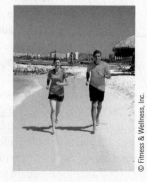

39 years has been approximately 3,042,000 calories
(15 miles × 100 calories/mile × 52 weeks × 37 years), or
the equivalent of 869 pounds of fat (3,042,000 ÷ 3,500). In
essence, without this 30-minute workout 5 times per week,
the authors would weigh 1,011 and 985 pounds, respectively!

Try It

Ask yourself whether a regular aerobic exercise program is
part of your long-term gratification and health enhancement program. If the answer is no, are you ready to change
your behavior? Use the Behavior Change Planner to help you
answer the question.

© Cengage Learning

40 percent of the caloric expenditure comes from fat. Overall, however, you can burn twice as many calories during vigorous-intensity exercise and, subsequently, more fat as well.

Let's look at a practical illustration. If you exercised for 30 to 40 minutes at light intensity and burned 200 calories, about 100 of those calories (50 percent) would come from fat. If you exercised at a vigorous intensity during those same 30 to 40 minutes, you could burn 400 calories, with 120 to 160 of the calories (30 percent to 40 percent) coming from fat. Thus, even though it is true that the percentage of fat used is greater during light-intensity exercise, the overall amount of fat used is still less during light-intensity exercise. Plus, if you were to exercise at a light intensity, you would have to do so twice as long to burn the same amount of calories.

Another benefit is that the metabolic rate remains at a slightly higher level longer after vigorous-intensity exercise, so you continue to burn a few extra calories following exercise. Very few calories are burned during recovery following a 45-minute moderate-intensity (50 percent or less of maximal capacity) exercise session, whereas when exercising at or above 70 percent of the maximal capacity for the same 45 minutes, nearly 40 percent of the total energy expenditure of the exercise bout is achieved during the recovery phase as the body returns to its pre-exercise baseline. A 500-calorie 45-minute vigorous exercise session will bring about another 200-calorie energy expenditure during the post-exercise recovery session.[20] Researchers believe that the extra caloric expenditure following vigorous exercise is because (a) the body uses more fat and less carbohydrates following a hard exercise session, (b) additional energy is required to replenish glycogen stores used during intense exercise, and (c) hormones released during vigorous exercise remain high, maintaining an elevated metabolism for several hours thereafter.

The previous discussion does not mean that light-intensity exercise is ineffective. Light-intensity exercise provides substantial health benefits, including a decrease in premature morbidity among overweight individuals. Additionally, beginners are more willing to participate and stay with light-intensity programs. The risk of injury when starting out is quite low with this type of a program. Light-intensity exercise does promote weight loss.

In terms of overall weight loss, there is controversy regarding the optimal exercise dose. Initial research indicated that vigorous-intensity exercise triggered more fat loss than light- to moderate-intensity exercise. Research conducted in the 1990s at Laval University in Quebec, Canada, using both men and women participants, showed that subjects who performed a high-intensity interval-training (HIIT) program lost more body fat than participants in a light- to moderate-intensity continuous aerobic endurance group.[21] Even more surprising, this finding occurred despite the fact that the vigorous-intensity group burned fewer total calories per exercise session. The researchers concluded that the "results reinforce the notion that for a given level of energy expenditure, vigorous exercise favors negative energy and lipid balance to a greater extent than exercise of low- to moderate-intensity. Moreover, the metabolic adaptations taking place in the skeletal muscle in response to the HIIT program appear to favor the process of lipid oxidation." If time constraints do not allow much time for exercise, to increase energy expenditure, a vigorous 20- to 30-minute exercise program is recommended.

Recently, it has been suggested that *when attempting to lose weight*, particularly for women, lengthy exercise sessions may not be helpful because they actually trigger greater food consumption following exercise, whereas shorter exercise sessions do not lead to a greater caloric intake. Thus, some people think that the potential weight reduction effect of lengthy exercise sessions may be attenuated because people end up eating more food when they exercise.

A recent 2009 study had postmenopausal women exercise at 50 percent of their maximal aerobic capacity for about 20 minutes, 40 minutes, or 60 minutes 3 to 4 times per week.[22] On average, the groups lost 3, 4.6, and, 3.3 pounds of weight, respectively. The data indicated that the 20- and 40-minute groups lost weight close to what had been predicted, whereas the 60-minute group lost significantly less than predicted. The researchers concluded that 60 minutes of exercise led this group of women to compensate with greater food intake, possibly triggered by an increase in ghrelin levels. All three groups, nonetheless, exhibited a significant decrease in waist circumference, independent of total weight lost. Researchers theorize that the biological mechanism to maintain fat stores in women is stronger than in men.

On the other hand, a 2010 study of more than 34,000 women who were followed for 13 years, starting at an average age of 54, found that on average the women gained 6 pounds of weight; but a small group of them who reported 60 minutes of almost daily exercise at a moderate intensity closely maintained their body weight.[23] The exercise routine of the latter group was not something new to them, but rather exercise that they had been doing for years. While the best exercise dose for optimal weight loss may not be a precise science, the research is quite clear that regular exercise is the best predictor of long-term weight maintenance. The data also indicate that even as little as 80 weekly minutes of aerobic or strength-training exercise prevents regain of the harmful visceral fat.

The take-home message from these studies is that when trying to lose weight, initial lengthy exercise sessions (longer than 60 minutes) may not be the best approach to weight loss, *unless* you carefully monitor daily caloric intake and avoid caloric compensation. The data show that people who carefully monitor caloric intake, instead of "guesstimating" energy intake, are by far more successful with weight loss.

Caloric compensation in response to extensive exercise in overweight individuals may be related to a low initial fitness level and the already low caloric intake. Overall, inactive people tend to eat fewer calories, and a lengthy exercise session may very well trigger a greater appetite due to the large negative caloric balance. Research confirms that energy deficit, and not exercise, is the most significant regulator of the hormonal responses seen in previously inactive individuals who begin an exercise program.[24] In active/fit individuals, lengthy exercise sessions are not at all counterproductive. If such were the case, health clubs and jogging trails would be full of overweight and obese people.

New research is beginning to look into the role of increasing light-intensity ambulation (walking) and standing activities (doing some of the work on your feet instead of sitting the entire time) on weight loss. In essence, the individual will increase light-intensity physical activity throughout the day. Light-intensity activities do not seem to trigger the increase in ghrelin levels seen in previously inactive individuals who undertake long moderate- or vigorous-intensity exercise sessions. The difference in energy expenditure from increasing light-intensity activities throughout the day can represent several hundred calories. As you achieve a higher fitness level, you can combine light-intensity activities performed throughout the day with moderate- and/or vigorous-intensity exercise.

The most important reason why physical activity and exercise are so vital for weight loss maintenance is because sedentary living expends no additional energy (calories) over the resting metabolic rate. With limited physical activity throughout the day, sedentary people cannot afford to eat very many calories, perhaps only 1,000 to 1,200 calories per day. And such a low level of energy intake is not sufficient to keep the person from constantly feeling hungry. The only choice they now have is to go hungry every day, an impossible task to sustain. After terminating the diet, in just a few short days energy intake climbs, with an end result of weight regain. Thus, the only logical way to increase caloric intake and maintain weight loss is by burning more calories through exercise and incorporating physical activity throughout daily living.

If you wish to engage in vigorous-intensity exercise to either maintain lost weight or for adequate weight management, a word of caution is in order: Be sure that it is medically safe for you to participate in such activities and that you build up gradually to that level. If you are cleared to participate in vigorous-intensity exercise, do not attempt to do too much too quickly because you may incur injuries and become discouraged. You must allow your body a proper conditioning period of 8 to 12 weeks or even longer.

Also keep in mind that vigorous intensity does not mean high impact. High-impact activities are the most common cause of exercise-related injuries. Additional information on proper exercise prescription is presented in Chapter 3. And remember, when on a weight loss program, *always* carefully monitor your daily caloric intake to avoid food overconsumption.

In addition to exercise and food management, sensible adjustments in caloric intake are recommended. Most research finds that a negative caloric balance is required to lose weight. Perhaps the only exception is with people who are eating too few calories. A nutrient analysis often reveals that "faithful" dieters are not consuming enough calories. These people actually need to increase their daily caloric intake (combined with an exercise program) to get their metabolism to kick back up to a normal level.

Overweight and Fit Debate

A hotly debated topic in the exercise and medical community is the topic most commonly referred to as "fit and fat." Can a person possibly be overweight/obese and still be fit?

Initially, the debate started with research indicating that the higher the aerobic fitness level, as measured by total treadmill-walking time, the lower the mortality rate, regardless of body weight. Most recently, fitness in these studies has been defined as "accumulating 30 minutes of moderate intensity activity on most days of the week." Some researchers believe that many overweight people who reach this goal are not predisposed to premature death. The data indicate that, on average, death rates for thin, but unfit, individuals are twice as high as that of obese and "fit" people. Furthermore, looking at every category of body composition, most "unfit" people have a higher rate of premature death than "fit" individuals. Thus, at least partially, lack of physical activity (fitness), and not the weight problem itself, may be the cause of premature death in most overweight people. However, it's not simply a matter of fitness or fatness, because both obesity and physical inactivity are independent risk factors for heart disease, type 2 diabetes, and other chronic ailments.

Fitness does offer substantial benefits, but regular physical activity in itself does not completely reverse chronic disease risks associated with excess body fat. Studies are encouraging because they show that many overweight/obese people who focus on healthy eating and become physically active can decrease the risk of premature mortality, regardless of whether they lose weight or not. Few obese people, however, eat healthy and exercise regularly for 30 minutes on most days of the week. Most obese people either choose not to exercise or are unable to do so because of functional limitations as a result of the excessive body weight.

The answer to the question as to whether a person can be fit and fat depends on the definition of fitness. If cardiorespiratory fitness is determined by "accumulating 30 minutes of moderate-intensity activity on most days of the week," then the answer is a definite "yes." If one measures fitness based on maximal oxygen uptake (VO_{2max}—see Chapter 2, page 36), the answer is a clear "no." Many fitness experts do not agree with the concept of fit and fat. Exercise by itself will not remove all of the heart risks of being overweight, but it can blunt them. According to Dr. JoAnn Manson of the Harvard Medical School, "it's a rare bird" to find someone who is truly overweight and yet truly fit from a cardiorespiratory standpoint.

Most nutritionists and exercise scientists agree that healthy eating and healthy exercise contribute to healthy body weight. There are more than 50 medical conditions—from type 2 diabetes, acid reflux, and arthritis to sleep apnea and some types of cancers that are directly related to excessive body weight. At this point, most fitness leaders do not support the notion that people can enjoy vibrant health and good quality of life while being overweight or obese.

6.5 *Designing Your Own Weight Loss Program*

Estimating Your Caloric Intake

With Activity 6.1 (pages 175–176) and Table 6.1 and Table 6.2, you can estimate your daily energy (caloric) requirement. Because this is only an estimated value, individual adjustments related to many of the factors discussed in this chapter may be necessary to establish a more precise value. Nevertheless, the estimated value does offer a beginning guideline for weight control or reduction.

The **estimated energy requirement (EER)** without additional planned activity and exercise is based on age, total body weight, height, and gender. Individuals who hold jobs that require a lot of walking or heavy manual

Table 6.1 Estimated Energy Requirement (EER) Based on Age, Body Weight, and Height (includes activities of independent living only and no moderate physical activity or exercise)

Men: EER = 662 − (9.53 × Age) + (15.91 × BW) + (539 × HT)
Women: EER = 354 − (6.91 × Age) + (9.36 × BW) + (726 × HT)

BW = body weight in kilograms (divide BW in pounds by 2.2046), HT = height in meters (multiply HT in inches by .0254).

SOURCE: National Academy of Sciences, Institute of Medicine, *Dietary Reference Intakes for Energy, Carbohydrates, Fiber, Fat, Protein and Amino Acids* (*Macronutrients*) (Washington, DC: National Academy Press, 2002).

labor burn more calories during the day than those who have sedentary jobs (such as working behind a desk). To estimate your EER, refer to Table 6.1. For example, the EER computation for a 20-year-old man 71 inches tall who weighs 160 pounds would be as follows:

1. Body weight in kilograms = 72.6 kg
   (160 lbs ÷ 2.2046)
   Height in meters = 1.8 m (71 × .0254)
2. EER = 662 − (9.53 × Age) + (15.91 × BW) + (539 × Ht)
   EER = 662 − (9.53 × 20) + (15.91 × 72.6) + (539 × 1.8)
   EER = 662 − 190.6 + 1,155 + 970
   EER = 2,596

Thus, the EER to maintain body weight for this individual would be 2,596 calories per day.

The second step is to determine the average number of calories this man burns daily as a result of exercise. To get this number, he must figure out the total number of minutes he exercises weekly and then figure the daily average exercise time. For instance, if he cycles at 10 miles per hour 5 times a week, 60 minutes each time, he exercises 300 minutes per week (5 × 60). The average daily exercise time is 42 minutes (300 ÷ 7, rounded off to the lowest unit).

Next, from Table 6.2, find the energy requirement for the activity (or activities) he has chosen for the exercise program. In the case of cycling (10 miles per hour), the requirement is .05 calories per pound of body weight per minute of activity (cal/lb/min). With a body weight of 160 pounds, this man would burn 8 calories each minute

GLOSSARY

Estimated energy requirement (EER) The average dietary energy (caloric) intake that is predicted to maintain energy balance in a healthy adult of defined age, gender, weight, height, and level of physical activity, consistent with good health.

Table 6.2 Caloric Expenditure of Selected Physical Activities

Activity*	Cal/lb/min	Activity*	Cal/lb/min	Activity*	Cal/lb/min
Aerobics	0.065	Elliptical training		Stationary cycling	
Moderate	0.095	Moderate	0.07	Moderate	0.055
Vigorous	0.070	Vigorous	0.09	Vigorous	0.07
Step aerobics	0.030	Golf	0.030	Strength training	0.05
Archery		Gymnastics		Swimming (crawl)	
Badminton	0.038	Light	0.03	20 yds/min	0.031
Recreation	0.065	Heavy	0.056	25 yds/min	0.04
Competition	0.031	Handball	0.064	45 yds/min	0.057
Baseball		High-intensity interval		50 yds/min	0.07
Basketball	0.046	training	0.120	Table tennis	0.03
Moderate	0.063	Hiking	0.04	Tennis	
Competition	0.030	Judo/karate	0.086	Moderate	0.045
Bowling	0.033	Jogging/running (on a level surface)		Competition	0.064
Calisthenics				Volleyball	0.03
Cross-country skiing	0.090	11.0 min/mile	0.070	Walking	
Moderate	0.120	8.5 min/mile	0.090	4.5 mph	0.045
Vigorous		7.0 min/mile	0.102	Shallow pool	0.09
Circuit training	0.070	6.0 min/mile	0.114	Water aerobics	
Moderate	0.100	Deep water**	0.100	Moderate	0.05
Vigorous		Racquetball	0.065	Vigorous	0.07
Cycling (on a level surface)	0.033	Rope jumping	0.06	Wrestling	0.085
5.5 mph	0.050	Rowing (vigorous)	0.09	Zumba	
10.0 mph	0.071	Skating (moderate)	0.038	Moderate	0.065
13.0 mph		Skiing		Vigorous	0.095
Dance	0.03	Downhill	0.06		
Moderate	0.055	Level (5 mph)	0.078		
Vigorous		Soccer	0.059		

*Values are for actual time engaged in the activity.

**Treading water.

Adapted from: P. E. Allsen, J. M. Harrison, and B. Vance, *Fitness for Life: An Individualized Approach* (Dubuque, IA: Wm. C. Brown, 1989). C. A. Bucher and W. E. Prentice, *Fitness for College and Life* (St. Louis: Times Mirror/Mosby College Publishing, 1989). C. F. Consolazio, R. E. Johnson, and L. J. Pecora, *Physiological Measurements of Metabolic Functions in Man* (New York: McGraw-Hill, 1963). R. V. Hockey, Physical Fitness: *The Pathway to Healthy Living* (St. Louis: Times Mirror/Mosby College Publishing, 1989). W. W. K. Hoeger et al., Research conducted at Boise State University, 1986–2009.

(body weight × .05, or 160 × .05). In 42 minutes, he burns approximately 336 calories (42 × 8).

The third step is to obtain the estimated total caloric requirement, with exercise, needed to maintain body weight. To do this, add the typical daily requirement (without exercise) and the average calories burned through exercise. In our example, it is 2,932 calories (2,596 + 336).

Therefore, this man has to consume fewer than 2,932 calories daily to lose weight. Because of the many factors that play a role in weight control, this is only an estimated daily requirement. Furthermore, to lose weight, we cannot predict that he will lose exactly 1 pound of fat in 1 week if he cuts his daily intake by 500 calories (500 × 7 = 3,500 calories, or the equivalent of 1 pound of fat).

The daily energy requirement is only a target guideline for weight control. Periodic readjustments are necessary because individuals differ and the estimated daily cost changes as you lose weight and modify your exercise habits.

To determine the target caloric intake to lose weight, multiply your current weight by 5 and subtract this amount from the total daily energy requirement (2,932 in our example) with exercise. For our moderately active male example, this would mean consuming only 2,132 calories per day to lose weight (160 × 5 = 800 and 2,932 − 800 = 2,132 calories).

This final caloric intake to lose weight should not be below 1,500 calories for most people. If distributed properly over the various food groups, 1,500 calories appears to be the lowest caloric intake that still provides the necessary nutrients the body needs. A multivitamin complex is recommended for diets that call for less than 1,500 calories. In terms of percentages of total calories, the daily distribution should be approximately 60 percent carbohydrates (mostly complex carbohydrates), less than 30 percent fat, and about 12 percent protein.

The time of day when food is consumed also may play a part in losing weight. When a person is attempting to lose weight, intake should consist of a minimum of 25 percent of the total daily calories for breakfast, 50 percent for lunch, and 25 percent or less at dinner. Breakfast, in particular, is a critical meal. Many people skip breakfast because it's the easiest meal to skip. Evidence, however, indicates that people who skip breakfast are hungrier later in the day and end up consuming more total daily calories than those who eat breakfast. If you find that breakfast is the easiest meal to skip, at least eat a small breakfast with some protein and a slight amount of fat to avoid excessive hunger pangs later in the morning.

Be aware that if most of the daily calories are consumed during one meal (as in the typical evening meal), the body may perceive that something is wrong and will slow down the metabolism so it can store more calories in the form of fat. Furthermore, eating most of the calories during one meal causes a person to go hungry the rest of the day, making it more difficult to adhere to the diet. Furthermore, try not to eat within 3 hours of going to bed. At this time of day, your metabolism is slowest; your caloric intake is less likely to be used for energy and more likely to be stored as fat.

Monitoring Your Diet Through Daily Food Logs

To help you monitor and adhere to your diet plan, you may use the daily food intake record form in Activity 6.2, pages 177–180. First make a master copy so you can make copies as needed in the future. Guidelines are provided for 1,200-, 1,500-, 1,800-, and 2,000-calorie diet plans. These plans were developed based on the MyPlate food plan and the Dietary Guidelines for Americans to meet the Recommended Dietary Allowances. The objective is to meet (not exceed) the number of servings allowed for each diet plan. Each time you eat a serving of any food, record it in the appropriate box. Evidence indicates that people who monitor daily caloric intake are more successful at weight loss than those who don't self-monitor.

To lose weight, you should use the diet plan that most closely approximates your target caloric intake. The plan is based on the following caloric allowances for these food groups:

- Grains: 80 calories per serving
- Fruits: 60 calories per serving

- Vegetables: 25 calories per serving
- Dairy (use low-fat products): 120 calories per serving
- Protein: Use low-fat (300 calories per serving) frozen entrees or an equivalent amount if you prepare your own main dish (see the following discussion)

As you start your diet plan, pay particular attention to food serving sizes. Take care with cup and glass sizes. A standard cup is 8 ounces, but most glasses nowadays contain between 12 and 16 ounces. If you drink 12 ounces of fruit juice, in essence you are getting two servings of fruit because a standard serving is ¾ cup of juice.

Read food labels carefully to compare the caloric value of the serving listed on the label with the caloric guidelines provided above. Here are some examples:

- One slice of standard whole-wheat bread has about 80 calories. A plain bagel may have 200 to 350 calories. Although it is low in fat, a 350-calorie bagel is equivalent to almost 4 servings in the grain group.
- The standard serving size listed on the food label for most cereals is 1 cup. As you read the nutrition information, however, you will find that for the same cup of cereal, one type of cereal has 120 calories and another cereal has 200 calories. Because a standard serving in the grain group is 80 calories, the first cereal would be 1½ servings and the second one 2½ servings.
- A medium-size fruit is usually considered to be 1 serving. A large fruit could provide as many as 2 or more servings.
- In the dairy group, 1 serving represents 120 calories. A cup of whole milk has about 160 calories, compared with a cup of skim milk, which contains 88 calories. A cup of whole milk, therefore, would provide 1⅓ servings in this food group.

Using Low-Fat Entrees

To be more accurate with caloric intake and to simplify meal preparation, use commercially prepared low-fat frozen entrees as the main dish for lunch and dinner meals (only one entree for the 1,200-calorie diet plan—see Activity 6.2, page 177). Look for entrees that provide about 300 calories and no more than 6 grams of fat per entree. These two entrees can be used as the protein group selections and will provide most of the daily requirement for the body. Along with each entree, supplement the meal with some of your servings from the other food groups. This diet plan has been used successfully in weight loss research programs.[25] If you choose not to use these low-fat entrees, prepare a similar meal using 3 ounces (cooked) of lean meat, poultry, or fish with additional beans, vegetables, rice, or pasta that will provide 300 calories with fewer than 6 grams of fat per dish.

As you record your food choices, be sure to write the precise amount for each serving. If you choose to do so, you then can run a computerized nutrient analysis to verify your caloric intake and food distribution pattern (percent of total calories from carbohydrate, fat, and protein).

Protein Intake

To minimize the loss of lean body mass and hunger pangs while dieting, it is extremely important that you consume sufficient protein with each meal. You need to ensure that you are consuming between 1.5 gram and 2.0 grams of protein per kilogram of body weight per day (more if you are doing vigorous aerobic exercise and strength training). As explained in Chapter 5 (Table 5.2, page 131), if you weigh 141 pounds (64 kg) and you are on a weight-loss program, your total daily protein intake would be between 96 and 128 grams per day (64 × 1.5 and 64 × 2.0) or the equivalent of 384 to 512 calories from protein every day (96 × 4 and 128 × 4), distributed in 32 to 43 grams of protein for each of your daily 3 meals. High-protein/low-calorie foods include fat-free or low-fat dairy products (milk, plain Greek yogurt, and cheese), eggs, lean meats and poultry, fish, soybeans and soy milk, tofu, quinoa, and beans. To help monitor your daily protein intake, you can calculate and record your daily intake in Activity 6.2 as well.

Effect of Food Choices on Long-Term Weight Gain

Although still in its infancy, research published in 2011 on more than 120,000 people who were evaluated every 4 years over a 20-year period showed that food choices have a significant effect on weight gain.[26] On average, study participants gained 17 pounds over the course of 20 years. Regardless of other lifestyle habits, individuals who consumed unhealthy foods gained the most weight, whereas those who made healthy food choices gained the least amount of weight. Although more research is needed, in this study, four-year weight change was most strongly associated with the consumption of potato chips, potatoes, sugar-sweetened beverages, unprocessed and processed red meats and inversely associated with the consumption of vegetables, whole grains, fruits, nuts, and yogurt. The take-home message: Consume more fruits, vegetables, whole grains, low-fat dairy products, and nuts (the last in moderation because of their high caloric content).

6.6 Behavior Modification and Adherence to a Lifetime Weight Management Program

Achieving and maintaining recommended body composition is by no means impossible, but it does require desire and commitment. If weight management is to become a priority in life, people must realize that they have to transform their behavior to some extent.

Modifying old habits and developing new, positive behaviors take time. Individuals who apply the management techniques provided in the Behavior Modification Planning box (pages 172–173) are more successful at changing detrimental behavior and adhering to a positive, lifetime weight control program. In developing a retraining program, people are not expected to use all of the strategies listed but should pick the ones that apply to them.

Critical Thinking

What behavioral strategies have you used to properly manage your body weight? • How do you think those strategies would work for others?

During the weight loss process, surround yourself with people who have the same goals as you do (weight loss). Data released in 2007 showed that obesity can spread through "social networks."[27] That is, if your friends, siblings, or spouse gain weight, you are more likely to gain weight as well. People tend to accept a higher weight standard if someone they are close to or care about gains weight.

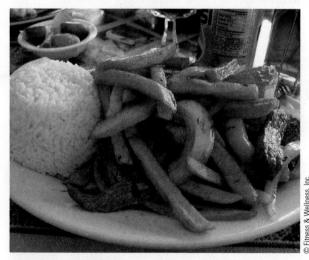

© Fitness & Wellness, Inc.

"Supersized" portion sizes at restaurants in the United States contribute to the growing epidemic of obesity.

Behavior Modification Planning

Weight Loss Strategies

1. *Make a commitment to change.* The first necessary ingredient is the desire to modify your behavior. You have to stop precontemplating or contemplating change and get going! You must accept that you have a problem and decide by yourself whether you really want to change. Sincere commitment increases your chances for success.

2. *Set realistic goals.* The weight problem developed over several years. Similarly, new lifetime eating and exercise habits take time to develop. A realistic long-term goal also will include short-term objectives that allow for regular evaluation and help maintain motivation and renewed commitment to attain the long-term goal.

3. *Monitor caloric intake.* Keep an accurate daily record of food consumption. *"If you eat it, record it."* People who keep accurate food logs are more successful at weight loss.

4. *Plan on three small meals and possibly one to two snacks each day.* Eating less but more often helps keep your blood sugar levels steady and avoid hunger pangs. Include adequate protein intake with each meal and use primarily high-volume, low-calorie foods. Space your meals and snacks so that you eat every three to four hours. Snacks need to be nutrient-rich, including fruits, vegetables, low-fat/plain yogurt, or a small amount of nuts. Avoid quick pick-me-up high-sugar and processed foods that tend to encourage overeating.

5. *Weigh yourself regularly*, preferably at the same time of day and under the same conditions. Do not adapt and accept a higher body weight as a new stable weight. Make dietary and physical activity adjustments accordingly.

6. *Incorporate exercise into the program.* Choosing enjoyable activities, places, times, equipment, and people to work out with will help you adhere to an exercise program (see Chapter 6 to Chapter 9). If time is a factor, you can easily create extra time in your day by recording your favorite TV programs and watching them later. You can then skip the commercials and end with extra time to fit in exercise.

7. *Differentiate hunger and appetite.* Hunger is the actual physical need for food. Appetite is a desire for food, usually triggered by factors such as stress, habit, boredom, depression, availability of food, or just the thought of food itself. Developing and sticking to a regular meal pattern will help control hunger.

8. *Select low-energy/high-volume foods.* Soups, salads, and vegetables are more effective in promoting fullness with a meal; plus, they are lower in calories.

9. *Increase fiber intake.* Whole grains, fruits, vegetables, and legumes help you feel more satisfied and for a longer time by increasing chewing time, saliva secretion, gastric juices, and absorption time; all of which helps reduce overall caloric intake.

10. *Eat less fat.* Each gram of fat provides nine calories, and protein and carbohydrates provide only four. In essence, you can eat more food by consuming primarily fruits, vegetables, and whole grains (complex carbohydrates) with each meal. Most of your fat intake should come from healthy unsaturated sources.

11. *Pay attention to calories.* Just because food is labeled "low-fat" does not mean you can eat as much as you want. When reading food labels—and when eating—don't just look at the fat content. Pay attention to calories as well. Many low-fat foods are high in calories.

12. *Cut unnecessary items from your diet.* Substituting water for a daily can of soda would cut 51,100 (140 × 365) calories yearly from the diet—the equivalent of 14.6 (51,000 ÷ 3,500) pounds of fat. If you always drink water instead of sugar-sweetened beverages when thirsty and with your meals, you can do even better and decrease caloric intake by an average of 300 daily calories. Several studies also indicate that liquid calories do not provide the same sense of satiety as a similar amount of calories from solid foods. An apple, for example, increases fullness more than a cup of apple juice. Research has shown that people who consume liquid calories do not account for those calories by eating less food during or in the subsequent meal. Liquid calories do little to suppress hunger.

13. *Maintain a daily intake of calcium-rich foods*, especially low-fat or nonfat dairy products.

14. *Add foods to your diet that reduce cravings*, such as eggs; small amounts of red meat, fish, poultry, tofu, oils, and fats; and nonstarchy vegetables such as

(Continued)

Behavior Modification Planning (continued)

lettuce, green beans, peppers, asparagus, broccoli, mushrooms, and Brussels sprouts. Also increasing the intake of low-glycemic carbohydrates with your meals helps you go longer before you feel hungry again.

15. *Avoid mindless eating.* Many people make food decisions based on psychological triggers, including family and friends, packages and containers, watching television and TV ads, watching movies, computer distractions, and reading. Most foods consumed in these situations lack nutritional value or are high in sugar and fat.

16. *Stay busy.* People tend to eat more when they sit around and do nothing. Occupying the mind and body with activities not associated with eating helps take away the desire to eat. Some options are walking; cycling; playing sports; gardening; sewing; or visiting a library, a museum, or a park. You also might develop other skills and interests not associated with food.

17. *Plan meals and shop sensibly.* Always shop on a full stomach, because hungry shoppers tend to buy unhealthy foods impulsively—and then snack on the way home. Always use a shopping list, which should include 100 percent whole grains (breads and cereals), fruits and vegetables, low-fat milk and dairy products, lean meats, fish, and poultry.

18. *Cook wisely:*
    - Use less fat and fewer refined foods in food preparation.
    - Trim all visible fat from meats and remove skin from poultry before cooking.
    - Skim the fat off gravies and soups.
    - Bake, broil, boil, or steam instead of frying.
    - Sparingly use butter, cream, mayonnaise, and salad dressings.
    - Avoid coconut oil, palm oil, and cocoa butter.
    - Prepare plenty of foods that contain fiber.
    - Include whole-grain breads and cereals, vegetables, and legumes in most meals.
    - Eat fruits for dessert.
    - Stay away from soda pop, fruit juices, fruit-flavored drinks, and sports and energy drinks.

- Use less sugar, and cut down on other refined carbohydrates, such as corn syrup, malt sugar, dextrose, and fructose.
- Stay hydrated with water—drink at least six glasses (6 to 8 ounces each) a day.

19. *Do not serve more food than you should eat.* Measure the food in portions and keep serving dishes away from the table. Do not force yourself or anyone else to "clean the plate" after they are satisfied (including children after they already have had a healthy, nutritious serving).

20. *Try "junior size" instead of "super size."* People who are served larger portions eat more, whether they are hungry or not. Use smaller plates, bowls, cups, and tall/thin glasses. Try eating half as much food as you commonly eat. Additionally, portions served on smaller plates appear bigger than they are, thus the tendency is to serve less on a small plate. People also drink less from tall/thin glasses than from large or even short/wide glasses. Watch for portion sizes at restaurants as well: Supersized foods create supersized people.

21. *Use smaller and different color dishes.* People tend to over-serve food on larger dinner plates. Reducing your standard dinner plate by two inches results in about 20 percent fewer calories served. Changing the contrast between the plate and the food, for example pasta with red marinara sauce over a white vs. a red plate, also reduces the amount of food served by a similar 20 percent.

22. *Use smaller serving spoons.* People tend to serve less food when given a smaller serving spoon.

23. *Eat out infrequently.* The more often people eat out, the more body fat they have. People who eat out 6 or more times per week consume about 300 extra calories per day and 30 percent more fat than those who eat out less often.

24. *Eat slowly and at the table only.* Eating on the run promotes overeating because the body doesn't have enough time to "register" consumption and people overeat before the body perceives the fullness signal. Eating at the table encourages people to take time out to eat and deters snacking between meals. After eating, do not sit around the table but, rather, clean up and put away the food to avoid snacking.

25. *Avoid social binges.* Social gatherings tend to entice self-defeating behavior. Use visual imagery to plan ahead. Do not feel pressured to eat or drink and don't rationalize in these situations. Choose low-calorie foods and entertain yourself with other activities, such as dancing and talking.

26. *Do not place unhealthy foods within easy reach.* Ideally, avoid bringing high-calorie, high-sugar, or high-fat foods into the house. If they are there already, store them where they are hard to get to or see—perhaps the garage or basement.

27. *Avoid evening food raids.* Most people do really well during the day but then "lose it" at night. Take control. Stop and think. To avoid excessive nighttime snacking, stay busy after your evening meal. Go for a short walk, floss and brush your teeth, and get to bed earlier. Even better, close the kitchen after dinner and try not to eat anything three hours prior to going to sleep.

28. *Practice stress management techniques* (discussed in Chapter 7). Many people snack and increase their food consumption in stressful situations.

29. *Get support.* People who receive support from friends, relatives, and formal support groups are much more likely to lose and maintain weight loss than those without such support. The more support you receive, the better off you will be.

30. *Monitor changes and reward accomplishments.* Being able to exercise without interruption for 15, 20, 30, or 60 minutes; swimming a certain distance; running a mile—all these accomplishments deserve recognition. Create rewards that are not related to eating: new clothing, a tennis racquet, a bicycle, exercise shoes, or something else that is special and you would not have acquired otherwise.

31. *Prepare for slip-ups.* Most people will slip and occasionally splurge. Do not despair and give up. Reevaluate and continue with your efforts. An occasional slip won't make much difference in the long run.

32. *Think positive.* Avoid negative thoughts about how difficult changing past behaviors might be. Instead, think of the benefits you will reap, such as feeling, looking, and functioning better, plus enjoying better health and improving the quality of life. Avoid negative environments and unsupportive people.

Try It

In your Online Journal or class notebook, answer the following questions: How many of the previous listed strategies do you use to help you maintain recommended body weight? Do you feel that any of these strategies specifically help you manage body weight more effectively? If so, explain why.

© Cengage Learning

In the study, the social ties of more than 12,000 were examined over 32 years. The findings revealed that if a close friend becomes obese, your risk of becoming obese during the next 2 to 4 years increases 171 percent. The risk also increases 57 percent for casual friends, 40 percent for siblings, and 37 percent for the person's spouse. The reverse was also found to be true. When a person loses weight, the likelihood of friends, siblings, or spouse to lose weight is also enhanced.

Furthermore, the research found that gender plays a role in social networks. A male's weight has a greater effect on the weight of male friends and brothers than on female friends or sisters. Similarly, a woman's weight has a far greater influence on sisters and girlfriends than on brothers or male friends. Thus, if you are trying to lose weight, choose your friendships carefully: Do not surround yourself with people who either have a weight problem or are still gaining weight.

6.7 *You Can Do It!*

The challenge of taking off excessive body fat and keeping it off for good has no simple solution. Weight management is accomplished through lifetime commitment to physical activity and proper food selection. When taking part in a weight reduction program, people have to decrease their caloric intake moderately and implement strategies to modify unhealthy eating behaviors.

Relapses into past negative behaviors are almost inevitable. Making mistakes is human and does not mean failure. Failure comes to those who give up and do not use previous experiences to build upon and, instead, develop skills that will prevent self-defeating behaviors in the future. Where there's a will, there's a way, and those who persist will reap the rewards.

Assess Your Behavior

· ·

1. Are you satisfied with your current body composition and quality of life? If not, are you willing to do something about it? If so, what do you plan to do to reach your goal?

2. Are physical activity, aerobic exercise, and strength training a regular part of your lifetime weight management program?

3. Do you weigh yourself regularly and make adjustments in energy intake and physical activity habits if your weight starts to slip upward?

4. Do you exercise portion control, watch your overall caloric intake, and plan ahead before you eat out or attend social functions that entice overeating?

Assess Your Knowledge

· ·

1. Obesity is defined as a body mass index equal to or above
   a. 10.
   b. 25.
   c. 30.
   d. 45.
   e. 50.

2. The second leading cause of preventable death in the United States is
   a. obesity.
   b. lack of cardiorespiratory fitness.
   c. diabetes caused by excessive weight.
   d. excessive body weight combined with physical inactivity.
   e. None of the above.

3. Obesity increases the risk for
   a. hypertension.
   b. congestive heart failure.
   c. atherosclerosis.
   d. type 2 diabetes.
   e. All are correct choices.

4. Tolerable weight is a body weight
   a. that is not ideal but one that you can live with.
   b. that will tolerate the increased risk of chronic diseases.
   c. with a BMI range between 25 and 30.
   d. that meets both ideal values for percent body fat and BMI.
   e. All are correct choices.

5. When the body uses protein instead of a combination of fats and carbohydrates as a source of energy,
   a. weight loss is very slow.
   b. a large amount of weight loss is in the form of water.
   c. muscle turns into fat.
   d. fat is lost very rapidly.
   e. fat cannot be lost.

6. One pound of fat represents
   a. 1,200 calories.
   b. 1,500 calories.
   c. 3,500 calories.
   d. 5,000 calories.
   e. None of the above choices is correct.

7. The mechanism that seems to regulate how much a person weighs is known as
   a. setpoint.
   b. weight factor.
   c. basal metabolic rate.
   d. metabolism.
   e. energy-balancing equation.

8. The key to successful weight management is
   a. frequent dieting.
   b. very low calorie diets when "normal" dieting doesn't work.
   c. a lifetime physical activity program.
   d. regular low-carbohydrate/high-protein meals.
   e. All are correct choices.

9. The daily amount of physical activity recommended for weight loss maintenance is
   a. 15 to 20 minutes.
   b. 20 to 30 minutes.
   c. 30 to 60 minutes.
   d. 60 to 90 minutes.
   e. Any amount is sufficient as long as it is done daily.

10. A daily energy expenditure of 300 calories through physical activity is the equivalent of approximately how many pounds of fat per year?
    a. 12
    b. 15
    c. 22
    d. 27
    e. 31

Correct answers can be found on page 307.

Activity 6.1 Caloric Requirement: Computation Form

Name _____ **Date** _____

Course _____ **Section** _____

A. Current body weight .... _____

B. Estimated energy requirement per day (use Table 6.1, page 167) .... _____

C. Selected physical activity (e.g., jogging)* .... _____

D. Number of exercise sessions per week .... _____

E. Duration of exercise session (in minutes) .... _____

F. Total weekly exercise time in minutes (D $\times$ E) .... _____

G. Average daily exercise time in minutes (F $\div$ 7) .... _____

H. Caloric expenditure per pound per minute (cal/lb/min) of selected physical
    activity (use Table 6.2, page 168) .... _____

I. Total calories burned per minute of exercise (A $\times$ H) .... _____

J. Average daily calories burned as a result of the exercise program (G $\times$ I) ... _____

K. Total daily caloric requirement with exercise to maintain body weight (B + J) ... _____

L. Number of calories to subtract from daily requirement to achieve a
    negative caloric balance (multiply current body weight by 5)** .... _____

M. Target caloric intake to lose weight (K − L) .... _____

*If more than one physical activity is selected, you will need to estimate the average daily calories burned as a result of each additional activity (steps C through J)
and add all of these figures to K above.

**This figure should not be below 1,500 calories, with the possible exception of 1,200 calories for small/petite women. See Activity 6.2 for the 1,200-, 1,500-, 1,800-,
and 2,000-calorie diet plans.

Activity 6.1 Caloric Requirement: Computation Form *(continued)*

1. How much effort are you willing to put into reaching your weight loss goal?

_____

_____

2. Indicate your feelings about participating in an exercise program.

_____

_____

3. Will you commit to be more physically active and to participate in a combined aerobic and strength-training program?
   Yes ☐   No ☐

   If your answer is "Yes," proceed to the next question; if you answered "No," please review Chapters 3 and 6 again.

4. Indicate your current number of daily steps: [   ]

5. List aerobic activities you enjoy or may enjoy doing.

_____

_____

6. Select one or two aerobic activities in which you will participate regularly.

   [   ]   [   ]

7. List facilities available to you where you can carry out the aerobic and strength-training programs.

_____

_____

8. Indicate days and times you will set aside for your aerobic and strength-training program (accumulate 60 to 90 minutes of physical activity 6 to 7 days per week, including 3 to 5 weekly sessions of aerobic exercise lasting about 30 minutes each and 2 to 3 weekly strength-training sessions).

   Monday: _____

   Tuesday: _____

   Wednesday: _____

   Thursday: _____

   Friday: _____

   Saturday: _____

   Sunday: _____

9. Conclusion: Briefly describe whether you think you can meet the goals of your physical activity, aerobic, and strength-training programs. What obstacles will you have to overcome, and how will you overcome them?

_____

_____

_____

Activity 6.2   Daily Food Intake Record Form

Name _____   **Date** _____

Course _____   **Section** _____

1,200 CALORIE DIET PLAN
Instructions:

The objective of the diet plan is to meet (not exceed) the number of servings allowed for the food groups listed. Each time that you eat a particular food, record it in the space provided for each group along with the amount you ate. Refer to the number of calories below to find out what counts as one serving for each group listed. Instead of the meat, poultry, fish, dry beans, eggs, and nuts group, you are allowed to have a commercially available low-fat frozen entree for your main meal (this entree should provide no more than 300 calories and less than 6 grams of fat). You can make additional copies of this form as needed.

Dairy: 2 servings
Grains: 6 servings
Fruits: 2 servings
Veggies: 3 servings
Protein: 1 low-fat frozen entree

ChooseMyPlate.gov

Daily grams of protein intake: Body weight in kg _____ × 1.5 and 2.0 = _____ g to _____ g

Grains (80 calories/serving): 6 servings   **Protein (g)**

1		
2		
3		
4		
5		
6		

Vegetables (25 calories/serving): 3 servings

1		
2		
3		

Fruits (60 calories/serving): 2 servings

| 1 | | |
| 2 | | |

Dairy (120 calories/serving, use low-fat milk and milk products): 2 servings

| 1 | | |
| 2 | | |

Low-fat Frozen Entree (300 calories and less than 6 grams of fat): 1 serving

| 1 | | |

Grams of protein consumed with each meal today: Breakfast: _____ g, Lunch: _____ g, Dinner: _____ g

Source: USDA 2011

Activity 6.2 **Daily Food Intake Record Form** *(continued)*

1,500 CALORIE DIET PLAN
Instructions:

The objective of the diet plan is to meet (not exceed) the number of servings allowed for the food groups listed. Each time that you eat a particular food, record it in the space provided for each group along with the amount you ate. Refer to the number of calories below to find out what counts as one serving for each group listed. Instead of the meat, poultry, fish, dry beans, eggs, and nuts group, you are allowed to have two commercially available low-fat frozen entrees for your main meal (these entrees should provide no more than 300 calories and less than 6 grams of fat). You can make additional copies of this form as needed.

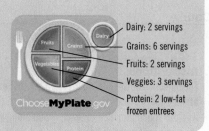

- Dairy: 2 servings
- Grains: 6 servings
- Fruits: 2 servings
- Veggies: 3 servings
- Protein: 2 low-fat frozen entrees

Daily grams of protein intake: Body weight in kg _____ × 1.5 and 2.0 = _____ g to _____ g

Grains (80 calories/serving): 6 servings   **Protein (g)**

1 ___
2 ___
3 ___
4 ___
5 ___
6 ___

Vegetables (25 calories/serving): 3 servings

1 ___
2 ___
3 ___

Fruits (60 calories/serving): 2 servings

1 ___
2 ___

Dairy (120 calories/serving, use low-fat milk and milk products): 2 servings

1 ___
2 ___

Two Low-fat Frozen Entrees (300 calories and less than 6 grams of fat): 2 servings

1 ___
2 ___

Grams of protein consumed with each meal today: Breakfast: _____ g, Lunch: _____ g, Dinner: _____ g

Source: USDA 2011

Activity 6.2 **Daily Food Intake Record Form** *(continued)*

1,800 CALORIE DIET PLAN
Instructions:
The objective of the diet plan is to meet (not exceed) the number of servings allowed for the food groups listed. Each time that you eat a particular food, record it in the space provided for each group along with the amount you ate. Refer to the number of calories below to find out what counts as one serving for each group listed. Instead of the meat, poultry, fish, dry beans, eggs, and nuts group, you are allowed to have two commercially available low-fat frozen entrees for your main meal (these entrees should provide no more than 300 calories and less than 6 grams of fat). You can make additional copies of this form as needed.

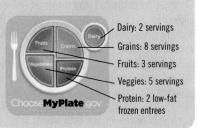

- Dairy: 2 servings
- Grains: 8 servings
- Fruits: 3 servings
- Veggies: 5 servings
- Protein: 2 low-fat frozen entrees

Daily grams of protein intake: Body weight in kg _____ × 1.5 and 2.0 = _____ g to _____ g

Grains (80 calories/serving): 8 servings   **Protein (g)**

1		
2		
3		
4		
5		
6		
7		
8		

Vegetables (25 calories/serving): 5 servings

1		
2		
3		
4		
5		

Fruits (60 calories/serving): 3 servings

1		
2		
3		

Dairy (120 calories/serving, use low-fat milk and milk products): 2 servings

1		
2		

Two Low-fat Frozen Entrees (300 calories and less than 6 grams of fat): 2 servings

1		
2		

Grams of protein consumed with each meal today: Breakfast: _____ g, Lunch: _____ g, Dinner: _____ g

Activity 6.2 Daily Food Intake Record Form *(continued)*

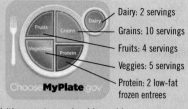

2,000 CALORIE DIET PLAN

Instructions:

The objective of the diet plan is to meet (not exceed) the number of servings allowed for the food groups listed. Each time that you eat a particular food, record it in the space provided for each group along with the amount you ate. Refer to the number of calories below to find out what counts as one serving for each group listed. Instead of the meat, poultry, fish, dry beans, eggs, and nuts group, you are allowed to have two commercially available low-fat frozen entrees for your main meal (these entrees should provide no more than 300 calories and less than 6 grams of fat). You can make additional copies of this form as needed.

Dairy: 2 servings
Grains: 10 servings
Fruits: 4 servings
Veggies: 5 servings
Protein: 2 low-fat frozen entrees

Daily grams of protein intake: Body weight in kg _____ $\times$ 1.5 and 2.0 = _____ g to _____ g

Grains (80 calories/serving): 10 servings   **Protein (g)**

1		
2		
3		
4		
5		
6		
7		
8		
9		
10		

Vegetables (25 calories/serving): 5 servings

1		
2		
3		
4		
5		

Fruits (60 calories/serving): 4 servings

1		
2		
3		
4		

Dairy (120 calories/serving, use low-fat milk and milk products): 2 servings

1		
2		

Two Low-fat Frozen Entrees (300 calories and less than 6 grams of fat): 2 servings

1		
2		

Grams of protein consumed with each meal today: Breakfast: _____ g, Lunch: _____ g, Dinner: _____ g

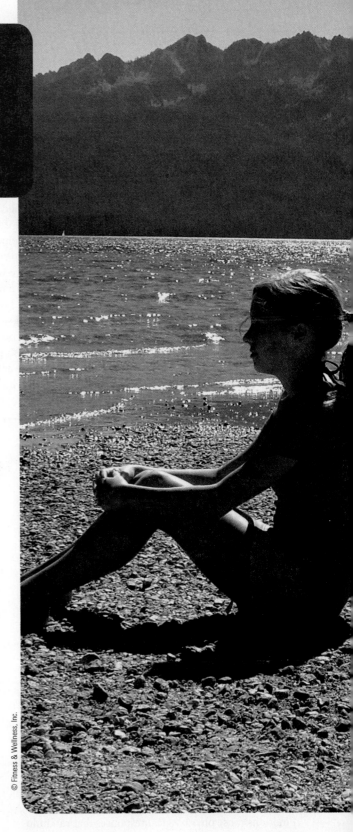

7

Stress Management

"Stress is the spice of life."
—Hans Selye

Objectives

> Define stress, eustress, and distress.
> Explain how stress affects health and optimal performance.
> Define the two major types of behavior patterns or personality types.
> Learn whether you have a hostile personality.
> Develop time management skills.
> Identify the major sources of stress in your life.
> Define the role of physical exercise in reducing stress.
> Learn to use various stress management techniques.

© Fitness & Wellness, Inc.

REAL LIFE STORY | Vicki's Fast-Paced Life

I have never been one to take life at a slow pace. In high school I danced on the drill team, took AP courses, and even worked part time for my brother. I was also on a local studio's dance team. I don't think I am a Type A person, but I certainly have led a very fast-paced life. To afford college, I needed to get a part-time job. I started out by taking 18 credit hours my first two semesters. I was getting by on 5 to 6 hours of sleep per night, I wasn't exercising, I was gaining weight, and I felt extremely stressed all the time. There were many times that I felt my heart racing even when quietly studying at the library. I checked my pulse once while lying in bed before going to sleep and my resting heart rate was 96 beats per minute. Near the end of my freshman year, I almost had a nervous breakdown. At the health center I was referred to the counseling center. It was there that I learned that I needed to slow down. The counselor helped me identify the main stressors in my life and we worked out a plan to help me slow down.

I realized that I only had one life to live and it was up to me to live life the best possible way that I could. I was also encouraged to start being more active and eating right. I took the summer off from school, except for one class: Lifetime Fitness and Wellness. I started to exercise and spent time learning how to manage stress effectively. For my sophomore year, I prioritized my activities—exercise, good nutrition, and 7 to 8 hours of sleep each night were at the top of my list. I eliminated time killers, planned short time-outs each day, and because of my part time job, I signed up for only 14 credits each semester. I feel much better, happier, and healthier now. My heart rate is down to 64, and my heart has not raced since summer, at the end of my freshman year.

Kurhan/Shutterstock.com

Learning to live and get ahead today is not possible without **stress**. To succeed in an unpredictable world that changes with every new day, working under pressure has become the rule rather than the exception for most people. As a result, stress has become one of the most common problems we face. Current estimates indicate that the annual cost of stress and stress-related diseases in the United States exceeds $300 billion, a direct result of health care costs, lost productivity, and absenteeism.

7.1 *The Mind/Body Connection*

A growing body of evidence indicates that virtually every illness known to modern humanity—from arthritis to migraine headaches, from the common cold to cancer—is influenced for good or bad by our emotions. To a profound extent, emotions affect our susceptibility to disease and our immunity. The way we react to what comes along in life can determine in great measure how we will react to the disease-causing organisms that we face. The feelings we have and the way we express them can either boost our immune system or weaken it.

Emotions cause physiological responses that can influence health. Certain parts of the brain are associated with specific emotions and specific hormone patterns. The release of certain hormones is associated with various emotional responses, and those hormones affect health. These responses may contribute to development of disease. Emotions have to be expressed somewhere, somehow. If they are suppressed repeatedly, as in stressful situations, and/or if a person feels conflict about controlling them, they often reveal themselves through physical symptoms. These physiological responses may weaken the immune system over time.

The immune system patrols and guards the body against attackers. This system consists of about a trillion cells called **lymphocytes** (the cells responsible for waging war against disease or infection) and many trillions of molecules called **antibodies**. The brain and the immune system are closely linked in a connection that allows the mind to influence both susceptibility and resistance to disease.

A fighting spirit also plays a major role in the recovery from illness. A fighting spirit involves the healthy expression of emotions, whether they are negative or positive. Many physicians believe that a patient's attitude, especially a fighting spirit, is the underlying factor in spontaneous remission from incurable illness. Fighters are not stronger or more capable than others—they simply do not give up easily. They enjoy better health and live longer, even when physicians and laboratory tests say they should not.

Sleep and Wellness

Sleep is a natural state of rest that is vital for good health and wellness. It is an anabolic process that allows the body to restore and heal itself. During sleep, we replenish depleted energy levels and allow the brain, muscles, organs, and various body tissues to repair themselves.

Sleep deprivation weakens the immune system, impairs mental function, and has a negative impact on physical, social, academic, and job performance. Lack of sleep also impacts stress levels, mood, memory, behavioral patterns, and cognitive performance. Cumulative long-term consequences include an increase in the risk for cardiovascular disease, high blood pressure, obesity, diabetes, and psychological disorders. People who get less sleep have a threefold increased risk of getting a cold, are more likely to develop coronary heart disease earlier in life, increase body-wide inflammation, and have higher blood levels of the stress hormone cortisol. What most people notice is a chronic state of fatigue, exhaustion, and confusion.

Stress-wise, getting to bed too late often leads to oversleeping, napping, missing classes, poor grades, and distress. It further increases tension, irritability, intolerance, and confusion, and may cause depression and life dissatisfaction. Not getting enough sleep can also lead to vehicle accidents with serious or fatal consequences as people fall asleep behind the wheel. More than 5,000 fatal crashes each year may be attributed to sleepy drivers. (Sleepy drivers are just as dangerous as drunken drivers.) Irregular sleep patterns, including sleeping in on weekends, also contribute to many of the aforementioned problems.

Although more than 100 sleep disorders have been identified, they can be classified into four major groups:

- Problems with falling and staying asleep
- Difficulties staying awake
- Difficulty adhering to a regular sleep schedule
- Sleep-disruptive behaviors (including sleepwalking and sleep terror disorder)

College students are some of the most sleep-deprived people of all. On average, they sleep about 6 and a half hours per night, and approximately 30 percent report chronic sleep difficulties. Only 8 percent report sleeping 8 or more hours per night. For many students, college is the first time they have complete control of their schedule, including when they go to sleep and how many hours they sleep.

Lack of sleep during school days and pulling all-nighters interferes with the ability to pay attention, learn, process, and retain new information. You may be able to retain the information in short-term memory, but it will most likely not be there for a cumulative exam or when you need it for adequate job performance. Deep sleep that takes place early in the night, and a large portion of the REM (rapid eye movement) dream sleep that occurs near the end of the night, have both been linked to learning. The brain has been shown to consolidate new information for long-term memory while you sleep. Convincing sleep-deprived students to get adequate sleep is a real challenge because they often feel overwhelmed by school, work, and family responsibilities. Students who go to sleep early and get about eight hours of sleep per night are more apt to succeed.

Compounding the problem is staying up late Friday and Saturday nights and crashing the next day. Doing so further disrupts the circadian rhythm, the biological clock that controls the daily sleep/wake schedule. Such disruption influences quantity and quality of sleep and keeps people from falling asleep and rising at the necessary times for school, work, or other required activities. In essence, the body wants to sleep and be awake at odd times of the 24-hour cycle.

A term used to describe the cumulative effect of needed sleep that you don't get is sleep debt. Crashing on weekends, although it may help somewhat, does not solve the problem. You need to address the problem behavior by getting sufficient sleep each night so that you can be at your best the next day.

The exact amount of sleep that each person needs varies among individuals. Most people require about eight hours. According to the National Sleep Foundation, most people get about seven hours of sleep per night. Experts believe that the last two hours of sleep are the most vital for well-being. Thus, if you need eight hours of sleep and you routinely get six, you may be forfeiting the most critical sleep hours for health and wellness. Most students do not address sleep disorders until they start to cause mental and physical damage.

While there is no magic formula to determine how much sleep you need, if you don't need an alarm clock to get up every morning, you wake up at about the same time, and you are refreshed and feel alert throughout the day, you most likely have a healthy sleeping habit.

To improve your sleep pattern, you need to exercise discipline and avoid staying up late to watch a movie or leaving your homework or studying for an exam until

---

GLOSSARY

Stress The mental, emotional, and physiological response of the body to any situation that is new, threatening, frightening, or exciting.

Lymphocytes Immune system cells responsible for waging war against disease or infection.

Antibodies Substances produced by the white blood cells in response to an invading agent.

the last minute. As busy as you are, your health and well-being are your most important assets. You only live once. Keeping your health and living life to its fullest potential include a good night's rest. Take the following steps to enhance the quality of your sleep:

- Exercise and be physically active (avoid exercise four hours prior to bedtime).
- Avoid eating a heavy meal or snacking two to three hours before going to bed (digestion increases your metabolism).
- Limit the amount of time that you spend (primarily in the evening) surfing and socializing on the Internet, texting, and watching television.
- Go to bed and rise at about the same time each day.
- Keep the bedroom cool, quiet, and dark.
- Develop a bedtime ritual (meditation, prayer, and white noise).
- Use your bed for sleeping only (do not watch television, do homework, or use a laptop in bed).
- Relax and slow down 15 to 30 minutes before bedtime.
- Do not drink coffee or caffeine-containing beverages several hours before going to bed.
- Do not rely on alcohol to fall asleep (alcohol disrupts deep sleep stages).
- Avoid long naps (a 20- to 30-minute "power nap" is beneficial during an afternoon slump without interfering with nighttime sleep).
- Have frank and honest conversations with roommates if they have different sleep schedules.
- Evaluate your mattress every five to seven years for comfort and support. If you wake up with aches and pains or you sleep better when you are away from home, it is most likely time for a new mattress.

7.2 *Stress*

Every person has an optimal level of stress that is most conducive to adequate health and performance. When stress levels reach mental, emotional, and physiological limits, however, stress becomes distress and the person no longer functions effectively.

The body's response to stress has been the same ever since humans were first put on the earth. Stress prepares the organism to react to the stress-causing event, called the **stressor**. The difference is the way in which we react to stress. Many people thrive under stress. Others under similar circumstances are unable to handle it. An individual's reaction to a stress-causing agent determines whether stress is positive or negative.

Chronic negative reactions to stress raise the risk for many health disorders, including coronary heart disease, hypertension, eating disorders, ulcers, diabetes, asthma,

depression, migraine headaches, sleep disorders, and chronic fatigue, and may even play a role in the development of certain types of cancer. Crucial in maintaining emotional and physiological stability is to recognize when stress has a negative effect and to overcome the stressful condition quickly and efficiently.

The good news is that stress can be self-controlled. Most people have accepted stress as a normal part of daily life, and even though everyone has to deal with it, few seem to understand it and know how to cope effectively. People should not try to avoid stress entirely, as a certain amount is necessary for optimum health, performance, and well-being. It is difficult to succeed and have fun in life without "hits, runs, and errors."

7.3 *The Body's Reaction to Stress*

Dr. Hans Selye, one of the foremost authorities on stress, defined it as "the nonspecific response of the human organism to any demand that is placed upon it."[1] "Nonspecific" indicates that the body reacts in a similar way regardless of the nature of the event that leads to the stress response. In simpler terms, stress is the body's mental, emotional, and physiological response to any situation that is new, threatening, frightening, or exciting.

The body responds to stress with a rapid-fire sequence of physical changes known as **fight** or **flight** (see Figure 7.1). The hypothalamus activates the sympathetic nervous system, and the pituitary gland triggers the release of catecholamines (hormones) from the adrenal glands. These hormonal changes increase heart rate, blood pressure, blood flow to active muscles and the brain, glucose levels, oxygen consumption, and strength—all necessary for the body to either fight or flee. In cases of both fight and flight, the body relaxes and stress dissipates. If the person is unable to take action, however, the muscles tense and tighten instead.

Stress isn't necessarily bad. Selye further defined stress as either **eustress** or **distress**. In both cases, the nonspecific response is almost the same. In eustress, health and performance continue to improve even as stress increases. With distress, health and performance begin to deteriorate.

Critical Thinking

Can you identify sources of eustress and distress in your personal life during this past year? • Explain your emotional and physical response to each stressor and how the two differ.

Figure 7.1 Physiological response to stress: Fight or flight.

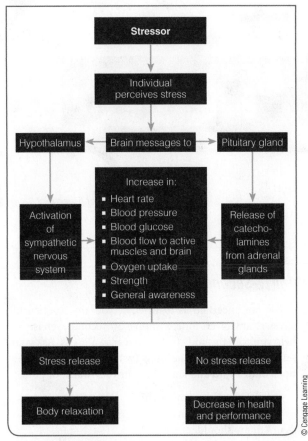

7.4 *Adaptation to Stress*

Human physiology is such that the body continuously strives to maintain a constant internal environment. This state of physiological balance, known as **homeostasis**, allows the body to function as effectively as possible. When a stressor triggers a nonspecific response, homeostasis is disrupted. This reaction to stressors, best explained by Selye through the **general adaptation syndrome (GAS)**, is composed of three stages: alarm reaction, resistance, and exhaustion/recovery.

Alarm Reaction

The alarm reaction is the immediate response to a stressor, whether positive or negative. During the alarm reaction, the body evokes an instant physiological reaction that involves the mobilization of systems and processes within the organism to minimize the threat to homeostasis (see "Coping with Stress," page 192). If the stressor subsides, the body recovers and returns to homeostasis.

Resistance

If the stressor persists, the body calls upon its limited reserves to build up resistance as it strives to maintain homeostasis. For a short while, the body copes effectively and meets the challenge of the stressor until it can be overcome (see Figure 7.2).

Exhaustion/Recovery

If stress becomes chronic and intolerable, the body spends its limited reserves and loses its ability to cope, entering the exhaustion/recovery stage. During this stage, the body functions at a diminished capacity while it recovers from stress. In due time, following an "adequate" recovery period, the body recuperates and is able to return to homeostasis. If chronic stress persists during the exhaustion stage, however, immune function is compromised, which can damage body systems and lead to disease.

An example of the stress response through the general adaptation syndrome can be illustrated in college test performance. As you prepare to take an exam, you experience an initial alarm reaction. If you understand the material, study for the exam, and do well (eustress), the body recovers and stress is dissipated. If, however, you are not adequately prepared and fail the exam, the resistance stage is triggered. You are now concerned about your grade, and you remain in the resistance stage until the next exam. If you prepare and do well, the body recovers. But if you fail once again and no longer can bring up your grade, exhaustion sets in, with possible physical and emotional breakdowns as a result. Exhaustion may be aggravated if you are struggling in other courses as well.

GLOSSARY

Stressor Stress-causing agent.

Fight or flight A series of physical responses activated automatically in response to environmental stressors.

Eustress Positive stress.

Distress Negative or harmful stress under which health and performance begin to deteriorate.

Homeostasis A natural state of equilibrium. The body attempts to maintain this equilibrium by constantly reacting to external forces that attempt to disrupt this fine balance.

General adaptation syndrome (GAS) A theoretical model that explains the body's adaptation to sustained stress; it includes three stages: alarm reaction, resistance, and exhaustion/recovery

Figure 7.2 General adaptation syndrome: The body's response to stress.

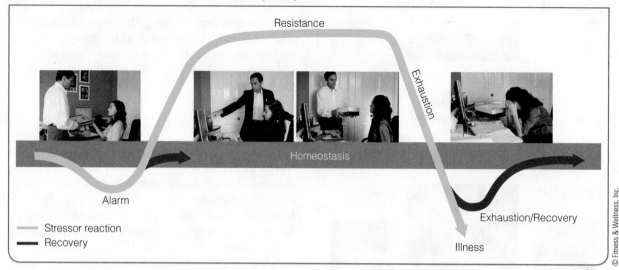

Resistance

Exhaustion

Homeostasis

Alarm

Exhaustion/Recovery

Illness

- - - Stressor reaction
—— Recovery

© Fitness & Wellness, Inc.

The exhaustion stage is often manifested in athletes and the most ardent fitness participants. Staleness is usually a consequence of overtraining. Peak performance can be sustained for only about two to three weeks at a time. Any attempts to continue intense training after peaking lead to exhaustion, diminished fitness, and mental and physical problems associated with overtraining. Thus, athletes and some fitness participants also need an active recovery phase following the attainment of peak fitness.

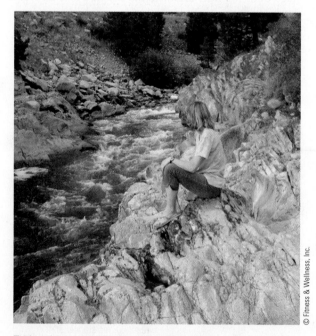

Taking time out during stressful life events is vital for good health and wellness.

© Fitness & Wellness, Inc.

Thirty-Second Body Scan

If you are uncertain as to whether you are experiencing stress at any given time, a simple 30-second exercise can help you scan the body to raise stress awareness. Ask yourself the following 10 questions (you can copy these questions onto a card and keep them in your wallet or purse):

- Am I clenching my teeth?
- Am I furrowing my brow?
- Are my shoulders tense?
- Am I breathing rapidly?
- Am I tapping my fingers?
- Do I feel knots in my stomach?
- Are my arms, thighs, or calves tight?
- Am I nervously bouncing my leg or foot?
- Am I curling my toes?
- Do I feel uneasiness anywhere else in my body?

The body scan can be performed daily or several times a day to help you learn to recognize when you are distressed. People are often unaware of stress signals and activities that are causing excessive stress. Increasing awareness allows you to initiate proper actions to more effectively manage stress. An example would be to breathe deeply for one to three minutes while doing the body scan and repeating positive affirmations (e.g., "I am at peace" or "I am calm and relaxed").

7.5 *Behavior Patterns*

All too often, individuals bring on stress as a result of their characteristic behavior patterns. The two main types of behavior patterns are **Type A** and **Type B**. Each

Behavior Modification Planning

Releasing Anger the Healthy Way

- Recognize the anger for what it is. Don't be afraid of it or try to suppress it.

- Figure out what made you so angry, then decide whether it's worth being so upset. Chances are that it's really a minor irritation or hassle.

- Stop before you act. Calm down first. Count to 10, take a deep breath, mentally recite the words to a favorite verse, or initiate some other distracting and relaxing activity. Then get ready to deal with the anger.

- If you're angry with somebody else, use calm tact to say why, without ripping into the other person. Tell him or her how you're feeling and try to negotiate some things.

- Be generous with the other person. Maybe he just failed an exam. Maybe she just heard bad news from home.

Maybe he's having a rotten day. Listen carefully to her side of things and try as much as you can to understand.

- When all else fails, forgive the other person. Everyone makes mistakes. Carrying a grudge will hurt you worse than it hurts the other person.

Try It

If you feel that anger is disrupting your health and relationships, the above actions can help you manage anger and restore a sense of well-being in your life. In your Online Journal or class notebook, list some strategies you can use to manage anger, study them each morning, and then evaluate yourself every night for the next day.

From Hoeger/Turner/Hafen, *Wellness*, 4E. © 2007 Cengage Learning.

---

type is based on several characteristics that are used to classify people into one of these behavioral patterns.

Type A behavior characterizes a primarily hard-driving, overly ambitious, aggressive, at times hostile, and overly competitive person. Type A individuals often set their own goals, are self-motivated, try to accomplish many tasks at the same time, are excessively achievement-oriented, and have a sense of time urgency. By contrast, Type B behavior is characteristic of calm, casual, relaxed, easygoing individuals. Type B people take one thing at a time, do not feel pressured or hurried, and seldom set their own deadlines.

Over the years, experts have indicated that individuals classified as Type A have a significantly higher incidence for disease, especially cardiovascular conditions.[2] Not all typical Type A people, however, are at higher risk for disease. Type A individuals who are chronically angry and hostile are at higher risk.[3] The questionnaire provided in Figure 7.3 can help you determine whether you have a hostile personality.

Some experts believe that emotional stress is far more likely than physical stress to trigger a heart attack. Especially vulnerable are people who are impatient and are readily annoyed when they have to wait for someone or something—an employee, a traffic light, in a restaurant line.

Research also is focusing on individuals who have anxiety, depression, and feelings of helplessness when they encounter setbacks and failures in life. People who lose control of their lives, those who give up on their dreams in life, knowing that they could and should be doing better, may be more likely to have heart attacks than hard-driving people who enjoy their work.

Many of the Type A characteristics are learned behaviors. Consequently, if people can learn to identify the sources of stress, they can change their behavioral responses. The main assessment tool to determine behavioral type is the structured interview, in which the interviewee is asked to reply to several questions that describe Type A and Type B behavior patterns. The interviewer notes the responses to the questions and also mental, emotional, and physical behaviors the individual exhibits as he or she replies to each question. Based on the answers and the associated behaviors, the interviewer rates the person along a continuum ranging from Type A to Type B.

7.6 *Vulnerability to Stress*

A number of factors affect the way in which people handle stress. How we deal with these factors actually can increase or decrease vulnerability to stress. The

---

GLOSSARY

Type A Behavior pattern characteristic of a hard-driving, overambitious, aggressive, at times hostile, and overly competitive person.

Type B Behavior pattern characteristic of a calm, casual, relaxed, and easygoing individual.

Figure 7.3 Hostility questionnaire.

Type A individuals with a hostile personality are at higher risk for disease. This questionnaire can help you identify if you have a hostile personality. Please circle the number of points that best represents your response to each statement.

	Never	Occasionally	Frequently	Always
1. I am impatient.	0	1	2	3
2. I am easily irritated.	0	1	2	3
3. I am argumentative.	0	1	2	3
4. I want to have the final word in every discussion.	0	1	2	3
5. I attack people verbally.	0	1	2	3
6. I am physically aggressive when angry.	0	1	2	3
7. I stop before I act when upset.	3	2	1	0
8. I manage anger at once—I do not let it build up.	3	2	1	0
9. I engage in healthy physical activity when upset or angry.	3	2	1	0
10. I am understanding of unplanned surprises.	3	2	1	0
11. I keep a journal and contemplate what caused me to be angry.	3	2	1	0
12. I give others the benefit of the doubt.	3	2	1	0
13. I am a forgiving person.	3	2	1	0
14. I use positive responses.	3	2	1	0
15. I schedule daily timeouts.	3	2	1	0
16. I sleep 7 to 8 hours per night.	3	2	1	0

Scoring.
Any number of points $\geq$ 1 obtained in items 5, 6, or 7 = _____   = Hostile Personality
Total points for items 1 to 3 and 8 to 16 = _____   A score $\geq$ 10 points = Hostile Personality

If the scores above indicate that you may have a hostile personality, professional counseling is recommended. The student counseling services at your institution may provide health services to help enhance personal growth, manage stress and hostile behavior, and develop personal effectiveness and resilience. You are strongly encouraged to take steps to control your responses to situations that trigger hostile behavior.

© Fitness & Wellness, Inc.

questionnaire provided in Figure 7.4 lists these factors so you can determine your vulnerability rating. Many of the items on this questionnaire are related to health, social support, self-worth, and nurturance (sense of being needed). All of the factors are crucial for a person's physical, social, mental, and emotional well-being. The questionnaire will help you identify specific areas in which you can make improvements to help you cope more efficiently.

The benefits of physical fitness are discussed extensively in this book. In addition, social support, self-worth, and nurturance are essential to cope effectively

with stressful life events. These factors play a supportive and protective role in people's lives. The more integrated people are in society, the less vulnerable they are to stress and illness.

Positive correlations have been found between social support and health outcomes. People can draw upon social support to weather crises. Knowing that someone else cares, that people are there to lean on, that support is out there, is valuable for survival (or growth) in times of need.[4]

As you complete the questionnaire, you will notice that many of the items describe situations and behaviors that

Figure 7.4 Stress vulnerability questionnaire.

Item	Strongly Agree	Mildly Agree	Mildly Disagree	Strongly Disagree
1. I try to incorporate as much physical activity* as possible in my daily schedule.	1	2	3	4
2. I exercise aerobically 20 minutes or more at least 3 times per week.	1	2	3	4
3. I regularly sleep seven to eight hours per night.	1	2	3	4
4. I take my time eating at least one hot, balanced meal a day.	1	2	3	4
5. I drink fewer than two cups of coffee (or equivalent) per day.	1	2	3	4
6. I am at recommended body weight.	1	2	3	4
7. I enjoy good health.	1	2	3	4
8. I do not use tobacco in any form.	1	2	3	4
9. I limit my alcohol intake to no more than one (women) or two (men) drinks per day.	1	2	3	4
10. I do not use hard drugs (chemical dependency).	1	2	3	4
11. I have someone I love, trust, and can rely on for help if I have a problem or need to make an essential decision.	1	2	3	4
12. There is love in my family.	1	2	3	4
13. I routinely give and receive affection.	1	2	3	4
14. I have close personal relationships with other people who provide me with a sense of emotional security.	1	2	3	4
15. There are people close by whom I can turn to for guidance in time of stress.	1	2	3	4
16. I can speak openly about feelings, emotions, and problems with people I trust.	1	2	3	4
17. Other people rely on me for help.	1	2	3	4
18. I am able to keep my feelings of anger and hostility under control.	1	2	3	4
19. I have a network of friends who enjoy the same social activities I do.	1	2	3	4
20. I take time to do something fun at least once a week.	1	2	3	4
21. My religious beliefs provide guidance and strength to my life.	1	2	3	4
22. I often provide service to others.	1	2	3	4
23. I enjoy my job (major or school).	1	2	3	4
24. I am a competent worker.	1	2	3	4
25. I get along well with coworkers (or students).	1	2	3	4
26. My income is sufficient for my needs.	1	2	3	4
27. I manage time adequately.	1	2	3	4
28. I have learned to say "no" to additional commitments when I am already pressed for time.	1	2	3	4
29. I take daily quiet time for myself.	1	2	3	4
30. I practice stress management as needed.	1	2	3	4

Total Points: [   ]

Scoring:

0–30 points	Excellent (great resistance to stress)
31–40 points	Good (little vulnerability to stress)
41–50 points	Average (somewhat vulnerable to stress)
51–60 points	Fair (vulnerable to stress)
≥61 points	Poor (highly vulnerable to stress)

*Walk instead of driving, avoid escalators and elevators, or walk to neighboring offices, homes, and stores.

© Fitness & Wellness, Inc.

Behavior Modification Planning

Changing a Type A Personality

- Make a contract with yourself to slow down and take it easy. Put it in writing. Post it in a conspicuous spot, then stick to the terms you set up. Be specific. Abstracts ("I'm going to be less uptight") don't work.

- Work on only one or two things at a time. Wait until you change one habit before you tackle the next one.

- Eat more slowly and eat only when you are relaxed and sitting down.

- If you smoke, quit.

- Cut down on your caffeine intake, because it increases the tendency to become irritated and agitated.

- Take regular breaks throughout the day, even as brief as 5 or 10 minutes, when you totally change what you're doing. Get up, stretch, get a drink of cool water, or walk around for a few minutes.

- Work on fighting your impatience. If you're standing in line at the grocery store, study the interesting things people have in their carts instead of getting upset.

- Work on controlling hostility. Keep a written log. When do you flare up? What causes it? How do you feel at the time? What preceded it? Look for patterns and figure out what sets you off. Then do something about it. Either avoid the situations that cause you hostility or practice reacting to them in different ways.

- Plan some activities just for the fun of it. Load a picnic basket in the car and drive to the country with a friend. After a stressful physics class, stop at a theater and see a good comedy.

- Choose a role model, someone you know and admire who does not have a Type A personality. Observe the person carefully, then try out some techniques the person demonstrates.

- Simplify your life so you can learn to relax a little. Figure out which activities or commitments you can eliminate right now, then get rid of them.

- If morning is a problem time for you and you get too hurried, set your alarm clock half an hour earlier.

- Take time out during even the most hectic day to do something truly relaxing. Because you won't be used to it, you may have to work at it at first. Begin by listing things you'd really enjoy that would calm you. Include some things that take only a few minutes: Watch a sunset, lie out on the lawn at night and look at the stars, call an old friend and catch up on news, take a nap, or sauté a pan of mushrooms and savor them slowly.

- If you're under a deadline, take short breaks. Stop and talk to someone for 5 minutes, take a short walk, or lie down with a cool cloth over your eyes for 10 minutes.

- Pay attention to what your own body clock is saying. You've probably noticed that every 90 minutes or so, you lose the ability to concentrate, get a little sleepy, and have a tendency to daydream. Instead of fighting the urge, put down your work and let your mind wander for a few minutes. Use the time to imagine and let your creativity run free.

- Learn to treasure unplanned surprises: a friend dropping by unannounced, a hummingbird outside your window, or a child's tightly clutched bouquet of wildflowers.

- Savor your relationships. Think about the people in your life. Relax with them and give yourself to them. Give up trying to control others and resist the urge to end relationships that don't always go as you'd like them to.

Try It

If Type A describes your personality, pick three of the above strategies and apply them in your life this week. At the end of each day, determine how well you have done that day and evaluate how you can improve the next day.

From Hoeger/Turner/Hafen, *Wellness*, 4E. © 2007 Cengage Learning.

are within your own control. To make yourself less vulnerable to stress, you will want to improve the behaviors that make you more vulnerable to stress. You should start by modifying the behaviors that are easiest to change before undertaking some of the most difficult ones.

7.7 Sources of Stress

Before addressing techniques that you can use to cope more effectively with stress, attempt to identify your current life stressors using the stress test provided in Figure 7.5. This

Figure 7.5 Stress test.

Take the Stress Test

To get a feel for the possible health impact of the various recent changes in your life, think back over the past year and circle the "stress points" listed for each of the events that you experienced during that time. Then add up your points. A total score of anywhere from about 250 to 500 or so would be considered a moderate amount of stress. If you score higher than that, you may face an increased risk of illness; if you score lower than that, consider yourself fortunate.

Health

An injury or illness that:	
kept you in bed a week or more, or sent you to the hospital	74
was less serious than that	44
Major dental work	26
Major change in eating habits	27
Major change in sleeping habits	26
Major change in your usual type or amount of recreation	28

Work

Change to a new type of work	51
Change in your work hours or conditions	35
Change in your responsibilities at work:	
more responsibilities	29
fewer responsibilities	21
promotion	31
demotion	42
transfer	32
Troubles at work:	
with your boss	29
with your coworkers	35
with persons under your supervision	35
other work troubles	28
Major business adjustment	60
Retirement	52
Loss of job:	
laid off from work	68
fired from work	79
Correspondence course to help you in your work	18

Home and Family

Major change in living conditions	42
Change in residence:	
move within the same town or city	25
move to a different town, city, or state	47
Change in family get-togethers	25
Major change in health or behavior of family member	55
Marriage	50
Pregnancy	67
Miscarriage or abortion	85
Gain of a new family member:	
birth of a child	66
adoption of a child	65
a relative moving in with you	59
Spouse beginning or ending work	46
Child leaving home:	
to attend college	41
due to marriage	41
for other reasons	45
Change in arguments with spouse	50
In-law problems	38
Change in the marital status of your parents:	
divorce	59
remarriage	50
Separation from spouse:	
due to work	53
due to marital problems	76
Divorce	96
Birth of grandchild	43
Death of spouse	119
Death of other family member:	
child	123
brother or sister	102
parent	100

Personal and Social

Change in personal habits	26
Beginning or ending school or college	38
Change of school or college	35
Change in political beliefs	24
Change in religious beliefs	29
Change in social activities	27
Vacation trip	24
New, close, personal relationship	37
Engagement to marry	45
Girlfriend or boyfriend problems	39
Sexual difficulties	44
"Falling out" of a close personal relationship	47
An accident	48
Minor violation of the law	20
Being held in jail	75
Death of a close friend	70
Major decision about your immediate future	51
Major personal achievement	36

Financial

Major change in finances:	
increased income	38
decreased income	60
investment or credit difficulties	56
Loss or damage of personal property	43
Moderate purchase	20
Major purchase	37
Foreclosure on a mortgage or loan	58

Total Score: [   ]

SOURCE: From Hoeger/Hoeger, Cengage Advantage Books: *Lifetime Physical Fitness and Wellness*, 12E. © 2016 Cengage Learning.

Figure 7.6 Stressors in the lives of college students.

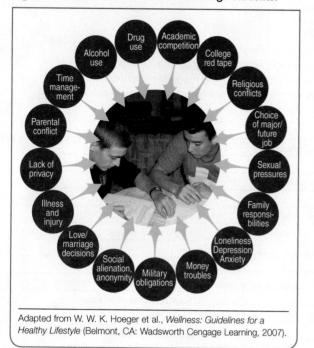

Adapted from W. W. K. Hoeger et al., *Wellness: Guidelines for a Healthy Lifestyle* (Belmont, CA: Wadsworth Cengage Learning, 2007).

test will help you determine stressors that you have encountered recently in your life. Think back over this past year and circle the "stress points" listed for each event that you experienced during this time. Then total the points and determine the amount of stress in your life during the past year.

Now, to help you cope more effectively, use the stress analysis form provided in Activity 7.1, pages 203–204. On this form, record the results of your stress questionnaires and list the stressors that affect you the most in your daily life. For each stressor, explain in the box provided the situation(s) under which it occurs, your response to it, the impact it is having in your life, and how you currently are handling the stressor. Based on what you have learned already, also indicate what you can do to either avoid the stressor or cope more effectively with it in the future. Common stressors in the lives of college students are depicted in Figure 7.6.

After completing the exercise in Activity 7.1, proceed to the discussion of relaxation techniques, pages 196–202. Once you have learned and mastered some of these techniques, return to your stress analysis and reevaluate your approach to cope with each stressor.

7.8 *Coping with Stress*

The ways in which people perceive and cope with stress seem to be more important in the development of disease than the amount and type of stress itself. If individuals perceive stress as a definite problem in their lives, when it interferes with their optimal level of health and performance, several techniques can help in coping more effectively.

First, of course, the person must recognize that a problem is present. Many people either do not want to believe they are under too much stress or they fail to recognize some of the typical symptoms of distress. Noting some of the stress-related symptoms will help a person respond more objectively and initiate an adequate coping response.

When people have stress-related symptoms, they first should try to identify and remove the stressor or stress-causing agent. This is not as simple as it may seem because in some situations eliminating the stressor is not possible or a person may not even know what has caused it. If the cause is unknown, keeping a log of the time and days when the symptoms arise, as well as the events preceding and following the onset of symptoms, might be helpful.

For instance, a couple noted that every afternoon around six o'clock, the wife became nauseated and had abdominal pain. After seeking professional help, both were instructed to keep a log of daily events. It soon became clear that the symptoms did not appear on weekends but always started just before the husband came home from work during the week. Following some personal interviews with the couple, it was determined that the wife felt a lack of attention from her husband and responded subconsciously by becoming ill to the point at which she required personal attention and affection from her husband. Once the stressor was identified, they initiated appropriate behavior changes to correct the situation.

In many instances, however, the stressor cannot be removed. Examples of situations in which little or nothing can be done to eliminate the stress-causing agent are the death of a close family member, first year on the job, an intolerable roommate, or a difficult college course. Nevertheless, stress can be managed through time management and relaxation techniques.

7.9 *Time Management*

The current "hurry-up" style of life is not conducive to wellness. The hassles involved in getting through a typical day often lead to stress-related illnesses. People who do not manage their time properly may experience chronic stress, fatigue, despair, discouragement, and illness.

Based on various national surveys, almost 80 percent of Americans report that time moves too fast for them. The younger the respondents, the more they struggled with lack of time. Almost half wished they had more time for exercise and recreation, hobbies, and family.

Common Time Killers

- Watching television or listening to the radio/music
- Excessive sleeping
- Surfing/socializing on the Internet
- Unnecessary texting and e-mailing
- Daydreaming
- Shopping
- Socializing/parties
- Excessive recreation
- Talking on the telephone
- Worrying
- Procrastinating
- Drop-in visitors
- Confusion (unclear goals)
- Indecision (what to do next)
- Interruptions
- Perfectionism (every detail must be done)

© Cengage Learning

Healthy and successful people are good time managers, able to maintain a pace of life within their comfort zone. In a survey of 1,954 Harvard graduates from the School of Business, only 27 percent had reached the goals they established in college. Upon graduation, all had rated themselves as a superior time manager, and now only 8 percent perceived themselves as superior time managers. The successful graduates attributed their success to "smart work," not necessarily "hard work."

Trying to achieve one or more goals in a limited time can create a tremendous amount of stress. The greatest demands on our time, nonetheless, frequently are self-imposed—trying to do too much, too fast, too soon.

Although some time killers such as eating, sleeping, and recreation are necessary for health and wellness, in excess they will cause stress. To make better use of your time:

1. **Find the time killers.** Many people do not know how they spend each part of the day. Keep a four- to seven-day log, and record your activities at half-hour intervals. As you go through your typical day, record the activities so you will remember all of them. At the end of each day, decide when you wasted time. You might be shocked by the amount of time you spent on the phone, sleeping (more than eight hours per night), or watching television.

2. **Set long-range and short-range goals.** Setting goals requires some in-depth thinking and helps put your life and daily tasks in perspective. Write down three goals that you want to accomplish (a) in life, (b) 10 years from now, (c) this year, (d) this month, and (e) this week. You may want to file this form and review it in years to come.

3. **Identify your immediate goals and prioritize them for today and this week.** Each day, sit down and determine what you need to accomplish that day and that week. Rank your "today" and "this week" tasks in three categories: (a) top priority, (b) medium priority, and (c) "trash." Top-priority tasks are clearly the most important ones. If you were to reap most of your productivity from 30 percent of your activities, which would they be? Medium-priority activities must be done but can wait a day or two. Trash activities are those that are not worth your time (for example, cruising the hallways).

4. **Use a daily planner to help you organize and simplify your day.** New digital tools have made it easier to have daily tasks and calendared items readily accessible for quick reference from laptops, smart phones, or other mobile devices. In this way you can access your priority list, appointments, notes, phone numbers, and addresses conveniently from your backpack, pocket, or purse. Many individuals think that planning daily and weekly activities is a waste of time. A few minutes to schedule your time each day, however, will pay off in hours saved.

As you plan your day, be realistic and find your comfort zone. Determine what is the best way to organize your day. Which is the most

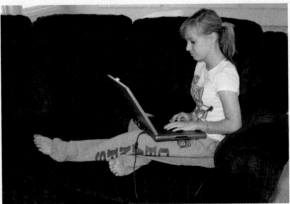

Planning and prioritizing your daily activities simplifies your days.

© Fitness & Wellness, Inc.

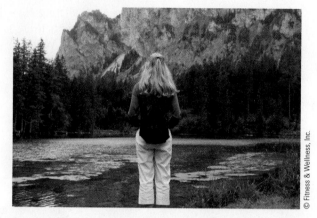

Regular leisure-time physical activity helps prevent psychological burnout.

productive time for work, study, or errands? Are you a morning person, or are you getting most of your work done when other people are quitting for the day? Pick your best hours for top-priority activities. Be sure to schedule enough time for

exercise and relaxation. Recreation is not necessarily wasted time. You need to take care of your physical and emotional well-being to ensure a balanced lifestyle.

5. **Take a few minutes each night to figure out how well you accomplished your goals that day.** Successful time managers evaluate themselves daily. This simple task will help you see the entire picture. Cross off the goals you accomplished, and carry over to the next day those you did not get done. You also may realize that some goals can be reclassified as low priority or be trashed.

In addition to the previous steps, the following general suggestions can help you make better use of your time:

- **Delegate.** When possible, delegate activities that someone else can do for you. Having another person type your paper while you prepare for an exam might be well worth the expense and your time.

Behavior Modification Planning

Common Symptoms of Stress

- Headaches
- Muscular aches (mainly in neck, shoulders, and back)
- Grinding teeth
- Nervous tic, finger tapping, or toe tapping
- Increased sweating
- Increase in or loss of appetite
- Insomnia
- Nightmares
- Fatigue
- Dry mouth
- Stuttering
- High blood pressure
- Tightness or pain in the chest
- Impotence
- Hives
- Dizziness
- Depression
- Irritation

- Anger
- Hostility
- Fear, panic, or anxiety
- Stomach pain or flutters
- Nausea
- Cold, clammy hands
- Poor concentration
- Pacing
- Restlessness
- Rapid heart rate
- Low-grade infection
- Loss of sex drive
- Rash or acne

Try It

If you regularly experience some of the above symptoms, use your Online Journal or class notebook to keep a log of when these symptoms occur and under what circumstances. You may discover that a pattern emerges when you experience distress in life.

© Cengage Learning

- **Say "no."** Learn to say no to activities that keep you from getting your top priorities done. You can do only so much in a single day. Many people are afraid to say no because they feel guilty if they do. Think ahead, and think of the consequences. Are you doing it to please others? What will it do to your well-being? Can you handle one more task? At some point you have to balance your activities and look at life and time realistically.

- **Avoid boredom.** Doing nothing can be a source of stress. People need to feel that they are contributing and that they are productive members of society. It also is good for self-esteem and self-worth. Set realistic goals, and work toward them each day.

- **Plan ahead for disruptions.** Even a careful plan of action can be disrupted. An unexpected phone call or visitor can ruin your schedule. Planning your response ahead of time will help you deal with these saboteurs.

- **Get it done.** Select only one task at a time, concentrate on it, and see it through. Many people do a little here, a little there, then do something else. In the end, nothing gets done. An exception to working on just one task at a time is when you are doing a difficult task. Rather than "killing yourself," interchange with another activity that is not as hard.

- **Eliminate distractions.** If you have trouble adhering to a set plan, remove distractions and trash activities from your eyesight. Television, radio, computers, magazines, open doors, or studying in a park might distract you and become time killers.

- **Set aside "overtimes."** Regularly schedule time you did not think you would need as overtime to complete unfinished projects. Most people underschedule rather than overschedule time. The result is usually late-night burnout! If you schedule overtimes and get your tasks done, enjoy some leisure time, get ahead on another project, or work on some of your trash priorities. Plan time for *you*.

- **Set aside special time for yourself daily.** Life is not meant to be all work. Use your time to walk, read, or listen to your favorite music.

- **Reward yourself.** As with any other healthy behavior, positive change or a job well done deserves a reward. We often overlook the value of rewards, even if they are self-given. People practice behaviors that are rewarded and discontinue those that are not.

7.10 *Technostress*

In today's fast-paced, 24-7 digital world, technology permeates every corner of our environment—not only in our computers, televisions, and handheld devices, but also in our cars, shopping centers, home appliances, and even some shoes and clothing. Students and workers are spending more time at the computer than ever before, and continue to spend downtime hours surfing the web, video gaming, texting, and socializing online.

Though innovation is meant to help improve the flow of work and daily life, technology has also been associated with feelings of anxiety and irritability, headaches, mental fatigue, lost productivity, and poor job performance. Tech-related stress has been termed "**technostress**," and as the name implies, refers to stress caused by the inability to adapt or cope with technology in a healthy way. The technology itself is not the source of stress, but how people handle and react to it. Distraction and lack of focus due to the never-ending interruption of incoming texts, emails, phone calls and social notifications has been called the epidemic of our digital age. People often feel stressed because they don't know how to manage the daily onslaught of resources and information made available on the web, leading to feelings of being overwhelmed with "information overload."

At school and on the job, working with technology can also cause frustration and a perceived lack of control when faced with errors and unexpected hiccups. Each new innovation—despite the promise of making work or life more efficient—comes with a learning curve that demands new skills and the ability to adapt to new programs and tools with faster reaction times. As a result, new technology can become a stressor in itself, causing many people to become resistant to technological advances. Constant connectivity can lead to overstimulation, blurred boundaries between work and play, isolation and/or increased distance in relationships, loss of concentration and attention span, and unhealthy attachment to technological devices. See "Tips to Manage Technostress" to learn ways to help reduce stress associated with modern technology.

GLOSSARY

Technostress Stress resulting from the inability to adapt or cope with digital technologies in a healthy way.

Tips to Manage Technostress

- **Turn it off.** Turn off your cell phone while at the movies, while enjoying dinner, or when wanting to spend uninterrupted quality time with family members and friends.

- **Slow down your reaction time.** Though technology often seems to run at hyper-speed, it doesn't mean you need to try and keep up at an impractical pace. Utilize email filters, and schedule set times during the day to check texts, emails, and phone messages.

- **Remove digital distractions.** Don't let your gadgets distract you from your school and work productivity, particularly in situations that require sustained attention and concentration, like studying for an exam, finishing a project, or writing creatively.

- **Avoid the urge to multi-task.** Research has found that multi-tasking actually lowers overall productivity, and students and employees who constantly switch between tasks are less likely to retain important information and more likely to make mistakes. Instead, practice focusing your energy on one task at a time through completion.

- **Take time to fully unplug.** Don't let technology dominate your life. Schedule regular gadget-free time away from your computer, cell phone, or other handheld devices to allow both your eyes and mind to rest.

© Cengage Learning

7.11 *Relaxation Techniques*

Stress management skills are essential to cope effectively and move forward in today's fast-paced world. Although you may reap benefits immediately after engaging in any of the several relaxation techniques described in this chapter, several months of regular practice may be necessary for total mastery. The relaxation exercises that follow should not be considered panaceas. In some instances a person's symptoms may not be caused by stress but, rather, may be related to an undiagnosed medical disorder.

Physical Activity

Physical exercise is one of the simplest tools to control stress. Exercise and fitness are thought to reduce the intensity of stress and recovery from a stressful event. The value of exercise in reducing stress is related to several factors, the main one being less muscular tension.

Imagine you are distressed after a miserable day at work. The job requires eight hours of work with a difficult boss. To make matters worse, it is late and on the way home the car in front of you is going much slower than the speed limit. The body's fight-or-flight mechanism is activated. Your heart rate and blood pressure shoot up, your breathing quickens and deepens, your muscles tense, and all systems say "go." Under the circumstances, you can take no action, and the stress will not be dissipated because you simply cannot hit your boss or the car in front of you. Instead, you could take action by "hitting" the tennis ball, the weights, the swimming pool, or the jogging trail. By engaging in physical activity, you are able to reduce the muscular tension and eliminate the physiological changes that triggered the fight-or-flight mechanism.

Further, during vigorous aerobic exercise lasting 30 minutes or longer, morphine-like substances referred to as endorphins are thought to be released from the pituitary gland in the brain. These substances not only act as painkillers but also seem to induce the soothing, calming effect often associated with aerobic exercise. Research has also shown that moderate-intensity exercise has an immediate effect on a person's mood and the effects last up to 12 hours following activity. Thus exercise mitigates the daily stress that leads to mood alterations. Exercise is free and easily accessible to everyone. Pick an activity that you enjoy and use it to combat stress, blue moods, anxiety, and depression.

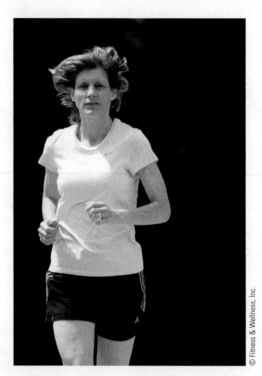

© Fitness & Wellness, Inc.

Physical activity is an excellent tool to control stress.

Behavior Modification Planning

Characteristics of Good Stress Managers

Good stress managers:

- are physically active, eat a healthy diet, and get adequate rest every day.
- believe they have control over events in their life (have an internal locus of control, see pages 16–17).
- understand their own feelings and accept their limitations.
- recognize, anticipate, monitor, and regulate stressors within their capabilities.
- control emotional and physical responses when distressed.
- use appropriate stress management techniques when confronted with stressors.
- recognize warning signs and symptoms of excessive stress.
- schedule daily time to unwind, relax, and evaluate the day's activities.
- control stress when called upon to perform.
- enjoy life despite occasional disappointments and frustrations.
- look success and failure squarely in the face and keep moving along a predetermined course.
- move ahead with optimism and energy and do not spend time and talent worrying about failure.
- learn from previous mistakes and use them as building blocks to prevent similar setbacks in the future.
- give of themselves freely to others.
- find deep meaning in life.

Try It

Change for many people is threatening but often required. Pick three of the above strategies and apply them in your life. After several days, determine the usefulness of these strategies in your physical, mental, social, and emotional well-being.

© Cengage Learning

Progressive Muscle Relaxation

One of the most popular methods used to dissipate stress is **progressive muscle relaxation**, which enables individuals to relearn the sensation of deep relaxation. Acute awareness of how it feels to progressively tighten and relax the muscles releases muscle tension and teaches the body to relax at will. Feeling the tension during the exercises also helps the person to be more alert to signs of distress because this tension is similar to that experienced in stressful situations. In everyday life, these feelings then can cue the person to do relaxation exercises.

Relaxation exercises should be done in a quiet, warm, well-ventilated room. The exercises should encompass all muscle groups of the body. Most important is to pay attention to the sensation you feel each time you tense and relax your muscles.

The instructions can be read to the person, memorized, or recorded. You should set aside at least 20 minutes to complete the entire sequence. Doing the exercises any faster will defeat their purpose. Ideally, you should complete the sequence twice a day.

First, stretch out comfortably on the floor, face up, with a pillow under your knees, and assume a passive attitude, allowing your body to relax as much as possible. Then contract each muscle group in sequence, taking care to avoid any strain. Tighten each muscle to only about 70 percent of the total possible tension to avoid cramping or some type of injury to the muscle itself.

To produce the relaxation effects, pay attention to the sensation of tensing and relaxing. Hold each contraction about five seconds, then allow the muscles to go totally limp. Take enough time to contract and relax each muscle group before going on to the next. An example of a complete progressive muscle relaxation sequence is as follows:

1. Point your feet, curling your toes downward. Study the tension in the arches and top of your feet. Hold and continue to note the tension, then relax. Repeat once again.
2. Flex the feet upward toward your face, and note the tension in your feet and calves. Hold and relax. Repeat once more.

GLOSSARY

Progressive muscle relaxation A relaxation technique that involves contracting, then relaxing muscle groups in the body in succession.

3. Push your heels down against the floor as if burying them in the sand. Hold and note the tension at the back of the thigh. Relax. Repeat once more.

4. Contract your right thigh by straightening your leg, gently raising your leg off the floor. Hold and study the tension. Relax. Repeat with the left leg. Hold and relax. Repeat each leg again.

5. Tense your buttocks by raising your hips ever so slightly off the floor. Hold and note the tension. Relax. Repeat once again.

6. Contract your abdominal muscles. Hold them tight and note the tension. Relax. Repeat one more time.

7. Suck in your stomach. Try to make it reach your spine. Flatten your lower back to the floor. Hold and feel the tension in the stomach and lower back. Relax. Repeat once more.

8. Take a deep breath and hold it, then exhale. Repeat. Note your breathing becoming slower and more relaxed.

9. Place your arms at the side of your body and clench both fists. Hold, study the tension, and relax. Repeat a second time.

10. Flex the elbows by bringing both hands to your shoulders. Hold tight and study the tension in the biceps. Relax. Repeat one more time.

11. Place your arms flat on the floor, palms up, and push the forearms hard against the floor. Note the tension in the triceps. Hold and relax. Repeat once more.

12. Shrug your shoulders, raising them as high as possible. Hold and note the tension. Relax. Repeat once again.

13. Gently push your head backward. Note the tension in the back of the neck. Hold and then relax. Repeat one more time.

14. Gently bring the head against the chest, push forward, hold, and note the tension in the neck. Relax. Repeat a second time.

15. Press your tongue toward the roof of your mouth. Hold, study the tension, and relax. Repeat once more.

16. Press your teeth together. Hold and study the tension. Relax. Repeat one more time.

17. Close your eyes tightly. Hold them closed and note the tension. Relax, leaving your eyes closed. Do this one more time.

18. Wrinkle your forehead and note the tension. Hold and relax. Repeat one more time.

When time is a factor during the daily routine and you are not able to go through the entire sequence, you may do only the exercises specific to the area that feels most tense. Performing a partial sequence is better than not doing the exercises at all. Completing the entire sequence, of course, yields the best results.

Breathing Techniques

How often do you pay attention to your breathing? Few people maintain a habit of breathing fully and properly. Proper breathing is vital to optimal health, as the process of inhaling air feeds life-sustaining oxygen to the lungs and in turn the cardiovascular system feeds it to virtually every part of the body, revitalizing organs, cells, and tissues.

Breathing exercises engage one of your body's most powerful mechanisms for naturally reducing stress. Studies have shown that students who practice deep breathing increase academic learning and achievement, and can help decrease levels of anxiety, nervousness, and loss of concentration. These exercises have been used for centuries in Asian countries to improve mental, physical, and emotional stamina. In breathing exercises, the person concentrates on "breathing away" the tension and inhaling fresh air to the entire body. Breathing exercises can be learned in only a few minutes and require considerably less time than the progressive muscle relaxation exercises.

As with any other relaxation technique, these exercises should be done in a quiet, pleasant, well-ventilated room. Any of the three examples of breathing exercises presented here will help relieve tension induced by stress.

Deep Breathing

Lie with your back flat against the floor, and place a pillow under your knees, feet slightly separated, with your toes pointing outward. (This exercise also may be done while sitting up in a chair or standing straight up.) Place one hand on your abdomen and the other hand on your chest. Breathe in and out slowly so the hand on your abdomen rises when you inhale and falls as you exhale. The hand on your chest should not move much at all. Repeat the exercise about 10 times. Then scan your body for tension, and compare your present tension with the tension you felt at the beginning of the exercise. Repeat the entire process once or twice more.

Sighing

Using the abdominal breathing technique, breathe in through your nose to a specific count (such as 4, 5, or 6). Now exhale through pursed lips to double the intake count (such as 8, 10, or 12, respectively). Repeat the exercise eight to ten times whenever you feel tense.

Complete Natural Breathing

Sit in an upright position or stand straight up. Breathing through your nose, fill your lungs gradually from the bottom up. Hold your breath for several seconds. Now exhale slowly by allowing your chest and abdomen to relax, and try to empty your lungs completely. Repeat the exercise 8 to 10 times.

Meditation

More than 700 scientific studies have verified that **meditation** induces relaxation and alleviates the harmful physiological effects of stress. Meditation is a mental exercise that can bring about psychological and physical benefits. Regular meditation has been shown to decrease blood pressure, stress, anger, anxiety, fear, negative feelings, and chronic pain, and increase activity in the brain's left frontal region—an area associated with positive emotions.[5] The objective of meditation is to gain control over one's attention by clearing the mind and blocking out the stressor(s) responsible for the higher tension.

Meditation "101"

Basic meditation techniques can be learned rather quickly and can be used frequently during times of increased stress. Initially, choose a room that is comfortable, quiet, and free of all disturbances (including telephones). After learning the technique, you will be able to meditate just about anywhere. A time block of approximately 15 minutes, twice a day, is suggested for meditation.

1. Sit in a chair or in a quiet place in an upright position with your hands resting either in your lap or on the arms of the chair. Close your eyes and focus on your breathing. Allow your body to relax as much as possible. Do not consciously try to relax because trying means work. Rather, assume a passive attitude and concentrate on your breathing.

2. Allow your body to breathe regularly, at its own rhythm, and repeat in your mind the word "one" every time you inhale and the word "two" every time you exhale. Paying attention to these two words keeps distressing thoughts from entering into your mind.

3. Continue to breathe in this way for about 15 minutes. Because the objective of meditation is to bring about a hypometabolic (slower metabolism) state leading to body relaxation, do not use an alarm clock to remind you that the 15 minutes have expired. The alarm will only trigger the stress response again, defeating the purpose of the exercise. Opening your eyes once in a while to keep track of the time is fine, but do not rush or anticipate the end of the 15 minutes. This time has been set aside for meditation, and you need to relax, take your time, and enjoy the exercise.

Critical Thinking

List the most significant stressor that you face as a college student. • What technique(s) have you used to manage this situation, and in what way has it helped you cope?

Mindfulness Meditation

Mindfulness can be defined as a mental state of heightened awareness of the present moment. In mindfulness meditation, you focus on becoming fully aware and accepting living in the present, paying particular attention to your feelings, thoughts, sensations, and emotions without passing judgment, dwelling in the past, or projecting yourself into the future. Important during mindfulness meditation is not to worry about things that you have no control over. To live in the present, you must understand that the most significant thing that you have control over is *your attitude*. While your confidence may be shaken because of life's challenges and stressors, you can control your attitude. Having a clear understanding that the "storm will pass" and that "there is light at the end of every tunnel" will allow you to navigate through life's stressors and ultimately overcome challenges and enjoy happiness while living in the present.

Mental training to work mindfully, eat mindfully, and enjoy daily life mindfully aims to prevent vulnerability to stress and illness through conscious living. Mindfulness has been successfully used in helping people adhere to medical treatment, improve hypertension and insomnia, more effectively handle pain, and manage anxiety and depression associated with illness. In college students, mindfulness has been shown to improve intellectual and academic performance, including better knowledge retention during lectures.

Yoga

Yoga is an excellent stress-coping technique. **Yoga** is a school of thought in the Hindu religion that seeks to help

GLOSSARY

Meditation A mental exercise in which the objective is to gain control over one's attention, clearing the mind and blocking out stressors.

Mindfulness A mental state of heightened awareness of the present moment.

Yoga A school of thought in the Hindu religion that seeks to help the individual attain a higher level of spirituality and peace of mind.

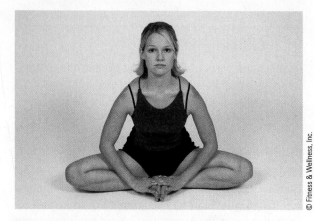

© Fitness & Wellness, Inc.

Yoga exercises help induce the relaxation response.

the individual attain a higher level of spirituality and peace of mind. Although its philosophical roots can be considered spiritual, yoga is based on principles of self-care.

Yoga practitioners adhere to a specific code of ethics and a system of mental and physical exercises that promote control of the mind and the body. In Western countries, many people are mainly familiar with the exercise portion of yoga. This system of exercises (postures) can be used as a relaxation technique for stress management. The exercises include a combination of postures, diaphragmatic breathing, muscle relaxation, and meditation that help buffer the biological effects of stress.

Western interest in yoga exercises gradually developed over the last century, particularly since the 1970s. People pursue yoga exercises for their potential to dispel stress by raising self-esteem, clearing the mind, slowing respiration, promoting neuromuscular relaxation, and increasing body awareness. In addition, the exercises help control involuntary body functions including heart rate, blood pressure, oxygen consumption, and metabolic rate. Doing yoga exercises can increase muscular flexibility, muscular strength and endurance, and balance and can lead to a better aligned musculoskeletal system.[6] Because yoga therapy has been shown to be clinically beneficial for rehabilitation after a stroke[7], yoga is also used in many hospital-based programs for cardiac patients to help manage stress and decrease blood pressure.

There are many different styles of yoga. Classes vary according to their emphasis. Some styles of yoga are athletic, and others are passive in nature. The most popular variety in the Western world is **hatha yoga**, which incorporates a series of static-stretching postures performed in specific sequences (also known as "asanas") that help induce the relaxation response. Participants hold the postures for several seconds while concentrating on breathing patterns, meditation, and body awareness.

Most yoga classes are now variations of hatha yoga, and many of the typical stretches used in flexibility exercises today have been adapted from hatha yoga. Examples include:

1. *Integral yoga* and *viniyoga* which focus on gentle/static stretches.
2. *Iyengar yoga*, which promotes muscular strength and endurance.
3. *Yogalates*, incorporating Pilates exercises to increase muscular strength.
4. *Power yoga* or *yogaerobics*, a high-energy form that links many postures together in a dancelike routine to promote cardiorespiratory fitness.

As with flexibility exercises, the stretches in hatha yoga should not be performed to the point of discomfort. Instructors should not push participants beyond their physical limitations. Similar to other stress management techniques, yoga exercises are best performed in a quiet place for about 15 to 60 minutes per session. Many yoga participants like to perform the exercises daily.

To appreciate yoga exercise, a person has to experience it. We are only introducing yoga here. Although participants can practice yoga exercises with the instruction of a book or video, most participants take classes. Many of the postures are difficult and complex, and few individuals can master the entire sequence in the first few weeks.

Individuals who are interested in yoga exercise should initially pursue it under qualified instruction. Many universities offer yoga courses, and you also can check online for a listing of yoga instructors or classes in your area. Yoga courses are offered at many health clubs and recreation centers. Because instructors and yoga styles vary, you may want to observe a class before enrolling. You should look for an instructor whose views on wellness parallel your own. There are no national certification standards for instructors. If you are new to yoga, you are encouraged to compare a couple of instructors before you select a class.

Tai Chi

Tai chi chuan (full name) originated in China centuries ago and is practiced today for defense training and for physical and mental health benefits. The martial side, however, is no longer the focus of its practice, so the activity can be performed by young and old, and even the very old. Many fitness practitioners use it in conjunction with aerobic and strength training.

Tai chi is often described as "meditation in motion" because it is performed with flowing, rhythmic movements that focus heavily on breathing and the slow execution of its movements. The main objective is to promote tranquility and reflection through postures that combine meditation and dance. The postures are performed in sequences known as "sets" that require concentration, coordination, controlled breathing, muscle relaxation, strength, flexibility, gait, and body balance.

Research has attributed many health benefits to tai chi, including diabetes management, arthritis relief, lower blood pressure, faster recovery from heart disease and injury, improved strength and flexibility, better sleep, and improved physical work capacity.

Tai chi is frequently used for stress management to relieve tension, stress, and anxiety. The mental aspect of having to concentrate on leading the movement and paying attention to detail through the gentle actions dissipates stress. The activity leaves no room to think or worry about other problems, thus calming and relaxing the mind and body.

To master tai chi, you need initial professional guidance. You are encouraged to join a group or a class available at many college campuses or community health clubs. The class should emphasize fitness and health benefits over combat techniques. Once you have mastered many of the sets available, you can practice the activity on your own.

Visual Imagery

Visual or mental **imagery** has been used as a healing technique for centuries in various cultures around the world. In Western medicine, the practice of imagery is relatively new and not widely accepted among health care professionals. Imagery induces a state of relaxation that rids the body of the stress that leads to illness. It improves circulation and increases the delivery of healing antibodies and white blood cells to the site of illness.[8]

Visual imagery involves the creation of relaxing visual images and scenes in times of stress to elicit body and mind relaxation. Imagery works by offsetting the stressor with the visualization of relaxing scenes such as a sunny beach, a beautiful meadow, a quiet mountaintop, or some other peaceful setting. If you are ill, you can also visualize your white blood cells attacking an infection or a tumor. Imagery is also used in conjunction with breathing exercises, meditation, and yoga.

As with other stress management techniques, imagery should be performed in a quiet and comfortable environment. You can either sit or lie down for the exercise. If you lie down, use a soft surface and place a pillow under your knees. Be sure that your clothes are loose and that you are as comfortable as you can be.

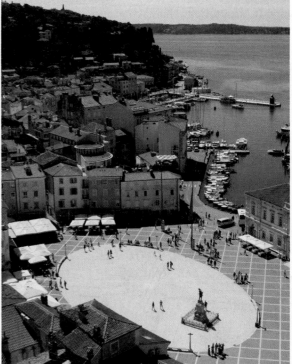

Visual imagery is an effective technique for coping with stress.

Close your eyes and visualize one of your favorite scenes in nature. Place yourself into the scene and visualize yourself moving about and experiencing nature to its fullest. Enjoy the people, the animals, the colors, the sounds, the smells, and even the temperature in your scene. After 10 to 20 minutes of visualization, open your eyes and compare the tension in your body and mind at this point with how you felt prior to the exercise. You can repeat this exercise as often as you deem necessary when you are feeling tension or stress.

Which Technique Is Best?

Because each person reacts to stress differently, the best strategy to alleviate stress depends mostly on the individual. Which technique you use does not matter as long as it works. You may want to experiment with several or all of

GLOSSARY

Hatha yoga A yoga style that incorporates a series of static-stretching postures performed in specific sequences.

Imagery Mental visualization of relaxing images and scenes to induce body relaxation in times of stress or as an aid in the treatment of certain medical conditions such as cancer, hypertension, asthma, chronic pain, and obesity.

© Fitness & Wellness, Inc.

the techniques presented here to find out which works best for you. Many people choose a combination of two or more.

All of the strategies discussed in this chapter help to block out stressors and promote mental and physical relaxation by diverting the attention to a different, non-threatening action. Some of the techniques are easier to learn and take less time per session. Regardless of which technique you select, the time you spend doing stress management exercises (several times a day, as needed) is well worth the effort when stress becomes a significant problem in your life.

People need to learn to relax and take time for themselves. What makes people ill is not stress itself but, instead, the way they react to the stress-causing agent. Individuals who are diligent and take control of themselves find that they enjoy a better, happier, and healthier life.

Assess Your Behavior

1. Are you able to channel your emotions and feelings to exert a positive effect on your mind, health, and wellness?

2. Do you use time management strategies on a regular basis?

3. Do you use stress management techniques, and do they allow you to be in control over the daily stresses of life?

Assess Your Knowledge

1. Positive stress is also referred to as
   a. eustress.
   b. poststress.
   c. functional stress.
   d. distress.
   e. physiostress.

2. Which of the following is not a stage of the general adaptation syndrome?
   a. alarm reaction
   b. resistance
   c. compliance
   d. exhaustion/recovery
   e. All are stages of the general adaptation syndrome.

3. Which of the following behaviors seems to have the greatest impact in increasing the risk for illness among Type A individuals?
   a. hard-driven
   b. overambitious
   c. chronic hostility
   d. overly competitive
   e. All increase the risk equally.

4. Effective time managers
   a. delegate.
   b. learn to say "no."
   c. avoid boredom.
   d. set aside "overtimes."
   e. do all of the above.

5. Hormonal changes that occur during a stress response
   a. decrease heart rate.
   b. increase blood pressure.
   c. diminish blood flow to the muscles.
   d. induce relaxation.
   e. sap the body's strength.

6. Exercise decreases stress levels by
   a. deliberately diverting stress to various body systems.
   b. metabolizing excess catecholamines.
   c. diminishing muscular tension.
   d. stimulating alpha-wave activity in the brain.
   e. doing all of the above.

7. Which of the following exercises is included in the progressive muscle relaxation technique?
   a. pointing the feet
   b. wrinkling the forehead
   c. contracting the abdominal muscles
   d. pressing the teeth together
   e. All of the above exercises are used.

8. The technique in which a person breathes in through the nose to a specific count and then exhales through pursed lips to double the intake count is known as
   a. sighing.
   b. deep breathing.
   c. meditation.
   d. autonomic ventilation.
   e. release management.

9. Meditation
   a. induces relaxation.
   b. alleviates the harmful physiological effects of stress.
   c. can be performed just about anywhere.
   d. incorporates breathing exercises.
   e. includes all of the above statements.

10. Yoga exercises have been used successfully to
    a. stimulate ventilation.
    b. increase metabolism during stress.
    c. help in rehabilitation after a stroke. .
    d. decrease body awareness.
    e. accomplish all of the above.

Correct answers can be found on page 307.

Activity 7.1   Stress Analysis

Name _____   Date _____

Course _____   Section _____

I. Record your results and stress categories for each questionnaire given in this chapter.

	Points	Category

Hostility (see Figure 7.3, page 188):   _____

Stress Vulnerability
(see Figure 7.4, page 189):   _____   _____   (0–30 = Excellent, 31–40 = Good, 41–50 = Average, 51–60 = Fair, ≥61 = Poor)

Stress Test (see Figure 7.5, page 191):   _____   _____   (≤249 = low risk, ≥250–500 = moderate risk, >500 = high risk)

II. Life stressor. In the space provided below, list a stressor you frequently encounter in life. Explain the situation(s) under which it occurs, your response to it, the impact it has on your life, and how you are presently handling the stressor. Also indicate what you can do to either avoid the stressor or cope with it more effectively in the future.

_____

_____

_____

_____

_____

_____

_____

_____

_____

_____

_____

Activity 7.1 **Stress Analysis** *(continued)*

III. In your own words, express how life stresses and your personality affect you in your daily life.

_____

_____

_____

_____

_____

_____

_____

_____

_____

_____

IV. In the space provided below, list, in order of priority, three behaviors that you would like to change to decrease your vulnerability to stress. Briefly indicate how you intend to accomplish these changes.

_____

_____

_____

_____

_____

_____

_____

_____

_____

_____

_____

_____

_____

_____

V. Number of current daily steps: _____

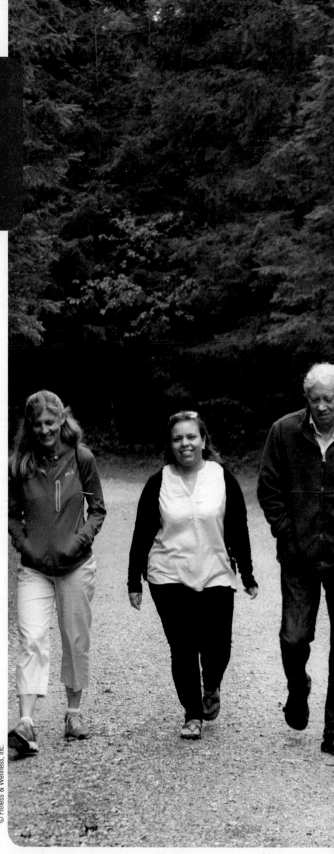

8

A Healthy Lifestyle Approach

"Exercise can be used as a vaccine to prevent disease and a medication to treat disease. If there were a drug with the same benefits as exercise, it would instantly be the standard of care."
—Robert Sallis

Objectives

> Understand the importance of implementing a healthy lifestyle program.

> Recognize the relationship between spirituality and wellness.

> Identify the major risk factors for coronary heart disease.

> Be able to differentiate physiological age and chronological age.

> Become acquainted with cancer-prevention guidelines.

> Learn the health consequences of chemical abuse and irresponsible sex.

© Fitness & Wellness, Inc.

REAL LIFE STORY | George's Health Status

I didn't go to college right out of high school. I worked full time for 20 years, but now at age 38, I have decided to pursue a degree in business administration. I wasn't very happy when I found out I had to take a Fitness and Wellness for Life course. I tried to get out of it, but the department chair would not waive or substitute the requirement. Of course, I didn't expect to do well on the fitness tests, but when the instructor encouraged us to have a blood lipid profile, I thought "at my age I should probably have one done." My total cholesterol was 280, the LDL-cholesterol was 220, and my HDL-cholesterol was only 30; worse yet, my triglycerides were 480! I was also a pack-a-day smoker. I realized then that I was a sure candidate for a heart attack. I saw my doctor, and when I told him

that I was in this fitness/wellness class, he asked that rather than medication, I try exercise and healthy eating first and see him again in three months. He also told me to give up smoking.

Suddenly my fitness/wellness course took on a whole new meaning. I went back and reviewed my aerobic exercise prescription and faithfully started to exercise five to seven days per week. I also conducted a nutrient analysis and kept the nutrition charts right on the kitchen counter. I learned to read labels and drastically cut down on saturated fat and trans fats. I also limited sweets and alcohol in my diet. It took me a

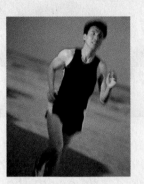

year, but I finally quit smoking.

At the follow-up blood test at three months, my total cholesterol was down to 225 and the triglycerides were at 180. I continued with my lifestyle changes and have even done a few 5K and 10K races. Now, four years later, I received the best graduation present I could get: total cholesterol 182, LDL-cholesterol 118, HDL-cholesterol 46, and triglycerides 96! To celebrate, I ran a 5K that weekend in 22:48. The fitness and wellness class is the best course I had in college, and it has truly given me a better chance at a healthier and longer life.

Purestock/Jupiter Images

Improving our health—the quality, and most likely the length, of our lives—is a matter of personal choice. The wellness approach—the combination of a fitness program and a healthy lifestyle program—can help accomplish these goals.

8.1 *A Wellness Lifestyle*

Wellness is the constant and deliberate effort to stay healthy and achieve the highest potential for well-being. Twelve simple lifestyle habits can increase longevity significantly:

1. Be physically active (exercise and avoid excessive sitting throughout the day).
2. Do not use tobacco.
3. Eat a healthy diet.
4. Avoid frequent high-sugar snacks between meals.
5. Maintain recommended body weight through healthy nutrition and physical activity.
6. Sleep seven to eight hours each night.
7. Lower stress levels.
8. Drink alcohol moderately or not at all.
9. Surround yourself with healthy relationships.
10. Be informed about the environment and avoid environmental risk factors.
11. Increase education (more educated people live longer).
12. Take personal safety measures.

Spiritual Well-Being

There appears to be a strong connection between the mind, the spirit, and the body. To enjoy a wellness lifestyle, a person has to practice behaviors that will lead to positive outcomes in all dimensions of wellness (see Chapter 1). These dimensions are interrelated; one dimension frequently affects the others. For example, a person who is emotionally "down" often has no desire to exercise, study, socialize with friends, or attend church and may be more susceptible to illness and disease. Because spirituality plays an important role and has not been discussed thus far, it merits some attention.

Figure 8.1 Components of spiritual well-being.

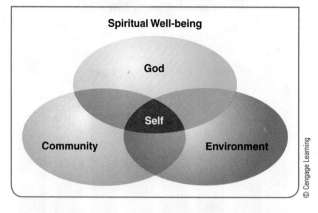

Figure 8.2 Underlying causes of death in the United States.

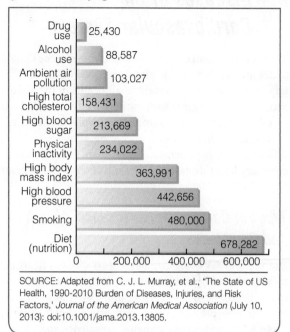

SOURCE: Adapted from C. J. L. Murray, et al., "The State of US Health, 1990-2010 Burden of Diseases, Injuries, and Risk Factors,' *Journal of the American Medical Association* (July 10, 2013): doi:10.1001/jama.2013.13805.

The definition of **spirituality** by the National Interfaith Coalition on Aging encompasses everyone because it assumes that all people are spiritual in nature. Spiritual health provides a unifying power that integrates the other dimensions of wellness (see Figure 8.1). Basic characteristics of spiritual people include a sense of meaning and direction in life, a relationship to a higher being, freedom, prayer, faith, love, closeness to others, peace, joy, fulfillment, and altruism.

Although not everyone claims an affiliation with a certain religion or denomination, most people in the United States believe in God or a universal spirit functioning as God. People, furthermore, believe to a varying extent that (a) a relationship with God is meaningful; (b) God can grant help, guidance, and assistance in daily living; and (c) mortal existence has a purpose. If we accept any or all of these statements, attaining spirituality will have a definite effect on our happiness and well-being.

The reasons why religious affiliation enhances wellness are difficult to determine. Possible reasons include the promotion of healthy lifestyle behaviors, social support, assistance in times of crisis and need, and counseling to overcome one's weaknesses. At least 200 studies have been conducted on the effects of prayer on health. About two-thirds of these studies have linked prayer to positive health outcomes—as long as these prayers are offered with sincerity, humility, love, empathy, and compassion. Some studies have shown faster healing time and fewer complications in patients who didn't even know they were being prayed for, compared with patients who were not prayed for.[1]

Altruism—a key attribute of spiritual people—seems to enhance health and longevity. Studies indicate that people who regularly volunteer live longer. Doing good for others is good for oneself, especially for the immune system.

The relationship between spirituality and wellness, therefore, is meaningful in our quest for a better quality of life. As with other parameters of wellness, optimum

spirituality requires development of the spiritual nature to its fullest potential.

8.2 *Causes of Death*

Of all deaths in the United States, approximately 53 percent are caused by cardiovascular disease (CVD) and cancer.[2] Close to 80 percent of these deaths could be prevented by following a healthy lifestyle. The third and fourth leading causes of death—chronic lower respiratory disease (CLRD) and accidents—also are preventable, primarily by abstaining from tobacco and other drugs, wearing seat belts, and using common sense. Most of the underlying causes of death in the United States are related to the lifestyle people choose to live (see Figure 8.2). Four factors: poor diet and nutrition, smoking, excessive body weight, and lack of physical activity, are responsible for more than 1.7 million deaths annually.

GLOSSARY

Spirituality A sense of meaning and direction in life, a relationship to a higher being; encompasses freedom, prayer, faith, love, closeness to others, peace, joy, fulfillment, and altruism.

Altruism True concern for and action on behalf of others (opposite of egoism); a sincere desire to serve others above one's personal needs.

8.3 *Diseases of the Cardiovascular System*

The most prevalent degenerative conditions in the United States are **cardiovascular diseases**. Based on current vital statistics, about 30 percent of all deaths in the United States were attributable to diseases of the heart and blood vessels.[3] More than 85 million people are afflicted by cardiovascular diseases, including some 80 million suffering with hypertension, more than 15 million with **coronary heart disease (CHD)**, and about 375,000 heart attack and 130,000 stroke deaths per year.

Types of Cardiovascular Disease and Prevalence

Examples of CVD are coronary heart disease, heart attack, peripheral vascular disease, congenital heart disease, rheumatic heart disease, atherosclerosis, strokes, high blood pressure, and congestive heart failure. Table 8.1 provides the estimated prevalence and annual number of deaths caused by the major types of CVD.

The American Heart Association estimated that the cost of heart and blood vessel disease in the United States exceeded $300 billion per year.[4] More than half of all heart attack deaths occur within an hour of the onset of symptoms, before the person reaches the hospital.

Although heart and blood vessel disease is still the number one health problem in the United States, the incidence declined by almost 46 percent between 1960 and 2010 (see Figure 8.3). The main reason for this dramatic decrease is health education. More people now are aware of the risk factors for CVD and are changing their lifestyle to lower their potential risk for these diseases.

Table 8.1 Estimated Prevalence and Yearly Number of Deaths from Cardiovascular Disease

	Prevalence	Deaths
All forms of cardiovascular diseases*	85,600,000	700,000
Coronary heart disease	15,500,000	**
Heart attack	7,600,000	375,000
Stroke	6,600,000	129,000
High blood pressure	80,000,000	65,000***

*Includes people with one or more forms of cardiovascular disease.

**Number of deaths included under heart attack.

***Mortality figures appear to be low because many heart attacks and stroke deaths are caused by high blood pressure.

SOURCE: American Heart Association, *Heart Disease and Stroke Statistics—2015 Update* (Dallas, TX: American Heart Association, 2014).

Figure 8.3 Incidence of cardiovascular disease in the United States for selected years, 1900–2010.

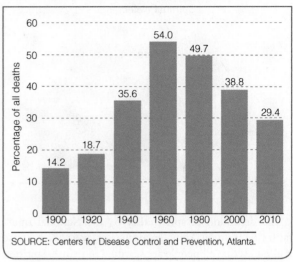

SOURCE: Centers for Disease Control and Prevention, Atlanta.

The heart and the coronary arteries are illustrated in Figure 8.4. The major form of CVD is CHD. In CHD, the arteries that supply the heart muscle with oxygen and nutrients are narrowed by fatty deposits such as cholesterol and triglycerides. Narrowing of the coronary arteries diminishes the blood supply to the heart muscle, which can precipitate a heart attack.

CHD is the single leading cause of death in the United States, accounting for approximately 15 percent of all deaths and about half of all cardiovascular deaths. More than half of the people who died suddenly from CHD had no previous symptoms of the disease. Further, the risk of death is greater in the least educated segment of the population.

Figure 8.4 The heart and its blood vessels.

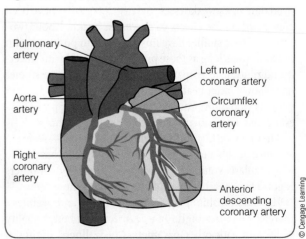

Risk Factors for CHD

Following are the leading **risk factors** for the development of CHD:

- Physical inactivity
- High blood pressure
- Excessive body fat
- Low HDL-cholesterol
- Elevated LDL-cholesterol
- Elevated triglycerides
- Elevated homocysteine
- Inflammation
- Diabetes
- Abnormal electrocardiograms (ECGs)
- Tobacco use
- Stress
- Personal and family history of CVD
- Age
- Gender

An important concept in CHD risk management is that many of the risk factors are preventable and reversible. Approximately 90 percent of CHD can be prevented if people practice healthy lifestyle habits. The above risk factors are discussed in the following pages.

Physical Inactivity

Improving cardiorespiratory endurance through aerobic exercise and avoiding excessive daily sitting has perhaps the greatest impact in reducing the overall risk for CVD. In this day and age of mechanized societies, we cannot afford *not* to be physically active. Research data on the benefits of aerobic exercise in reducing CVD are too impressive to be ignored.

For habitually sedentary people, sudden heavy-duty physical activity, such as shoveling snow or strenuous yard work, can trigger a cardiovascular event. The research shows that unaccustomed physical exertion increases the risk for a cardiovascular incident 50- to 100-fold.

As shown in Figure 8.5, work conducted at the Aerobics Research Institute in Dallas showed a much higher incidence of cardiovascular deaths in low-fit people as compared to moderate- and high-fit people.[5] Scientific studies indicate that, when feasible, vigorous-intensity

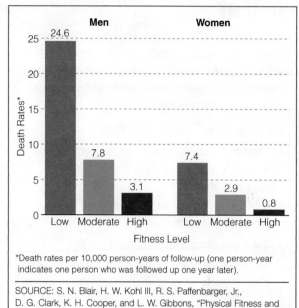

Figure 8.5 Relationship between fitness levels and cardiovascular mortality.

*Death rates per 10,000 person-years of follow-up (one person-year indicates one person who was followed up one year later).

SOURCE: S. N. Blair, H. W. Kohl III, R. S. Paffenbarger, Jr., D. G. Clark, K. H. Cooper, and L. W. Gibbons, "Physical Fitness and All-Cause Mortality: A Prospective Study of Healthy Men and Women," *Journal of the American Medical Association* 262 (1989): 2395–2401.

activity is preferable because of greater improvements in aerobic fitness, blood pressure, and glucose control, and a larger reduction in CHD risk.

A regular aerobic exercise program helps to control most of the major risk factors that lead to heart and blood vessel disease. Aerobic exercise will

- increase cardiorespiratory endurance.
- decrease and control blood pressure.
- reduce body fat.
- lower blood lipids (cholesterol and triglycerides).
- improve high-density lipoprotein (HDL) cholesterol (see "Abnormal Cholesterol Profile" on pages 211–214).
- decrease low-grade (hidden) inflammation in the body.
- help control or decrease the risk for diabetes.

---GLOSSARY---

Cardiovascular diseases The array of conditions that affect the heart and blood vessels.

Coronary heart disease (CHD) Condition in which the arteries that supply the heart muscle with oxygen and nutrients are narrowed by fatty deposits such as cholesterol and triglycerides.

Risk factors Lifestyle and genetic variables that may lead to disease.

Warning Signals of a Heart Attack and Stroke

Any or all of the following signs may occur during a heart attack or a stroke. If you experience any of these and they last longer than a few minutes, call 911 and seek medical attention immediately. Failure to do so may cause irreparable damage and even result in death.

Warning Signs of a Heart Attack

- Chest pain, discomfort, pressure, or squeezing that lasts for several minutes. These feelings may go away and return later.
- Pain that radiates to the shoulders, neck, or arms or between the shoulder blades.
- Chest discomfort with shortness of breath, lightheadedness, sweating, nausea, or fainting

Warning Signs of Stroke

The acronym **FAST** is commonly used to help recognize and enhance responsiveness for a stroke victim.

- **F**acial dropping. Part of the face is dropping, weak, numb, or hard to move.
- **A**rm weakness. An inability to completely raise one arm.
- **S**peech difficulties. The inability to understand or repeat a simple sentence.
- **T**ime. Time is of the essence when suffering a stroke.
- Other symptoms may include a sudden severe headache, confusion, dizziness, difficulty walking, loss of balance or coordination, or sudden visual difficulty.

© Cengage Learning

- increase and maintain good heart function, sometimes improving certain ECG abnormalities.
- encourage smoking cessation.
- alleviate stress.
- counteract a personal history of heart disease.

Also try to minimize total daily sitting time. Research data indicate that excessive daily sitting (at a desk, commuting to and from work, eating meals, and watching television) increases the risk for cardiovascular disease, obesity, some chronic disorders, and premature mortality. The risk is increased even among people who complete 30 minutes of moderate-intensity physical activity on most days of the week but still spend a large part of the day sitting.

People who commute and have a desk job can easily spend the majority of their day in the seated position, with the only change being the chair beneath them. If your job (as most now do) requires that a large portion of the day be spent in a sitting position, at least make yourself get up and take frequent breaks. Small, creative lifestyle changes such as always answering the phone standing; walking to the office next door instead of texting, emailing, or using the phone; taking a few moments to stretch or do an occasional strength exercise such as a squat; and using stairs instead of elevators and escalators all make a difference. Be especially proactive about uninterrupted sitting during leisure time.

Physical activity and exercise even exceed the benefits of prescription medications in reducing premature mortality in people suffering from heart disease, diabetes, and stroke. Cardiac patients who exercise require less medication, are less likely to have follow-up surgeries or bypasses, and have a much lower risk of dying from a subsequent heart attack than their physically inactive counterparts. People with chronic conditions, however, should not stop taking their medications, but because of its effectiveness, they should add daily physical activity and regular exercise to their drug-treatment therapy.

In terms of life expectancy, in 2012 research involving 654,827 individuals looking at leisure time physical activity of moderate to vigorous intensity and their effects on mortality, the results indicated that higher levels of physical activity are associated with greater gains in life expectancy. People at the highest level of physical activity gained 4.5 years in life expectancy, and being active and of normal weight (BMI of 18.5 to 24.9) yielded a gain of 7.2 years of life as compared to being inactive and obese.[6]

High Blood Pressure (Hypertension)

Blood pressure should be checked regularly, regardless of whether it is elevated or not. **Blood pressure** is measured in milliliters of mercury (mm Hg) and usually is expressed in two numbers. The higher number reflects the **systolic blood pressure**, the pressure exerted during the forceful contraction of the heart. The lower value, **diastolic blood pressure**, is taken during the heart's relaxation phase, when no blood is being ejected.

Ideally, blood pressure is 120/80 or below (see Table 8.2). Blood pressures ranging from 120/80 to 139/89 are referred to as prehypertension. All blood pressures above 140/90 are considered to be **hypertension**. High blood pressure can be controlled with different types of medications, along with the lifestyle changes described below for people with mild hypertension.

Table 8.2 Blood Pressure Guidelines (expressed in mm Hg)

Rating	Systolic	Diastolic
Normal	≤120	≤80
Prehypertension	121–139	81–89
Hypertension	≥140	≥90

SOURCE: National Heart, Lung, and Blood Institute.

Recommended treatment for people with mild hypertension includes regular aerobic exercise, weight control, a low-salt/low-fat and high-potassium/high-calcium diet, lower alcohol and caffeine intake, smoking cessation, and stress management. People with high blood pressure should follow their physician's advice and stay on any prescribed medication.

Adequate potassium intake seems to regulate water retention and lower blood pressure slightly. According to the Institute of Medicine of the National Academy of Sciences, we need to consume at least 4,700 mg of potassium per day. Most Americans get only half that amount. Food items high in potassium include vegetables (especially leafy green), citrus fruit, dairy products, fish, beans, and nuts.

In terms of salt (sodium) intake, data indicate that to either prevent or postpone the onset of hypertension, and to help some hypertensives control their blood pressure, we should consume less sodium than previously recommended. The recommendation now is less than 1,500 mg of sodium daily for people between 19 and 50 years of age. The current upper limit (UL) has been set at 2,300 mg per day. Among Americans and Canadians, about 95 percent of men and 75 percent of women exceed this limit.

Regular physical activity plays a large role in managing blood pressure. On the average, fit individuals have lower blood pressure than unfit people. Aerobic exercise of moderate intensity supplemented by strength training is recommended for individuals with high blood pressure.[7] Data show that strength training provides similar reductions in blood pressure as aerobic exercise. Individuals who discontinue exercise do not maintain the benefits. Even in the absence of any significant decrease in resting blood pressure, hypertensive individuals who exercise have a lower risk of all-cause mortality as compared to hypertensive/sedentary individuals.

Excessive Body Fat

Excessive body fat has been recognized as a factor contributing to coronary heart disease. Furthermore, when abdominal fat is stored primarily around internal organs (visceral fat), disease risk is greater than when abdominal fat is stored subcutaneously (beneath the skin).

The best approach to prevent increases in visceral fat is through regular exercise. Data on men and women who were followed for 6 months showed no visceral fat gains in groups that either walked (178 min/week) or jogged (120 min/week) an average of 12 miles per week.[8] A sedentary group in this same study actually gained almost 9 percent visceral fat during the 6 months, while a 20-mile-per-week jogging group (173 min/week) lost 7 percent visceral fat. Thus, it appears that 30 minutes of vigorous exercise 6 times per week is best to properly manage visceral fat. Of significant concern, just six months of inactivity further increased visceral fat, subsequently increasing disease risk.

The causes of obesity are complex, including an individual's combination of genetics, behavior, and lifestyle factors. Studies, however, have shown reduction in chronic disease risk factors with only a 2 percent to 3 percent weight loss.

Abnormal Cholesterol Profile

The term **blood lipids** is used mainly with reference to cholesterol and triglycerides. If you never have had a blood lipid test, it is highly recommended. The blood test measures total **cholesterol**, **high-density lipoprotein (HDL)** cholesterol, **low-density lipoprotein (LDL)** cholesterol, and triglycerides. A significant elevation in blood lipids has been linked to heart and blood vessel disease.

The general recommendation is to keep total cholesterol levels below 200 mg/dL (see Table 8.3). The risk for

---GLOSSARY---

Blood pressure A measure of the force exerted against the walls of the vessels by the blood flowing through them.

Systolic blood pressure Pressure exerted by the blood against the walls of the arteries during the forceful contraction (systole) of the heart.

Diastolic blood pressure Pressure exerted by the blood against the walls of the arteries during the relaxation phase (diastole) of the heart.

Hypertension Chronically elevated blood pressure.

Blood lipids (fat) Cholesterol and triglycerides.

Cholesterol A waxy substance, technically a steroid alcohol, found only in animal fats and oil; used in making cell membranes, as a building block for some hormones, in the fatty sheath around nerve fibers, and in other necessary substances.

High-density lipoprotein (HDL) Cholesterol-transporting molecules in the blood (good cholesterol).

Low-density lipoprotein (LDL) Cholesterol-transporting molecules in the blood (bad cholesterol).

Table 8.3 Recommended Blood Lipid Levels

Total cholesterol	<200 mg/dL
LDL cholesterol	<100 mg/dL
HDL cholesterol	≥40 mg/dL
Triglycerides	≤150 mg/Dl

Source: National Cholesterol Education Program and National Heart, Lung and Blood Institute.

heart attack increases 2 percent for every 1 percent increase in total cholesterol.[9] Approximately 32 million American adults have total cholesterol values at or above 240 mg/dL.[10]

Although the average adult in the United States consumes around 500 mg of cholesterol daily, the body actually manufactures more than that. Saturated fats and trans fats (trans-fatty acids) raise cholesterol levels more than anything else in the diet. The average saturated fat intake in the American diet produces approximately 1,000 mg of cholesterol per day.[11] Because of individual differences, some people can have a higher-than-normal intake of saturated fats and still maintain normal levels. Others, who have a lower intake, can have abnormally high levels.

Unsaturated fats are mainly of plant origin and cannot be converted to cholesterol. Saturated fats are found primarily in meats and dairy products. Poultry and fish contain less saturated fat than beef does but should be eaten in moderation (about 3 ounces per day). In a 10-year study of more than 500,000 men and women over the age of 50, those who ate the most red meat (an average of 4.5 ounces per day), had a much higher risk of dying from heart disease and cancer.[12] Of the highest red meat eaters, men had a 31 percent higher risk of dying during the study period, whereas women had a 50 percent higher risk of dying from heart disease during this time. Cancer risk was about 20 percent higher among men and women who consumed the most red meat.

Omega-3 polyunsaturated fatty acids are of particular importance in preventing heart disease. Omega-3-rich fish meals (found in salmon, tuna, and mackerel) not only help lower LDL-cholesterol and triglycerides, but they also help raise HDL-cholesterol.[13] Because of the cardioprotective benefits of omega-3 fatty acids, the American Heart Association recommends eating oily fish at least twice per week.

As important as total cholesterol is, many heart attacks occur in people who have only slightly elevated total cholesterol. More significant is the way in which cholesterol is carried in the bloodstream. Cholesterol is transported primarily in the form of low-density lipoprotein (LDL) cholesterol and high-density lipoprotein (HDL) cholesterol. LDL-cholesterol ("bad" cholesterol) tends to release cholesterol, which then may penetrate the lining of the arteries and speed up the process of **atherosclerosis**. An LDL-cholesterol value below 100 mg/dL is optimal.

Foods that contain trans fats, hydrogenated fat, or partially hydrogenated vegetable oil should be avoided. Studies indicate that these foods elevate cholesterol as much as saturated fats do, but even worse, they decrease the cardioprotective HDL-cholesterol (see discussion that follows). Hydrogen is frequently added to monounsaturated and polyunsaturated fats to increase shelf life and to solidify them so they are more spreadable. French fries, doughnuts, apple fritters, baked foods, pastries, biscuits, crackers, pie crusts, pizza crust, stick margarine, and spreads often contain trans fats. The label "partially hydrogenated" and "trans fat" indicates that the product carries a health risk just as high as that of saturated fat.

The American Heart Association recommends that people limit trans fat intake to less than 1 percent of the total daily caloric intake. This amount represents about 2 grams of trans fats a day for a 2,000-calorie diet. Because the Food and Drug Administration (FDA) requires that all food labels list the trans fat content, you can keep better track of your daily trans fat intake by paying attention to food labels.

Unfortunately, the FDA allows food manufacturers to label any product that has less than half a gram of trans fat per serving as having zero. Be aware that if you eat 3 or 4 servings of a particular food with near half a gram of trans fat, you may be getting your maximum daily allowance (1 gram per 1,000 calories of daily caloric intake). Thus, you are encouraged to look at the list of ingredients and search for the words "partially hydrogenated" as an indicator of hidden trans fats.

In a process known as reverse cholesterol transport, HDL particles act as "scavengers," removing cholesterol from the body and preventing plaque from forming in the arteries. For this reason, HDL-cholesterol is referred to as the "good" cholesterol. The more HDL-cholesterol, the better, as it offers some protection against heart disease. Low levels of HDL-cholesterol could be the best predictor of CHD and may be more significant than the total cholesterol value.

The recommended HDL-cholesterol values to minimize the risk for CHD are a minimum of 40 mg/dL. For the most part, HDL-cholesterol is determined genetically and women have higher levels than men. The female sex hormone estrogen tends to raise HDL, so premenopausal women have a much lower incidence of heart disease. African American adult men have higher HDL values than whites. HDL-cholesterol also decreases with age.

In late 2013 the American Heart Association and the American College of Cardiology released new recommendations for heart disease and stroke prevention. The guidelines focus on cholesterol, lifestyle, obesity, and risk assessment. In terms of cholesterol, numeric targets are deemphasized and now focus on treating people who are deemed to be at high risk for cardiovascular disease (CVD), with complete emphasis on statin therapy. The LDL cholesterol number is no longer the main consideration in treatment. Some experts strongly disagree with these new guidelines. They feel that the recommendations will increase the number of people on statin medications and will not be more effective than the previous target-based guidelines (see Cholesterol Guidelines in Table 8.3, page 212). The new recommendations specifically target four high-risk groups for whom statin drugs are recommended:

1. People with pre-existing CVD (those who have suffered angina, a heart attack, stroke, or a transient ischemic attack or mini stroke, and anyone who has had a cardiovascular procedure such as angioplasty to widen arteries).
2. Type 2 diabetics between 40 and 75 years of age.
3. People with very high LDL cholesterol (190 mg/dl or above).
4. People between 40 and 75 without CVD or diabetes who have a 10-year risk of CVD of at least 7.5 percent based on a new *online risk calculator* (see Risk assessment below).

Lowering LDL cholesterol, however, is still important. The new guidelines encourage people to consume no more than 5 to 6 percent of total daily calories from saturated fat and less than 1 percent from trans fats.

The healthy lifestyle guidelines incorporate adequate physical activity, weight management, and dietary patterns that emphasize vegetables, fruits, whole grains, low-fat dairy products, fish, poultry, and nuts. People should limit red meat, processed foods, saturated and trans fats, sodium, and sugary foods and beverages. Physical activity performed on a regular basis, 40 minutes of exercise 3 to 4 days a week, is also encouraged in the guidelines.

Increasing HDL-cholesterol. Increasing HDL-cholesterol lessens the risk for CHD. Habitual aerobic exercise, weight loss, niacin, and quitting smoking help raise HDL-cholesterol. HDL-cholesterol and a regular aerobic exercise program clearly are related (vigorous intensity or above 6 METs, for at least 20 minutes 3 times per week—see Chapter 3 and Chapter 4). Individual responses to aerobic exercise differ, but generally, the greater the exercise volume, the higher the HDL-cholesterol level.

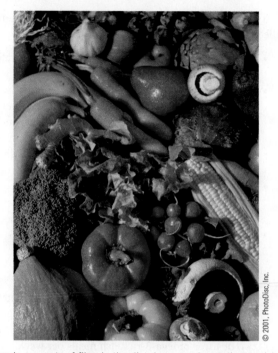

Ample amounts of fiber in the diet decreases heart disease risk.

Lowering LDL-cholesterol. If LDL-cholesterol is higher than ideal, it can be lowered with proper nutrition, by losing body fat, by taking medication, and by participating in a regular aerobic exercise program.

To decrease LDL-cholesterol, the diet should be low in saturated fat, trans fats, and cholesterol. It should also be high in fiber. A top priority in the American diet is to replace saturated fat with monounsaturated and polyunsaturated fats because the latter tend to decrease LDL-cholesterol. Exercise is important, as dietary manipulation by itself is not as effective in lowering LDL-cholesterol as a combination of diet plus aerobic exercise.

Total daily fiber intake must be in the range of 25 to 38 grams per day (see the discussion of fiber in Chapter 5, pages 126–128). The incidence of heart disease is low in populations in which daily fiber intake exceeds 30 grams per day. The fiber intake of most people in the United States averages less than 15 grams per day. Fiber, in particular the soluble type, has been shown to lower cholesterol. This statement is made on the second bullet of the very next page.

GLOSSARY

Atherosclerosis Fatty/cholesterol deposits in the walls of the arteries leading to formation of plaque.

To lower LDL-cholesterol levels, the following general dietary guidelines are recommended:

- Minimize the use of simple and refined carbohydrates (including sugars) and processed foods.
- Consume between 25 and 38 grams of fiber daily, including a minimum of 10 grams of soluble fiber (good sources are oats, fruits, barley, legumes, and psyllium).
- Increase consumption of vegetables, fruits, whole grains, and beans.
- Do not consume more than 200 mg of dietary cholesterol a day (this recommendation is to be followed while trying to lower LDL cholesterol).
- Consume red meats (three ounces per serving) fewer than three times per week and no organ meats (such as liver and kidneys).
- Do not eat commercially baked foods.
- Avoid foods that contain trans fats, hydrogenated fat, or partially hydrogenated vegetable oil.
- Increase intake of omega-3 fatty acids by eating two or three omega-3-rich fish meals per week.
- Consume 25 grams of soy protein a day.
- Drink low-fat milk (1 percent or less fat, preferably) and use low-fat dairy products.
- Do not use coconut oil, palm oil, or cocoa butter.
- Use margarines and salad dressings that contain stanol ester instead of butter and regular margarine.
- Bake, broil, grill, poach, or steam food instead of frying.
- Refrigerate cooked meat before adding to other dishes. Remove fat hardened in the refrigerator before mixing the meat with other foods.
- Avoid fatty sauces made with butter, cream, or cheese.
- Maintain recommended body weight.

Saturated Fat Replacement in the Diet

Once people learned that saturated fats were unhealthy, instead of consuming more fruits, vegetables, legumes, and grains, many increased consumption of "low-fat" simple carbohydrates and refined sugars (low-fat varieties of breads, rolls, cereals, cookies, ice cream, cakes, and desserts). Unknown to most consumers is the fact that desserts are among the top saturated fat contributors in the American diet. Using simple carbohydrates for saturated fat doesn't lower LDL cholesterol as effectively as unsaturated fats or even proteins from plant sources with small amounts of fish. Although low in fat, simple carbohydrates and refined sugars are high in calories that lead to weight gain. The data show that exchanging refined carbohydrates for saturated fat exacerbates blood lipid problems,

including a higher LDL cholesterol, a reduction in HDL cholesterol, and higher triglycerides. Scientists believe that high refined-carbohydrate diets increase palmitoleic acid, a minor monounsaturated fatty acid that actually behaves like a saturated acid, increasing LDL-cholesterol. Data also indicate that each additional daily serving of sugar-sweetened drinks increases heart disease risk by up to 19 percent. Complex carbohydrates (e.g., whole grains), on the contrary, help lower LDL-cholesterol.

Very low-fat diets (less than 25 percent fat) are not recommended to lower LDL-cholesterol because they also tend to lower HDL-cholesterol and increase triglycerides. Replacing saturated fat with monounsaturated and polyunsaturated fats is preferable because it provides greater cardioprotective benefits.[14] The recommendation is not to limit fat consumption in the diet to an absolute minimum, but to maintain total fat intake around 25 percent to 35 percent of total calories, with a primary shift toward polyunsaturated fats. To do so, choose fish, nuts, seeds, and vegetable oils that are liquid at room temperature (with the exception of tropical oils including coconut, palm, and palm kernel oils). Olive, canola, corn, and soybean oils and nuts are sample food items that are high in monounsaturated fats and polyunsaturated fats. A specialized nutrition book should be consulted to determine food items that are high in monounsaturated and polyunsaturated fats.

At present, it is unknown whether the cardioprotective benefits are the result of limiting saturated fat intake or increasing polyunsaturated fat consumption. Another review found that consumption of polyunsaturated fat in place of saturated fat reduced the incidence of heart attacks and cardiac deaths.[15] Thus, moderate fat intake (not low fat), along with decreased refined carbohydrates and decreased caloric intake is encouraged.

Elevated Triglycerides

Triglycerides, also known as free fatty acids, make up most of the fat in our diet and most of the fat that circulates in the blood. In combination with cholesterol, triglycerides speed up formation of plaque in the arteries. Triglycerides are carried in the bloodstream primarily by very low-density lipoproteins (VLDLs) and **chylomicrons**.

Although they are found in poultry skin, lunch meats, and shellfish, these fatty acids are manufactured mainly in the liver from refined sugars, starches, and alcohol. High intake of alcohol and sugars (honey and fruit juices included) significantly raises triglyceride levels. To lower triglycerides, avoid pastries, candies, soft drinks, fruit juices, white bread, pasta, and alcohol. In addition, cutting down on overall fat consumption, quitting smoking, reducing weight (if overweight), and doing aerobic exercise are helpful measures. Omega-3 fatty acids also help, but doses higher than those found in fish are required. A desirable blood triglyceride level is less than 150 mg/dL (see Table 8.3, page 212).

Medications to lower blood lipids. Effective medications are available to treat elevated cholesterol and triglycerides. Most notable among them are the statins group (Lipitor, Mevacor, Pravachol, Lescol, Crestor, and Zocor), which slow down cholesterol production and increase the liver's ability to remove blood cholesterol. They also decrease triglycerides and produce a small increase in HDL levels.

High doses (1.5 to 3 grams per day) of nicotinic acid or niacin (a B vitamin) also help lower LDL-cholesterol and triglycerides and increase HDL-cholesterol. A fourth group of drugs, known as fibrates, is primarily used to lower triglycerides.

The guidelines by the American Heart Association and the American College of Cardiology recommend that people at high risk for CVD disease be treated with statin therapy. Unless at high risk, many experts feel that in general, it is better to lower LDL-cholesterol without medication because drugs can often cause undesirable side effects. People with heart disease often must take cholesterol-lowering medication, but it is best if medication is combined with lifestyle changes to augment the cholesterol-lowering effect. In 2012 the FDA added safety alerts to the prescribing information of statins. Although rare among the millions of people who take these medications, the adverse effects include memory loss, cognitive impairment like forgetfulness and confusion, higher blood sugar levels that may lead to a diagnosis of diabetes, and muscle pain. Anyone starting treatment with statin drugs should be aware of these side effects.

Elevated Homocysteine

Clinical data indicating that many heart attack victims have normal cholesterol levels have led researchers to look for other risk factors that may contribute to atherosclerosis. Although it is not a blood lipid, a high concentration of **homocysteine** in the blood is thought to enhance the formation of plaque and subsequently lead to blockage of the arteries. The body uses homocysteine to help build proteins and carry out cellular metabolism. Homocysteine forms during an intermediate step in the creation of another amino acid. This process requires the presence of folate and vitamins B_6 and B_{12}.

Typically, homocysteine is metabolized rapidly, so it does not accumulate in the blood or damage the arteries. Many people, however, have high blood levels of homocysteine. This might be attributable to either a genetic inability to metabolize homocysteine or a deficiency in the vitamins required for its conversion.

Homocysteine is typically measured in micromoles per liter (μmol/L). A level below 9.0 μmol/L is desirable, while a level above 13.0 μmol/L is viewed as elevated. Homocysteine accumulation is theorized to be toxic because it may

1. damage the inner lining of the arteries (the initial step in the process of atherosclerosis).
2. stimulate the proliferation of cells that contribute to plaque formation.
3. encourage clotting that may completely obstruct an artery.

Keeping homocysteine from accumulating in the blood seems to be as simple as eating the recommended daily servings of vegetables, fruits, grains, and some meat and legumes. Increasing evidence that folate can prevent heart attacks has led to the recommendation that people consume 400 mcg per day of folate. Most Americans, however, do not get 400 daily mcg of folate. Five daily servings of fruits and vegetables can provide sufficient levels of folate and vitamin B_6 to remove and clear homocysteine from the blood.

Vitamin B_{12} is found primarily in animal flesh and animal products. Vitamin B_{12} deficiency is rarely a problem, as one cup of milk or an egg provides the daily requirement. The body also recycles most of this vitamin; therefore, it takes years to develop a deficiency.

Inflammation

For years it has been known that chronic low-grade inflammation plays a role in CHD and that inflammation hidden deep in the body is a common trigger of heart attacks, even when cholesterol levels are normal or low and arterial plaque is minimal. Chronic low-grade inflammation can occur in a variety of places throughout the body. It leads to continued elevated levels of toxins and most people are unaware of its existence until damage occurs. It persists for years or decades in people with unhealthy lifestyles. Physical inactivity, smoking, excessive body weight, a diet high in saturated fat, chronic

GLOSSARY

Triglycerides Fats formed by glycerol and three fatty acids.

Chylomicrons Molecules that transport triglycerides in the blood.

Homocysteine Intermediate amino acid in the interconversion of two other amino acids: methionine and cysteine.

Figure 8.6 Relationships among C-reactive protein, cholesterol, and risk for cardiovascular disease.

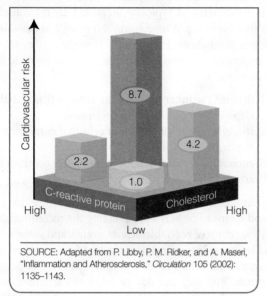

SOURCE: Adapted from P. Libby, P. M. Ridker, and A. Maseri, "Inflammation and Atherosclerosis," *Circulation* 105 (2002): 1135–1143.

Table 8.4 High-Sensitivity CRP Guidelines

Amount	Rating
<1 mg/L	Low risk
1–3 mg/L	Average risk
>3 mg/L	High risk

SOURCE: T. A. Pearson, et al, "Markers of Inflammation and Cardiovascular Disease," *Circulation* 107 (2003): 499–511.

stress, periodontal disease, and infections that produce no outward symptoms can all cause inflammation.

To evaluate ongoing inflammation, physicians have turned to **C-reactive protein (CRP)**, a protein whose level in the blood increases with inflammation. The evidence shows that CRP blood levels elevate years before a first heart attack or stroke and that individuals with elevated CRP have twice the risk of a heart attack. The risk of a heart attack is even higher in people with both elevated CRP and cholesterol, resulting in an almost ninefold increase in risk (see Figure 8.6).

CRP levels are measured with the high-sensitivity CRP (hs-CRP) test, which measures inflammation in the blood vessels. The term "high-sensitivity" was derived from the test's capability to detect small amounts of CRP in the blood. Test results provide a good measure of the probability of plaque rupturing within the arterial wall. The two main types of plaque are soft and hard. Soft plaque is the most likely to rupture. Ruptured plaque releases clots into the bloodstream that can completely block an artery and lead to a heart attack or stroke. Other evidence has linked high CRP levels to high blood pressure and colon cancer. Guidelines for hs-CRP levels are given in Table 8.4.

CRP increases with obesity, excessive alcohol intake, and high-protein diets. Evidence further indicates that high-fat, fast-food meals increase CRP levels for several hours following the meals. Cooking meat and poultry at high temperatures creates damaged proteins (AGEs or advanced glycation end products) that trigger inflammation. CRP levels decrease with statin drugs, exercise, proper nutrition, weight loss, quitting smoking, and aspirin therapy. Omega-3 fatty acids (found in salmon, tuna, and mackerel fish) inhibit proteins that cause inflammation.

A new test approved by the FDA that assesses risk for both CHD and strokes associated with atherosclerosis is the **PLAC blood test**. The test measures the level of Lp-PLA$_2$ (Lipoprotein-associated Phospholipase A$_2$), an enzyme produced inside the plaque when the arteries are inflamed and which indicates risk for plaque rupture. If the Lp-PLA$_2$ level is high, the plaque is more likely to rupture through the inside lining of the artery into the bloodstream where it may cause a clot that could lead to a heart attack or stroke.

Diabetes

In people who have **diabetes mellitus**, the pancreas stops producing insulin (or does not produce enough to meet the body's needs) or the cells become resistant to the effects of insulin. The role of insulin is to "unlock" the cells and escort glucose into the cell. Diabetes affects about 30 million people in the United States, and about 1 million new cases are diagnosed each year. More than 75 percent of people with diabetes mellitus die from CVD. Diabetics may have problems metabolizing fats, which can make them more susceptible to atherosclerosis, coronary disease, heart attacks, high blood pressure, and strokes. Diabetics also tend to have lower HDL-cholesterol and higher triglyceride levels.

Chronic high blood sugar can also lead to nerve damage, vision loss, kidney damage, and lower immune function (making the individual more susceptible to infections). Diabetics are four times more likely to become blind and 20 times more likely than nondiabetics to develop kidney failure. Nerve damage in the lower extremities makes the person less aware of injury and infection. A small untreated sore can lead to severe infection, gangrene, and even amputation.

An 8-hour fasting blood glucose level of 126 mg/dL or higher on two separate tests confirms a diagnosis of diabetes. A level of 126 or higher should be brought to the attention of a physician. This guideline has changed from previous years, in which a level above 140 had been used to diagnose diabetes.

Behavior Modification Planning

American Heart Association Diet and Lifestyle Recommendations for Cardiovascular Disease Risk Reduction

- Balance caloric intake and physical activity to achieve or maintain a healthy body weight.
- Consume a diet rich in vegetables and fruits.
- Consume whole-grain, high-fiber foods.
- Consume fish, especially oily fish, at least twice a week.
- Limit your intake of saturated fat to less than 6 percent and trans fat to less than 1 percent of total daily caloric intake.
- Limit cholesterol intake to less than 300 mg per day.
- Minimize your intake of beverages and foods with added sugars.
- Choose and prepare foods with little or no salt.
- If you consume alcohol, do so in moderation.
- When you eat food that is prepared outside of the home, follow the above recommendations.
- Avoid use of and exposure to tobacco products.
- Be physically active.
- Aim for recommended levels of LDL-cholesterol, HDL-cholesterol, and triglycerides.
- Aim for a normal blood pressure.
- Aim for normal blood glucose levels.

Try It

In your Online Journal or class notebook, record which of the above recommendations you fall short on and propose at least one thing you could do to improve.

© Cengage Learning

Types of diabetes. The two types of diabetes are **type 1,** or **insulin-dependent diabetes mellitus (IDDM),** and **type 2,** or **non-insulin-dependent diabetes mellitus (NIDDM).** Type 1 has also been known as "juvenile diabetes" because it afflicts mainly young people. With type 1, the pancreas produces little or no insulin. With type 2, the pancreas either does not produce sufficient insulin or produces adequate amounts but the cells become insulin-resistant, thereby keeping glucose from entering the cell. Type 2 accounts for 90 percent to 95 percent of all diabetes cases.

Although diabetes has a genetic predisposition, type 2 diabetes is related closely to overeating, obesity, and lack of physical activity. More than 80 percent of type 2 diabetics are overweight or have a history of excessive weight.

Aerobic exercise helps prevent type 2 diabetes. The protective effect is even greater in those with risk factors such as obesity, high blood pressure, and family propensity. The preventive effect is attributed to less body fat and to better sugar and fat metabolism resulting from the regular exercise program. At 3,500 calories of energy expenditure per week through exercise, the risk is cut in half versus that of a sedentary lifestyle.

Strength training is also increasingly used to help prevent and treat diabetes. During strength training, muscles use glucose exclusively to perform their work. Following a good strength-training workout, muscles will use more glucose during the next 48 hours. And as muscle mass increases with training, so does the body's ability to utilize blood glucose. The key to increase and maintain proper insulin sensitivity is regularity of the aerobic and strength-training programs. Failure to maintain habitual physical activity voids the benefits.

GLOSSARY

C-reactive protein (CRP) A protein whose level in the blood increases with inflammation (which may be hidden deep in the body); elevation of this protein is an indicator of potential cardiovascular events.

PLAC blood test A blood test that measures the level of Lipoprotein-associated Phospholipase A2, an enzyme produced inside the plaque when the arteries are inflamed and indicates risk for plaque rupture.

Diabetes mellitus A condition in which blood glucose is unable to enter the cells because the pancreas either stops producing insulin or does not produce enough to meet the body's needs.

Insulin-dependent diabetes mellitus (IDDM or type 1) A form of diabetes in which the pancreas produces little or no insulin.

Non-insulin-dependent diabetes mellitus (NIDDM or type 2) A form of diabetes in which the pancreas either does not produce sufficient insulin or produces adequate amounts but the cells become insulin-resistant, keeping glucose from entering the cell.

Accumulating evidence indicates that increasing physical activity, losing excess weight, and improving nutrition is more effective to control diabetes and lower CVD risk than relying on drugs to manage the disease. Furthermore, research suggests that diabetic patients are worse off when medications are used to decrease blood sugar levels and blood pressure to *normal* or *below normal* levels. Accordingly, diabetic patients are strongly encouraged to adopt healthy lifestyle factors even if glucose levels are controlled with medication. Medications are recommended for diabetic patients with a systolic blood pressure above 140 mm Hg, but it is only necessary to drive it down to about 130 mm Hg.

Metabolic syndrome. As the cells resist the action of insulin, the pancreas releases even more insulin in an attempt to keep the blood glucose level from rising. A chronic rise in insulin seems to trigger a series of abnormalities referred to as **metabolic syndrome**. These abnormal conditions include low HDL-cholesterol, high triglycerides, and an increased blood-clotting mechanism. Many individuals with metabolic syndrome also have high blood pressure. All of these conditions increase the risk for CHD and other diabetic-related conditions (blindness, infection, nerve damage, and kidney failure). More than 50 million Americans are afflicted by metabolic syndrome.

Individuals with metabolic syndrome have an abnormal insulin response to carbohydrates, in particular those that are absorbed rapidly (high-glycemic foods). Metabolic syndrome research indicates that a low-fat/high-carbohydrate dietary plan may not be the best for prevention of CHD and actually could increase the risk for this disease in people with high insulin resistance and glucose intolerance. It might be best for these people to distribute their daily caloric intake so they derive 45 percent of their calories from carbohydrates (primarily low-glycemic), 35 to 40 percent from fat, and 15 percent from protein.[16] Of the 35 to 40 percent fat calories, 30 percent to 35 percent should come from mono- and polyunsaturated fats and less than 6 percent from saturated fat.

People with metabolic syndrome also benefit from weight loss (if overweight), exercise, and smoking cessation. Insulin resistance drops by about 40 percent in overweight people who lose 20 pounds. Forty-five minutes of daily aerobic exercise enhances insulin efficiency by 25 percent. Smoking, on the other hand, increases insulin resistance.

Abnormal Electrocardiograms

The **electrocardiogram (ECG or EKG)** is a recording of the electrical impulses that stimulate the heart to contract. ECGs are taken at rest, during the stress of exercise, and during recovery. An exercise or **stress ECG** also is known as a graded exercise stress test or a maximal exercise tolerance test. A stress ECG reveals the heart's tolerance to vigorous-intensity activities. Based on the findings, ECGs may be interpreted as normal, equivocal, or abnormal.

A stress ECG frequently is used to diagnose coronary heart disease. It also is administered to determine cardiorespiratory fitness levels, to screen individuals for preventive and cardiac rehabilitation programs, to detect abnormal blood pressure response during exercise, and to establish actual or functional maximal heart rate for purposes of participation in exercise.

Most adults who wish to start or continue an exercise program don't need a stress ECG. No set of guidelines can cover all cases when a stress electrocardiogram is recommended prior to exercise participation. The test, however, is recommended for individuals who are at high risk or are known to have cardiovascular, pulmonary, renal, or metabolic disease. Moreover, people feeling unusually winded in response to normal exertion, unexplained fatigue, or chest pain should have the test done.

Tobacco Use

Approximately 57 million adults and 3.5 million adolescents in the United States smoke cigarettes. Each day, an additional 3,000 people under the age of 18 smoke their first cigarette. Cigarette smoking is the single largest preventable cause of illness and premature death in the United States. If we include all related deaths, tobacco is responsible for more than 480,000 unnecessary deaths per year. Smoking has been linked to CVD, cancer, bronchitis, emphysema, and peptic ulcers.

More than 42,000 of those yearly deaths are nonsmokers who were exposed to secondhand smoke in their daily life. Both fatal and nonfatal cardiac events increase greatly in people who are exposed to passive smoking. Some 34,000 yearly deaths from heart disease are attributed to secondhand smoke. Even in regular smokers, adaptations to the harmful effects of smoking are slight, so the adverse effects are much greater to nonsmokers.

In relation to coronary disease, smoking speeds up the process of atherosclerosis and also produces a threefold increase in the risk of sudden death following a **myocardial infarction**. Smoking increases heart rate and blood pressure and irritates the heart, which can trigger fatal cardiac **arrhythmias**. As far as the extra load on the heart is concerned, giving up one pack of cigarettes per day is the equivalent of losing between 50 and 75 pounds of excess body fat! Another harmful effect is

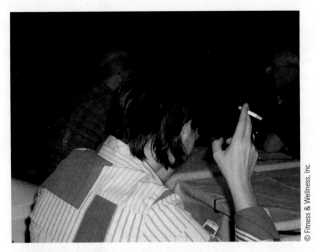

Cigarette smoking is the single largest preventable cause of illness and premature death in the United States.

a decrease in HDL-cholesterol, the "good" type that helps control blood lipids.

Pipe and cigar smoking and chewing tobacco also increase the risk for heart disease. Even if no smoke is inhaled, toxic substances are absorbed through the membranes of the mouth and end up in the bloodstream.

Quitting tobacco use is not easy. The addictive properties of nicotine make quitting difficult, and physical and psychological withdrawal symptoms set in. Figure 8.7 presents a six-step plan to help people stop smoking. The risk for CVD starts to decrease the moment a person quits smoking. One year after quitting, the risk of CHD decreases by half, and within 15 years, the relative risk of dying from CVD and cancer approaches that of a lifetime nonsmoker.

> **! Critical Thinking**
>
> Cigarette smoking is the largest preventable cause of premature illness and death in the United States. • Do you think the government should outlaw the use of tobacco in all forms? • Or does the individual have the right to engage in self-destructive behavior?

The most important factor in quitting cigarette smoking is a desire to do so. Most successful ex-smokers have been able to quit on their own, either by quitting cold turkey or by using self-help kits available from organizations such as the American Cancer Society, the American Heart Association, and the American Lung Association. Only 3 percent of ex-smokers quit as a result of formal cessation programs.

Stress

Stress has become a part of life. People have to deal daily with goals, deadlines, responsibilities, and pressures. The **stressor** itself is not what creates the health hazard but, rather, the individual's response to it.

The human body responds to stress by producing more catecholamines to prepare the body for **fight or flight**. If the person fights or flees, the body metabolizes the higher levels of catecholamines and is able to return to a normal state. If, however, a person is under constant stress and is unable to take action (as in the death of a close relative or friend, loss of a job, trouble at work, or financial insecurity), the catecholamines remain elevated in the bloodstream.

People who are not able to relax place a constant low-level strain on the cardiovascular system that could manifest itself in heart disease. Higher levels of the hormones epinephrine and cortisol in highly stressed people may raise blood pressure, elevate blood glucose levels, and increase cholesterol by 20 percent to 50 percent.[17] Even without a large amount of plaque, small deposits on the arterial wall can rupture during stressful events, tearing the blood vessel lining and triggering a clot that causes a heart attack.

─GLOSSARY─

Metabolic syndrome An array of metabolic abnormalities that contribute to the development of atherosclerosis triggered by resistance to insulin; these conditions include low HDL-cholesterol, high triglycerides, high blood pressure, and an increased blood-clotting mechanism.

Electrocardiogram (ECG or EKG) A recording of the electrical activity of the heart.

Stress electrocardiogram (stress ECG) An exercise test during which the workload is gradually increased (until the subject reaches maximal fatigue), with blood pressure and 12-lead electrocardiographic

monitoring throughout the test.

Myocardial infarction Heart attack; damage or death of an area of the heart muscle as a result of an obstructed artery to that area.

Arrhythmias Irregular heart rhythms.

Stress The mental, emotional, and physiological response of the body to any situation that is new, threatening, frightening, or exciting.

Stressor Stress-causing event.

Fight or flight A series of physical responses activated automatically in response to environmental stresses.

Figure 8.7 Six-step smoking cessation approach.

The following six-step plan has been developed as a guide to help you quit smoking. The total program should be completed in four weeks or less. Steps one through four should take no longer than two weeks. A maximum of two additional weeks are allowed for the rest of the program.

Step One. Decide positively that you want to quit. Now prepare a list of the reasons why you smoke and why you want to quit.

Step Two. Initiate a personal diet and exercise program. Exercise and decreased body weight cause a greater awareness of healthy living and increase motivation for giving up cigarettes.

Step Three. Decide on the approach you will use to stop smoking. You may quit cold turkey or gradually decrease the number of cigarettes smoked daily. Many people have found that quitting cold turkey is the easiest way to do it. Although it may not work the first time, after several attempts, all of a sudden smokers are able to overcome the habit without too much difficulty. Tapering off cigarettes can be done in several ways. You may start by eliminating cigarettes that you do not necessarily need, you can switch to a brand lower in nicotine or tar every couple of days, you can smoke less of each cigarette, or you can simply decrease the total number of cigarettes smoked each day.

Step Four. Set the target date for quitting. In setting the target date, choosing a special date may add a little extra incentive. An upcoming birthday, anniversary, vacation, graduation, family reunion—all are examples of good dates to free yourself from smoking.

Step Five. Stock up on low-calorie foods—carrots, broccoli, cauliflower, celery, popcorn (butter- and salt-free), fruits, sunflower seeds (in the shell), sugarless gum, and plenty of water. Keep such food handy on the day you stop and the first few days following cessation. Replace it for cigarettes when you want one.

Step Six. This is the day that you will quit smoking. On this day and the first few days thereafter, do not keep cigarettes handy. Stay away from friends and events that trigger your desire to smoke. Drink large amounts of water and fruit juices and eat low-calorie foods. Replace the old behavior with new behavior. You will need to replace smoking time with new positive substitutes that will make smoking difficult or impossible. When you desire a cigarette, take a few deep breaths and then occupy yourself by doing a number of things such as talking to someone else, washing your hands, brushing your teeth, eating a healthy snack, chewing on a straw, doing dishes, playing sports, going for a walk or bike ride, going swimming, and so on.

If you have been successful and stopped smoking, a lot of events still can trigger your urge to smoke. When confronted with such events, people rationalize and think, "One won't hurt." It will not work! Before you know it, you will be back to the regular habit. Be prepared to take action in those situations. Find adequate substitutes for smoking. Remind yourself of how difficult it has been and how long it has taken you to get to this point. As time goes on, it will only get easier rather than worse.

© Cengage Learning

Chronic stress also causes an increase of the brain chemical neuropeptide Y that promotes storage of visceral fat, further increasing the risk for type 2 diabetes, heart disease, some cancers, and body-wide inflammation. In addition, when a person is in a stressful situation, the coronary arteries that feed the heart muscle constrict, reducing the oxygen supply to the heart. If the blood vessels are largely blocked by atherosclerosis, abnormal heart rhythms or even a heart attack may follow.

As outlined in Chapter 7, individuals who are under a lot of stress and do not cope well with it need to take measures to counteract the effects of stress in their lives. Identifying and learning how to cope with the sources of stress will improve health and quality of life.

Physical activity is one of the best ways to relieve stress. During exercise the nervous system shifts from the sympathetic or stress tone to the parasympathetic or rest tone, a benefit that lasts several hours following exercise. When a person takes part in physical activity, the body metabolizes excess catecholamines and is able to return to a normal state. Exercise also steps up muscular activity, which contributes to muscular relaxation.

Personal and Family History

Individuals who have a family history of, or already have experienced, cardiovascular problems are at higher risk than those who never have had a problem. A series of genetic tests are now available that help identify individuals at risk for heart disease, even though they lead a healthy lifestyle and no other visible signs or symptoms of the disease are present. People with a family or personal history are encouraged strongly to keep all risk factors as low as possible. Because most risk factors are reversible, the risk for future problems decreases significantly.

Age and Gender

Age becomes a risk factor for men over age 45 and women over age 55. The greater incidence of heart disease may stem in part from lifestyle changes as we get older (less physical activity, poor nutrition, obesity, and so on). Earlier in life, men are at greater risk for CVD than women are. Following menopause, the risk for women increases. Currently, more women (401,495) than men (386,436) die from CVD.[18]

Young people should not think they are immune from heart disease. The process begins early in life. Autopsies conducted in people who have died in their 20s reveal that many of them already exhibit early stages of atherosclerosis. Other studies have found elevated blood cholesterol levels in children as young as 10 years old.

Even though the aging process cannot be stopped, it certainly can be slowed. The concept of **chronological age,** versus **physiological age** is important in longevity. Research indicates a physiological age difference of about 25 years between physically active and sedentary individuals. That is, an active 60-year-old person can have the body of an average 35-year-old. And 35-year-olds often are in such poor condition and health that they almost seem to have the body of a 60-year-old. Managing risk factors and developing positive lifestyle habits are the best ways to slow natural aging.

8.4 *Cancer*

Cancer causes about 23 percent of all deaths in the United States. More than 1.6 million new cases were reported in 2015 and about 589,439 million people died from cancer the same year.[19] Cancer is not a single disease, but a category of diseases that share similar traits including gene mutation and uncontrolled cell growth. More than 100 types of cancer can develop in the body.

An individual starts life with every cell in the body having identical DNA. Under normal conditions, the 100 trillion cells in the human body reproduce themselves in an orderly way. Cell growth (cell reproduction) takes place to repair and replace old, worn-out tissue. Cell growth is controlled by **deoxyribonucleic acid (DNA)** and **ribonucleic acid (RNA),** found in the nucleus of each cell. Normally, the DNA molecule is duplicated perfectly during cell division. In a few cases the DNA molecule is not replicated exactly but specialized enzymes repair it quickly. Occasionally, however, a cell will divide without being repaired. The two new cells will both carry the resulting defect.

The mutations of precancerous cells make them proliferate faster than healthy cells. Thus, it becomes more likely that future cell divisions will result in an additional mutation and pass along both mutations. It is not known how many mutations are necessary, but eventually, after several generations of cells have passed on a collection of accumulated mutations, a cancerous cell will develop. That cell will grow and multiply uncontrollably and ultimately form a small tumor.

A tumor can be either **benign** or **malignant.** Benign tumors do not invade other tissues. Although they can interfere with normal bodily functions, they rarely cause death. A malignant tumor is a cancer. The rate at which cancer cells grow varies from one type to another; some types grow fast, and others take years. A decade or more might pass between the initial mutations (as a result of carcinogenic exposure, chance, or genetics) and the time that cancer is diagnosed.

While cancer starts with the abnormal growth of one cell, it can multiply into billions of cancerous cells. A critical turning point in the development of cancer is when a tumor reaches about a million cells. At this stage it is referred to as **carcinoma in situ**, when it has not spread. Such an undetected tumor may go for months or years without any significant growth.

While encapsulated, a tumor does not pose a serious threat to human health. As the tumor continues to grow it invades and destroys normal tissue. To grow, the tumor requires more oxygen and nutrients. In time, a few of the cancer cells start producing chemicals that enhance **angiogenesis**. Cells break away from a malignant tumor and, in a process called **metastasis**, migrate through the

---

GLOSSARY

Chronological age Calendar age.

Physiological age Age based on the individual's functional and physical capacity.

Deoxyribonucleic acid (DNA) Genetic substance of which genes are made; molecule that bears a cell's genetic code.

Ribonucleic acid (RNA) Genetic material involved in the formation of cell proteins.

Benign Noncancerous.

Malignant Cancerous.

Cancer Group of diseases characterized by uncontrolled growth and spread of abnormal cells into malignant tumors.

Carcinoma in situ Encapsulated malignant tumor that is found at an early stage and has not spread.

Angiogenesis Capillary (blood vessel) formation into a tumor.

Metastasis Movement of bacteria or body cells from one part of the body to another.

new blood vessels to other parts of the body, where they can cause new cancer.

Although the immune system and the blood turbulence destroy most cancer cells, only one abnormal cell lodging elsewhere can start a new cancer. These cells also will grow and multiply uncontrollably, destroying normal tissue. New tumors anywhere in the body are referred to by the name of the original site of the first tumor. Once cancer cells metastasize, treatment becomes more difficult. Therapy can kill most cancer cells, but a few cells may become resistant to treatment. These cells then can grow into a new tumor that will not respond to the same treatment.

Most adults have precancerous or cancerous cells in their bodies. Adults have had more time to be exposed to carcinogens or the occasional accidental mutations during some of the trillions of cell divisions that take place over a person's lifetime.

As with CVD, cancer is largely preventable. As much as 80 percent of all human cancer is related to lifestyle or environmental factors (including diet, tobacco use, excessive use of alcohol, sexual and reproductive activity, and exposure to environmental hazards). Equally important is that more than 13.7 million Americans with a history of cancer were alive in 2012. Currently, almost 7 in 10 people diagnosed with cancer are expected to be alive 5 years from the initial diagnosis.

Guidelines for Preventing Cancer

The biggest factor in fighting cancer today is health education. A survey conducted by the American Institute for Cancer Research (AICR) published in 2014 revealed alarming results about our understanding of the link between lifestyle and cancer risk. Fewer than half of respondents were aware that body weight is linked to cancer risk or of the link between processed meat consumption and cancer development. Worse, only one in five respondents agreed that genetics is not the main cause of developing cancer. People need to be informed about the risk factors for cancer and the guidelines for early detection. The most effective way to protect against cancer is to change negative lifestyle habits and behaviors. Activity 8.1, page 238, includes a questionnaire regarding the risk factors and preventive measures discussed next.

Research sponsored by the American Cancer Society and the National Cancer Institute showed that individuals who have a healthy lifestyle have some of the lowest cancer mortality rates ever reported in scientific studies. In a landmark study, a group of about 10,000 members of the Church of Jesus Christ of Latter-day Saints in California was reported to have only about one-third

(men) to one-half (women) the rate of cancer mortality of the general white population.[20] In this study, the investigators looked at three general health habits in the participants: lifetime abstinence from smoking, regular physical activity, and sufficient sleep. Healthy lifestyle guidelines include abstaining from all forms of tobacco, alcohol, and drugs, and adhering to a well-balanced diet based on grains, fruits, and vegetables, and moderate amounts of poultry and red meat.

Additional 2009 data from more than 23,000 German participants indicated that people who never smoked, had a BMI less than 30, exercised at least 3.5 hours per week, and consumed a diet rich in fruits and vegetables and low in meat, had a 36 percent lower risk of cancer.[21] The conclusion of the latter two studies is that lifestyle is definitely an important factor in the risk for cancer.

Making Dietary Changes

The American Cancer Society estimates that one-third of all cancer in the United States is related to nutrition and lack of physical activity. A healthy diet, therefore, is crucial to decrease the risk for cancer. The diet should be predominantly vegetarian. **Cruciferous vegetables** (cauliflower, broccoli, cabbage, kale, Brussels sprouts, and kohlrabi), tea, vitamin D, soy products, calcium, and omega-3 fats are encouraged. The many components of a healthful diet—especially dietary fiber, nutrients, and phytonutrients—appear to work in synergy during metabolic processes to prevent and slow cancer development at various stages. If alcohol is used, it should be used in moderation. Obesity should be avoided.

Brightly colored fruits and vegetables are also encouraged. These fruits and vegetables contain **carotenoids** and vitamin C. Lycopene, one of the many carotenoids (a phytonutrient—see discussion that follows), has been linked to lowered risk of cancers of the prostate, colon, and cervix. Lycopene is especially abundant in cooked tomato products.

The evidence for vitamin D in protecting against cancer continues to be the focus of research. Vitamin D appears to be the most powerful regulator of cell growth and appears to keep cells from becoming malignant. Researchers are still working to understand the cause and effect relationship between health and vitamin D levels, but the protective effect of vitamin D appears to be strongest against breast, colon, and prostate cancers and possibly lung and digestive cancers. You should strive for "safe sun" exposure, that is, 10 to 20 minutes of unprotected sun exposure, on most days of the week between the hours of 10:00 a.m. and 4:00 p.m. For people living north of the 35th parallel (above the states of Texas and Georgia) in the United States and in Canada, with limited sun exposure during the winter months, a vitamin D_3 supplement of up to 2,000 IUs per day is strongly recommended. The cancer-protective benefits of this vitamin have already been discussed in detail in Chapter 5 (see "Vitamin D," pages 141–143).

Some researchers also believe that the antioxidant effect of vitamins helps protect the body from **free radicals**. Proteins that require the mineral selenium also appear to have a protective effect. Antioxidants are thought to absorb free radicals before they can cause damage, and they also interrupt the sequence of reactions once damage has begun. Research is still required in this area because a clear link has not been established.

Grains are high in fiber and contain vitamins and minerals—folate, selenium, and calcium—that seem to decrease the risk for colon cancer. Selenium also protects against prostate cancer and possibly lung cancer. Calcium may protect against colon cancer by preventing rapid growth of cells in the colon, especially in people with colon polyps.

Phytonutrients, antioxidant compounds found exclusively in abundance in fruits and vegetables, seem to exert a powerful effect in preventing cancer by blocking the formation of cancerous tumors and disrupting the process at almost every step of the way. New phytonutrients are continually being discovered and our understanding of the way combinations of phytonutrients work in synergy with each other and with dietary fiber and nutrients is continually growing. To obtain the highest possible protection, fruits and vegetables should be consumed several times throughout the day (instead of in one meal) to maintain effective phytonutrient levels throughout the day. Phytonutrient blood levels drop within three hours of consuming the produce.

Polyphenols (a phytonutrient) are cancer-fighting antioxidants found in tea. They are known to block the formation of **nitrosamines** and quell the activation of carcinogens. Polyphenols specifically have been shown to cause some types of cancer cells to die much like normal cells do, preventing tumor formation, reducing cancer cell proliferation, and possibly suppressing angiogenesis. Different types of tea contain different mixtures of polyphenols. White tea appears to have the highest amount, followed by green and black tea. These three teas are derived from the same plant during different times or by using different processing methods. Teas derived from some other plants, such as red tea, appear to have benefits as well. Herbal teas do not provide the same benefits as regular tea.

Observational data on tea-drinking habits in China showed that people who regularly drank green tea had about half the risk for chronic gastritis and stomach cancer, and the risk decreased further as the number of years of drinking green tea increased. In Japan, where people drink green tea regularly but smoke twice as much as people in the United States, the incidence of lung cancer is half that of the United States.

The antioxidant effect of one of the polyphenols in green tea—epigallocatechin gallate, or EGCG—is at least 25 times more effective than vitamin E and 100 times more effective than vitamin C at protecting cells and the DNA from damage believed to cause cancer, heart disease, and other diseases associated with free radicals.[22] EGCG is also twice as strong as the red wine antioxidant resveratrol, which helps prevent heart disease.

Research is also uncovering cancer-fighting phytonutrients in many common spices. Ginger, turmeric (a member of the ginger family), garlic, oregano, curry, pepper, cloves, fennel, rosemary, and black pepper are all encouraged for use in cooking and at the table.

Although previously viewed as a risk factor, minimal evidence exists that total fat intake affects cancer risk. There is far greater evidence that being overweight or obese increases cancer risk. Excessive caloric intake leads to weight gain and high-fat foods are typically calorie dense. Thus, indirectly, a high-fat diet can increase cancer risk through excessive body weight. Fat intake should consist primarily of monounsaturated and omega-3 fats. Omega-3 fats, found in many types of fish, flaxseeds, and flaxseed oil, seem to offer protection against colorectal, pancreatic, breast, oral, esophageal, and stomach cancers. Omega-3 fats block the synthesis of prostaglandins, bodily compounds that promote growth of tumors.

GLOSSARY

Cruciferous vegetables Plants that produce cross-shaped leaves (cauliflower, broccoli, cabbage, Brussels sprouts, and kohlrabi); these seem to have a protective effect against cancer.

Carotenoids Pigment substances (more than 600) in plants, about 50 of which are precursors to vitamin A; the most potent carotenoid is beta-carotene.

Free radicals Oxygen compounds produced in normal metabolism.

Phytonutrients Compounds found in fruits and vegetables that block formation of cancerous tumors and disrupt the process of cancer.

Nitrosamines Potentially cancer-causing compounds formed when nitrites and nitrates—which are used to prevent the growth of harmful bacteria in processed meats—combine with other chemicals in the stomach.

Foods high in vitamin C may deter some cancers. Salt-cured, smoked, and nitrite-cured foods have been associated with cancers of the esophagus and stomach. Processed meats should be consumed sparingly and always with orange juice or other foods rich in vitamin C. Vitamin C seems to discourage the formation of nitrosamines.

Cooking protein at high temperature should be avoided or done so only occasionally. The data suggest that grilling, broiling, or frying meat, poultry, or fish at high temperatures to "medium-well" or "well-done" leads to the formation of carcinogenic substances known as heterocyclic amines (HCAs) and polycyclic aromatic hydrocarbons (PAHs). Cancer risk seems to correlate to the amount of well-done meat an individual consumes, but even small amounts each day add up. Individuals who prefer their meat "medium-well" or "well-done" have a much higher risk for colorectal, stomach, breast, and prostate cancers.

Cooking proteins at high temperatures changes amino acids into HCAs that collect on the surface of meats. Charring meat increases their formation to an even greater extent. PAHs are formed when fat drips onto the rocks or coals of the grill. The subsequent fire flare-up releases smoke that coats the food with PAHs.

An electric contact grill such as a George Foreman grill is preferable when cooking meats because cooking temperatures are easily controlled. When cooking on an outdoor grill, line the grill with foil to keep the drippings off the rocks or coals. Microwaving the meat for a couple of minutes before barbecuing also decreases the risk, as long as the fluid released by the meat is discarded. Most of the potential **carcinogens** collect in this solution. For an occasional outdoor barbecue, trim off excess fat to avoid flare-ups and turn meats over frequently to decrease HCA formation. Removing the skin before serving and cooking at lower heat to "medium" also lowers the risk.

Mixing soy protein in powder form with meats also seems to decrease the formation of carcinogens when cooking meats. Soy foods may help because soy contains chemicals and active compounds that prevent cancer. Among these are isoflavones (phytonutrients), which are structurally similar to estrogen and may prevent breast, prostate, lung, and colon cancers. Isoflavones, frequently referred to as "phytoestrogens" or "plant estrogens," also block angiogenesis. Other phytonutrients and compounds in soy may prevent cancer by regulating cell growth and death, by discouraging metastasis, and by helping at other various stages of cancer development. Add soy to your diet with soy milk and whole foods such as tofu, miso, and edamame.

Based on the traditional diets of people in China and Japan, including children, who regularly consume soy foods, there doesn't seem to be an unsafe level of consumption. Soy protein powder supplementation, however, may not be safe because this may elevate soy protein intake to an unnaturally high level.

People who consume alcohol should do so in moderation. Alcohol use has been cited as one of the least emphasized causes for increased cancer risk. In the United States 3.5 percent of all cancer deaths are a result of alcohol consumption, with substantially higher numbers for some cancers. The National Toxicology Program classifies excessive alcohol consumption in the category "known to be a human carcinogen." Among other cancer-promoting effects, alcohol can damage DNA and proteins while it is being metabolized, with the extent of the damage depending on the individual's genetic inheritance.

Of breast cancer deaths, 15 percent are attributed to alcohol, with increased risk across all levels of alcohol consumption. Breast cancer risk begins with less than one drink per day and increases by 12 percent with each additional 10 ounces consumed per day. For other forms of cancers, alcohol becomes a serious danger at around 50 grams per day, where risk for cancers of the mouth, larynx, throat, and esophagus double or triple. The danger is also higher for people who use tobacco in any form, especially concerning cancers of the mouth, larynx, throat, esophagus, and liver. The odds of developing cancer of the oral cavity are fifteen times higher for those who use tobacco and drink alcohol. Excessive alcohol use is also a risk factor for colorectal cancer and a primary cause for liver cancer.

A 2009 study on almost 1.3 million women between the ages of 45 and 75, for example, indicated that as little as one drink of alcohol per day increases a woman's risk of cancer by 13 percent, including cancers of the breast, esophagus, larynx, rectum, and liver.[23] The researchers concluded that even the risks of low to moderate alcohol consumption outweigh any potential cardioprotective benefits. Based on these data, it is estimated that about 30,000 yearly female cancers in the United States are due to these low levels of alcohol consumption.

Maintaining recommended body weight also is encouraged. Adult weight gain increases the risk for many cancers, including those of the breast, prostate, colon and rectum, endometrium, esophagus, pancreas, and kidney. Obesity may also increase the risk for pancreatic, gallbladder, liver, prostate, ovarian, thyroid, and cervical cancers. For each of these types of cancer, the American Institute for Cancer Research has released the number of cases that could be prevented by diet, physical activity, and weight management. For example, 39,554 cases of breast cancer and 21,961 cases of colorectal cancer in the United States would have never occurred. Investigators theorize that excess weight raises hormone levels in the body that stimulate tumor growth.

Abstaining from Tobacco

Cigarette smoking by itself is a major health hazard. The World Health Organization estimates that smoking causes 6 million deaths worldwide annually, and that figure is expected to reach 8 million by 2030. Nonsmokers exposed to second hand smoke represent roughly one in ten deaths from smoking. The average life expectancy for a chronic smoker is about 10 years less than for a nonsmoker. The most prevalent carcinogenic exposure in the workplace is cigarette smoke. At least 27 percent of all cancer is tied to smoking, and 87 percent of lung cancer is tied to smoking. Use of smokeless tobacco can lead to nicotine addiction and dependence as well as increased risk for mouth, larynx, throat, and esophageal cancers.

Avoiding Excessive Sun Exposure

Near daily "safe sun" exposure, that is, 10 to 20 minutes of unprotected exposure during peak hours of the day (between 10:00 a.m. and 4:00 p.m.) is beneficial to health, but too much exposure to ultraviolet radiation (both UVB and UVA rays) is a major contributor to skin cancer. The most common sites of skin cancer are those exposed to the sun most often (face, neck, and back of the hands). There are three main types of skin cancer, each named after the type of cell from which they originate:

1. Basal cell carcinoma. Basal cells form the base, or the innermost layer of the epidermis.
2. Squamous cell carcinoma. Squamous originates from the word "scale." These flatter cells form the outside layer of the epidermis and shed as new cells form.
3. Malignant melanoma. Melanoma originates in cells that create melanin, which gives color to skin.

Nearly 90 percent of the almost 1 million cases of basal cell or squamous cell skin cancers reported yearly in the United States could have been prevented by protecting the skin from the sun's rays. Basal and squamous cell carcinoma require treatment but in the majority of cases do not spread to other parts of the body. **Melanoma,** the most deadly type of skin cancer, can appear quickly and metastasize in as little as six months. In 2015 it caused approximately 9,940 deaths in the United States. One in every five Americans will develop some type of skin cancer eventually.

One to two blistering sunburns can double the lifetime risk of melanoma, even more so if the sunburn took place prior to age 18, when cells divide at a much faster rate than later in life. A person can easily become overexposed during a day in the sun sooner than they expect and not realize until later in the day when the sunburn becomes painful and the damage is already done. Overexposure can be tricky to predict because sun exposure is strong or weak depending on time of year, a location's latitude and elevation, the sun's reflection off of snow or water, and several other factors. Furthermore, nothing is healthy about a "healthy tan." Tanning of the skin is the body's natural reaction to permanent and irreversible damage from too much exposure to the sun. Even brief exposures to sunlight add up to a greater risk for skin cancer and premature aging. The tan fades at the end of the summer season, but the underlying skin damage does not disappear. People with sensitive skin in particular should be extremely careful with sun exposure between 10:00 a.m. and 4:00 p.m.

The stinging sunburn comes from ultraviolet B (UVB) rays, which also are thought to be the main cause of premature wrinkling and skin aging, roughened/leathery/sagging skin, and skin cancer. Unfortunately, the damage may not become evident until up to 20 years later. In contrast, skin that has not been overexposed to the sun remains smooth and unblemished, and, over time, shows less evidence of aging.

Sun lamps and tanning parlors provide mainly ultraviolet A (UVA) rays. Once thought to be safe, they, too, are now known to be damaging and have been linked to melanoma. As little as 15 to 30 minutes of exposure to UVA can be as dangerous as a day spent in the sun. Similar to excessive exposure to sun, excessive exposure to recreational tanning at a salon causes DNA alterations that can lead to skin cancer.

Sunscreen lotion should be applied about 30 minutes before lengthy exposure to the sun because the skin takes that long to absorb the protective ingredients. Select sunscreens labeled "broad-spectrum," as these products block both UVA and UVB rays. A **sun protection factor (SPF)** of at least 15 is recommended. SPF 15 means that the skin takes 15 times longer to burn than it would with no lotion. If you ordinarily get mild sunburn after

---

GLOSSARY

Carcinogens Substances that contribute to the formation of cancers.

Melanoma The most virulent, rapidly spreading form of skin cancer.

Sun protection factor (SPF) Degree of protection offered by ingredients in sunscreen lotion; at least SPF 15 is recommended.

Behavior Modification Planning

Tips for a Healthy Cancer-Fighting Diet

Increase intake of phytonutrients, fiber, cruciferous vegetables, and more antioxidants by

- eating a predominantly vegetarian diet.
- eating more fruits and vegetables every day (six to eight servings per day maximize anticancer benefits).
- increasing the consumption of broccoli, cauliflower, kale, turnips, cabbage, kohlrabi, Brussels sprouts, hot chili peppers, red and green peppers, carrots, sweet potatoes, winter squash, spinach, garlic, onions, strawberries, tomatoes, pineapple, and citrus fruits in your regular diet.
- eating vegetables raw or quickly cooked by steaming or stir-frying.
- substituting tea and fruit and vegetable juices for coffee and soda.
- eating whole-grain breads.
- including calcium in the diet (or from a supplement).
- including soy products in the diet.
- using whole-wheat flour instead of refined white flour in baking.
- using brown (unpolished) rice instead of white (polished) rice.

Decrease daily fat intake by

- limiting consumption of beef and poultry to no more than three to six ounces (about the size of a deck of cards) once or twice a week.
- trimming all visible fat from meat and removing skin from poultry prior to cooking.
- decreasing the amount of fat and oils used in cooking.
- substituting low-fat for high-fat dairy products.
- using salad dressings sparingly.
- using only half to three-quarters of the amount of fat required in baking recipes.
- limiting fat intake to mostly monounsaturated (olive oil, canola oil, nuts, and seeds) and omega-3 fats (fish, flaxseed, and flaxseed oil).
- eating fish twice a week.
- including flaxseed oil in the diet.

Try It

Make a copy of these "Cancer-Fighting Diet" tips and each week incorporate into your lifestyle two additional dietary behaviors from the above list.

© Cengage Learning

20 minutes of noonday sun, an SPF 15 allows you to remain in the sun about 300 minutes before burning. Sunscreens with stronger SPF factors are not necessarily better. They should be applied just as often and they block only an additional 3 percent to 4 percent of ultraviolet rays. An SPF 15 is adequate for most people. During peak hours, reapplication is vital. For face protection on an average day, it is probably most realistic for the majority of people to apply sunscreen in the morning and then wear a protective hat when outdoors the remainder of the day. When swimming or sweating especially, you should reapply waterproof sunscreens more often because all sunscreens lose strength when they are diluted.

Warning Signals for Cancer

Everyone should become familiar with the following warning signs of cancer and bring them to a physician's attention if any are present:

- Change in bowel or bladder habits
- Sore that does not heal
- Unusual bleeding or discharge
- Thickening or lump in breast or elsewhere
- Indigestion or difficulty in swallowing
- Obvious change in wart or mole
- Nagging cough or hoarseness

© Cengage Learning

! Critical Thinking

You have learned about many of the risk factors for major cancer sites. • How will this information affect your health choices in the future? • Will it be valuable to you, or will you quickly forget all you have learned and remain in a contemplation stage at the end of this course?

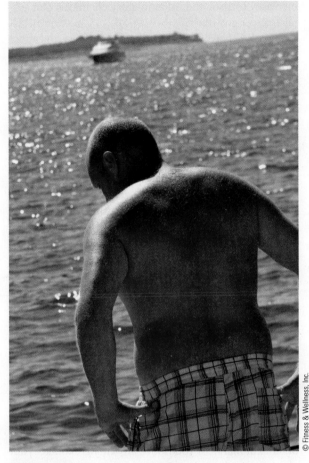

Sunburns and tanning pose a risk for skin cancer from overexposure to the sun's ultraviolet rays.

© Fitness & Wellness, Inc.

If you plan on being out in the sun for a lengthy period of time, even better than sunscreen is wearing protective clothing, including long-sleeved shirts, long pants, and a hat with a two- to three-inch brim all the way around. This sun-protection strategy is even more critical for fair-skinned individuals who burn readily or turn red after only a few minutes of unprotected sun exposure, have a large number of moles, or have a personal or family history of skin cancer risk.

Monitoring Estrogen, Radiation Exposure, and Potential Occupational Hazards

Estrogen use has been linked to endometrial and breast cancer in some studies. Estrogen produced by excess fat in women after menopause is of particular concern. As for exposure to radiation, although X-rays increase the risk for cancer, their benefits may outweigh the risk involved, and most medical facilities use the lowest dose possible to keep the risk to a minimum. Occupational hazards—such as exposure to asbestos fibers, nickel and

uranium dusts, chromium compounds, vinyl chloride, and bischlormethyl ether—increase the risk for cancer. The National Toxicology Program updates a list of environmental exposures every two years. The current list includes over 243 substances, some of which you may be familiar with, while others are more obscure and specific to certain industries. While each carcinogen should be considered individually, it is important to keep in mind that each person will have an individualized reaction to the combined exposures of their genetic expression and their lifetime environment. Cigarette smoking magnifies the risk from occupational hazards.

Physical Activity

An active lifestyle has been shown to have a protective effect against cancer. Although the mechanism is not clear, physical fitness and cancer mortality in men and women may have a graded and consistent inverse relationship. A daily 30-minute, moderate-intensity exercise program lowers the risk for colon, breast, and uterine cancers between 20 percent and 50 percent, and vigorous physical activity may lower the risk of more aggressive and fatal types of prostate cancer.[24]

Research among 38,410 men followed for an average period of 17.2 years indicated a strong inverse relationship between cardiorespiratory fitness and cancer mortality; that is, the lower-fit men had greater cancer death rates than the higher-fit men.[25] A 2009 study on more than 2,200 men 49 years of age and older that were followed up for more than 35 years found that at least 30 minutes a day of moderate- to high-intensity physical activity is inversely associated with the risk of premature death from cancer in men.[26] The researchers concluded that the activity needed to be at least of moderate intensity to achieve the benefit of reducing overall cancer mortality. After 10 years, men who switched from low or medium to high physical activity (greater than 5.2 METs) were found to have half the risk of dying from cancer. There were no changes in mortality rate when switching from a low to a medium level of physical activity. Other data suggest that in men 65 or older, exercising vigorously at least 3 times per week decreases the risk for advanced or fatal prostate cancer by 70 percent.[27]

Data on more than 6,300 women indicate that regular exercise lowers the risk for breast cancer by up to 40 percent, regardless of race or ethnicity.[28] Other studies have found similar results. Women who are active throughout life also cut their risk for endometrial cancer by about 40 percent. Those who started exercise in adulthood cut their risk by about 25 percent.[29] Among women diagnosed with breast cancer, those who walk 2 to 3 miles per hour 1 to 3 times per week are 20 percent less likely to die of the disease. Those who walk three to five times per week cut their risk in half.[30] Researchers believe that the decreased levels of circulating ovarian hormones through physical activity decrease breast cancer risk.

Regular strength training also contributes to lower cancer mortality. A total of 8,677 men between the ages of 20 and 82 were tracked for more than two decades. The data indicated that men who regularly worked out with weights and had the highest muscle strength were up to 40 percent less likely to die from cancer, even among men with a higher waist circumference and BMI.[31]

The risk for other forms of cancer may also decrease, but additional research is necessary before definite statements can be made. Growing evidence suggests that the body's autoimmune system may play a role in preventing cancer and that moderate exercise improves the autoimmune system.

Other Risk Factors for Cancer

Contributions to cancer of many of the other much publicized factors are not as significant as those just pointed out. Intentional food additives, saccharin, processing agents, pesticides, and packaging materials currently used in the United States and other developed countries seem to have minimal consequences. High levels of tension and stress and poor coping may affect the autoimmune system negatively and render the body less effective in dealing with the various cancers. Chronic stress increases cortisol and inflammatory chemicals that sustain cancer growth.[32]

Genetics plays a role in susceptibility in about 10 percent of all cancers. Most of the effect is seen in the early childhood years. Some cancers are a combination of genetic and environmental liability; genetics may add to the environmental risk of certain types of cancers. "Environment" means more than pollution and smoke. It incorporates diet, lifestyle-related events, viruses, and physical agents such as x-rays and exposure to the sun.

Early Detection

Fortunately, many cancers can be controlled or cured through early detection. The real problem comes when cancerous cells spread because they are then difficult to wipe out. Therefore, effective prevention and early detection are crucial. Herein lies the importance of periodic screening. At home, once a month, women should practice breast self-examination (BSE), and men, testicular self-examination (TSE). Men should pick a regular day each month (for example, the first day of the month) to practice TSE, and women should perform BSE two or three days after the menstrual period is over. Once a month you should also conduct a skin self-examination to detect possible skin cancers. Pay particular attention to areas that are constantly exposed to the sun. Note any changes in the size, texture, or color of moles, warts, or other skin marks. If you notice any change, contact your physician.

Behavior Modification Planning

Lifestyle Factors That Decrease Cancer Risk

Factor	Function
Physical activity	Controls body weight, may influence hormone levels, strengthens the immune system
Fiber	Contains anticancer substances, increases stool movement, blunts insulin secretion
Fruits and vegetables	Contain phytonutrients and vitamins that thwart cancer
Recommended weight	Helps control hormones that promote cancer
Healthy grilling	Prevents formation of heterocyclic amines (HCAs) and polycyclic aromatic hydro-carbons (PAHs), both carcinogenic substances
Tea	Contains polyphenols that neutralize free radicals, including epigallocatechin gallate (EGCG), which protects cells and DNA from damage believed to cause cancer
Spices	Provide phytonutrients and strengthen the immune system
Vitamin D	Disrupts abnormal cell growth
Monounsaturated fat	May contribute to cancer cell destruction

Try It

In your Online Journal or class notebook, note ways you can incorporate all of these factors into your everyday lifestyle.

Scientific evidence and testing procedures for prevention and early detection of cancer do change. Studies continue to provide new information. The intent of cancer prevention programs is to educate and guide individuals toward a lifestyle that will help prevent cancer and enable early detection of malignancy. Regular physical examinations by your doctor should include screenings recommended by the ACSM for the early detection of cancer in asymptomatic people.

Treatment of cancer always should be left to specialized physicians and cancer clinics. Current treatment modalities include surgery, radiation, radioactive substances, chemotherapy, hormones, targeted therapies, and immunotherapy.

8.5 *Chronic Lower Respiratory Disease*

Chronic lower respiratory disease (CLRD) encompasses diseases that limit airflow, such as chronic obstructive pulmonary disease, emphysema, and chronic bronchitis (all diseases of the respiratory system). The incidence of CLRD increases proportionately with cigarette smoking (and other forms of smoked tobacco) and exposure to certain types of industrial pollution. In the case of emphysema, genetic factors also may play a role.

8.6 *Accidents*

Accidents rank as the fourth leading cause of death in the United States, affecting the total well-being of millions of Americans each year. Automobile accidents are the number one cause of death for teens in the United States. Accident prevention and personal safety also are part of a health enhancement program aimed at achieving a higher quality of life. Proper nutrition, exercise, abstinence from cigarette smoking, and stress management are of little help if the person is involved in a disabling or fatal accident caused by distraction, a single reckless decision, or not wearing safety belts properly.

Accidents do not always just happen. We sometimes cause accidents. Other times we are victims of accidents. Although some factors in life—earthquakes and tornadoes, for example—are beyond our control, more often than not personal safety and accident prevention are a matter of common sense. Many accidents result from poor judgment and a confused mental state. Frequently accidents happen when we are upset, mentally spent, not paying attention to the task with which we are involved, trying to do too much at once, or abusing alcohol and other drugs.

Fatal accidents are often related to abusing drugs and not wearing seat belts. Furthermore, with the advent of cell phones, automobile accidents have increased. On an average day in the United States, nine people are killed as a result of distracted driving and 1,153 people are injured. As the Senior Director of Transportation Strategic Initiatives for the National Safety Council, David Teater, put it, "You never think it will happen to you — until it does." Teater's research on accident prevention has been motivated by the loss of his 12-year-old son in a cellphone related accident.

New research has utilized brain imaging on distracted drivers in real time. Results have revealed that cognitive workload is too high when holding a phone conversation to also drive safely. The collision risk is the same for hands free devices as for hand held phones—both increase risk of collision by four times. Texting while driving increases collision risk by sixteen times. Study results have also confirmed that multitasking is a myth. Rather than managing two tasks simultaneously, the brain switches between the tasks of conversing and driving, often placing conversation as the primary task and driving as the secondary. It is not uncommon for switching time to be tenths of a second, the difference of several car lengths when breaking. This lag is termed "reaction time switching costs." The minds of distracted drivers have also been shown to automatically screen out 50 percent of visual cues and proceed as if these cues didn't exist. Distracted drivers may experience this "attention blindness" to stop signs, cars attempting to merge or pass across intersections ahead of them, pedestrians, and so on. Making a left turn while talking on a phone is particularly problematic, and is among the most dangerous driving activities.

Alcohol intoxication is the leading cause of fatal automobile accidents, taking the lives of 28 people in the United States every day. Other drugs commonly abused in society alter feelings and perceptions, cause mental confusion, and impair judgment and coordination, greatly increasing the risk for accidental morbidity and mortality.

GLOSSARY

Chronic lower respiratory disease (CLRD) A group of diseases that limits airflow, such as chronic obstructive pulmonary disease, emphysema, and chronic bronchitis (all diseases of the respiratory system)

8.7 *Substance Abuse*

Chemical dependencies encompass some of the most self-destructive behaviors in society today. Abused substances include alcohol, hard drugs, and cigarettes (the latter has been discussed already in this chapter). Problems associated with substance abuse include driving while impaired, mixing drug prescriptions, family difficulties, and partaking of drugs to improve athletic performance (anabolic steroids). Although all forms of substance abuse are recognized to be unhealthy, the following information focuses on alcohol and on the illegal drugs marijuana, cocaine, methamphetamine, heroin, MDMA (ecstasy), and synthetic cannabinoids (fake pot or spice).

Alcohol

Alcohol use represents one of the most significant health-related drug problems in the United States today. Estimates indicate that 7 in 10 adults, or more than 100 million people 18 years and older, are drinkers. Approximately 17 million of them abuse alcohol or are alcohol dependent and will struggle with **alcoholism** throughout life. Currently, almost 79,000 yearly deaths in the United States are due to excessive drinking.

Alcohol is the number one drug problem among college students. According to national surveys, about 60 percent of full-time college students report using alcohol and 39 percent have engaged in binge drinking (consumed five or more drinks in a row). Data indicate that more than 1,800 college students between the ages of 18 and 24 die yearly from alcohol-related unintentional injuries, almost 700,000 are assaulted by another student who had been drinking, 400,000 have unprotected sex, more than 100,000 were too intoxicated to know if they'd consented to having sex, and 29 percent admitted to driving while intoxicated.

Alcohol intake impedes peripheral vision, impairs the ability to see and hear, decreases reaction time, hinders concentration and motor performance (including increased swaying), and causes impaired judgment of distance and speed of moving objects. Further, it lessens fear, increases risk-taking behaviors, stimulates urination, and induces sleep. A single large dose of alcohol also may decrease sexual function. One of the most unpleasant, dangerous, and life-threatening effects of drinking is the **synergistic action** of alcohol when combined with other drugs, particularly central nervous system depressants.

Long-term manifestations of alcohol abuse can be serious and life-threatening. These conditions include cirrhosis of the liver (often fatal); greater risk for oral, esophageal, and liver cancer; **cardiomyopathy**; high blood pressure; greater risk for strokes; inflammation of the esophagus, stomach, small intestine, and pancreas; stomach ulcers; sexual impotence; malnutrition; brain cell damage and consequent loss of memory; and depression, psychosis, and hallucinations.

Illegal Drugs

Approximately two-thirds of the world's production of illegal drugs is consumed in the United States. More than 24.6 million people in the United States use illegal drugs. Each year we spend more than $100 billion on illegal drugs.

According to the U.S. Department of Education, today's drugs are stronger and more addictive, posing a greater risk than ever before. Drugs lead to physical and psychological dependence. If used regularly, they integrate into the body's chemistry, raising drug tolerance and forcing the person to increase the dosage constantly for similar results. In addition to the serious health problems caused by drug abuse, more than half of all adolescent suicides are drug-related.

Furthermore, more than 53 million Americans report nonmedical use of psychotherapeutic drugs at some point in their lifetime. In 2013, about 15 million Americans abused prescription drugs, leading to 23,000 deaths due to an overdose of these drugs. Drug poisoning is now the leading cause of unintentional injury deaths in the United States, killing more Americans than car accidents. Psychotherapeutic drugs include any prescription pain reliever, tranquilizer, stimulant, or sedative, not including over-the-counter drugs. The risks associated with psychotherapy drug misuse or abuse varies depending on the drug. Some of the risks include respiratory depression or cessation, decreased or irregular heart rate, high body temperature, seizures, and cardiovascular failure. Abuse of prescription drugs, or using them in a manner other than exactly as prescribed, can lead to addictive behavior.

Marijuana

Marijuana (pot or weed) is the most widely used illegal drug in the United States. Studies in the 1960s indicated that the potential effects of marijuana were exaggerated and that the drug was relatively harmless. The drug as it is used today, however, is as much as 10 times stronger than it was when the initial studies were conducted. Long-term harmful effects of marijuana use include atrophy of the brain leading to irreversible brain damage, as well as decreased resistance to infectious diseases, chronic bronchitis, lung cancer, and possible sterility and impotence. Though the sale and possession of marijuana continues to be illegal under federal law, as of January 2015, marijuana has been legalized under individual state laws in twenty-three states—for medical use in nineteen states and Washington D.C., and for both medical and recreational use in Colorado, Washington, Oregon, and Alaska.

Cocaine

Similar to marijuana, for many years cocaine was thought to be a relatively harmless drug. This misconception came to an abrupt halt when two well-known athletes, Len Bias (basketball) and Don Rogers (football), died suddenly following cocaine overdose.

Sustained cocaine snorting can lead to a constant runny nose, nasal congestion and inflammation, and perforation of the nasal septum. Long-term consequences of cocaine use in general include loss of appetite, digestive disorders, weight loss, malnutrition, insomnia, confusion, anxiety, and cocaine psychosis (characterized by paranoia and hallucinations). Large overdoses of cocaine can end in sudden death from respiratory paralysis, cardiac arrhythmias, and severe convulsions. For individuals who lack an enzyme used in metabolizing cocaine, as few as two to three lines of cocaine may be fatal.

Methamphetamine

Methamphetamine or "meth" is a more potent form of amphetamine. Typically it comes as a white, odorless, bitter-tasting powder that dissolves readily in water or alcohol. The drug is a potent central nervous system stimulant that produces a general feeling of well-being, decreases appetite, increases motor activity, and decreases fatigue and the need for sleep.

Methamphetamine is easily manufactured with over-the-counter ingredients in clandestine "meth labs." The risk of injury in a meth lab is high because potentially explosive environmental contaminants are discarded during production of the drug. Users of methamphetamine experience increases in body temperature, blood pressure, heart rate, and breathing rate; a decrease in appetite; hyperactivity; tremors; and violent behavior. High doses produce irritability, paranoia, irreversible damage to blood vessels in the brain (causing strokes), and risk of sudden death from hyperthermia and convulsions if not treated at once.

Chronic abusers experience insomnia, confusion, hallucinations, inflammation of the heart lining, schizophrenia-like mental disorder, and brain-cell damage similar to that caused by strokes. Physical changes to the brain may last months or perhaps permanently. In addition, users frequently are involved in violent crime, homicide, and suicide. Using methamphetamines during pregnancy may cause prenatal complications, premature delivery, and abnormal physical and emotional development of the child.

Heroin

Heroin use has increased in recent years. Common nicknames for heroin include diesel, dope, dynamite, white death, nasty boy, china white, H. Harry, gumball, junk, brown sugar, smack, tootsie roll, black tar, and chasing the dragon. The most serious health threat to heroin users today is that they have no way of determining the strength of the drug purchased on the street, thus placing them at a constant risk for overdose and death. An estimated 15 percent of all drug-related hospital emergency room cases involve heroin use.

A heroin overdose can cause convulsions, coma, and death. During an overdose, heart rate, breathing, blood pressure, and body temperature drop dramatically. These physiological responses can induce vomiting, tighten the muscles, and cause breathing to stop. Death is often the result of lack of oxygen or choking to death on vomit.

Within four to five hours after the drug is taken, withdrawal sets in. Heroin withdrawal is painful and may last up to two weeks but could go on several months. Symptoms of withdrawal for long-term users include red/raw nostrils, bone and muscle pains, muscle spasms and cramps, sweating, hot and cold flashes, runny nose and eyes, drowsiness, sluggishness, slurred speech, loss of appetite, nausea, diarrhea, restlessness, and violent yawning. Symptoms of long-term use of heroin include hallucinations, nightmares, constipation, sexual difficulties, impaired vision, reduced fertility, boils, collapsed veins, and significantly elevated risk for lung, liver, and cardiovascular diseases, including bacterial infections in blood vessels and heart valves. Sudden infant death syndrome (SIDS) is seen more frequently in children born to addicted mothers. Heroin use also can kill a developing fetus or cause a spontaneous abortion.

GLOSSARY

Alcoholism Disease in which an individual loses control over drinking alcoholic beverages.

Synergistic action The result of mixing two or more drugs, the effects of which can be much greater than the sum of two or more drugs acting by themselves.

Cirrhosis A disease characterized by scarring of the liver.

Cardiomyopathy A disease affecting the heart muscle.

MDMA (Ecstasy)

MDMA, also known as "ecstasy," is named for its chemical structure: 3,4-methylenedioxymethamphetamine. Besides ecstasy, other street names for the drug are X-TC, E, Adam, Molly, and love drug.

Although MDMA usually is swallowed in the form of 1 or 2 pills in doses of 50 to 240 mg, it also can be smoked, snorted, or occasionally injected. Because the drug is often prepared with other substances, users have no way of knowing the exact potency of the drug or additional substances found in each pill.

MDMA has a reputation among young people for being fun and harmless as long as it is used sensibly. MDMA, however, is not a harmless drug. Users may experience rapid eye movement, faintness, blurred vision, chills, sweating, nausea, muscle tension, and teeth grinding. Individuals with heart, liver, or kidney disease or high blood pressure are especially at risk because MDMA increases blood pressure, heart rate, and body temperature; thus, it may lead to kidney failure, a heart attack, a stroke, and seizures.

Other evidence suggests that a pregnant woman using MDMA may find long-term learning and memory difficulties in her child. Other long-term side effects, lasting for weeks after use, include confusion, depression, sleep disorders, anxiety, aggression, paranoia, and impulsive behavior. Verbal and visual memory may be significantly impaired for years after prolonged use.

Synthetic Cannabinoids (Fake Pot or Spice)

Synthetic cannabinoids are currently the most widely used synthetic drugs in the United States and worldwide. More commonly known as "fake pot," synthetic cannabinoids are man-made chemicals that have compounds similar to the chemical THC found in the natural *Cannabis sativa* plant used for marijuana, though synthetic versions are generally more potent. Users claim that the substances provide a marijuana-like high and are popular among teenagers and young adults. The 2014 Monitoring the Future survey of youth drug-use trends found that 5.8 percent of high school seniors used synthetic cannabinoids in the past year, placing it as the second most common illicit drug used by seniors after marijuana.

Synthetic cannabinoids are often sprayed onto a mixture of herbs and are sold as Spice, K2, Moon Rocks, Skunk, Kind, Genie, Summit, potpourri, herbal incense, Yucatan Gold, Purple Passion, Train Wreck, or Ultra (among other names). According to the federal Drug Enforcement Agency (DEA), the adverse effects of synthetic cannabinoids are far more dangerous than the side effects of marijuana, including seizures, high blood pressure, anxiety attacks, hallucinations, nausea, loss of consciousness, and chemical dependency. Some samples tested have been shown to be 100 times more potent than marijuana.

Treatment for Chemical Dependency

Recognizing the hazards of chemical use, families, teams, and communities can assist each other in preventing problems, as well as help those who already have problems with chemical use. Treating chemical dependency (including alcohol) seldom is accomplished without professional guidance and support. To secure the best available assistance, people in need should contact a physician, their institution's counseling center, or obtain a referral from a local mental health clinic.

8.8 *Sexually Transmitted Infections*

As the name implies, **sexually transmitted infections (STIs)** are infections spread through sexual contact. STIs have reached epidemic proportions in the United States. Of the more than 30 known STIs, some are still incurable. More than half of all Americans will acquire at least one STI during their lifetime. Each year, about 20 million people in the United States are newly infected with STIs, and almost half of STIs afflict young people under 25.

Among the leading bacterial STIs in the United States are chlamydia, gonorrhea, syphilis, and trichomoniasis, which can be readily treated and cured if diagnosed early. Human immunodeficiency virus (HIV), human papillomavirus/genital warts (HPV), genital herpes (HSV), and hepatitis B (HBV), often referred to as the four "H"s, are STIs caused by viruses and currently have no cure, though hepatitis B and HPV can be prevented if a person is vaccinated before being exposed to the virus. If you are sexually active, it is important to be regularly screened for STIs as several STIs can cause infertility, genital cancers, and irreversible damage to the reproductive system.

HIV/AIDS

Human immunodeficiency virus (HIV) is the most frightening of all STIs because in most cases it is fatal if left untreated. There is still no known cure and without appropriate treatment, HIV infection leads to **AIDS or acquired immunodeficiency syndrome**—the end stage of HIV infection. **HIV** spreads among individuals who engage in risky behavior such as having unprotected sex

Cold Sores and Genital Herpes

One of the most common STIs, genital herpes, is caused by the herpes simplex virus (HSV). There are several types of HSV that produce different ailments, including genital herpes, oral herpes, shingles, and chicken pox. The two most common forms of HSV are types 1 and 2. In type 1—the HSV most often known to cause oral herpes—cold sores or fever blisters appear on the lips and mouth. HSV-2 is better known as the virus that causes genital herpes.

Unknown to most people, HSV-1 can also cause genital herpes and an increasing number of genital herpes caused by HSV-1 has been found worldwide. Approximately 100 million Americans older than the age of 12 are infected with HSV-1. Most of these individuals acquired the virus as children. Another 40 million are infected with HSV-2.

HSV is a highly contagious virus. Victims are most contagious during an outbreak and the virus is spread by direct skin to skin contact. HSV, nonetheless, can also spread through "asymptomatic viral shedding;" that is, when there are no visible signs or symptoms of an outbreak. Individuals infected with HSV (oral or genital) may shed the virus up to 20 percent of the time when they have no other symptoms of infection or visible lesions. In the case of HSV-2,

transmission often occurs from an infected person who does not have a visible sore and may not even be aware of such an infection. Presently, herpes is incurable and its victims remain infected for life.

Society typically labels HSV-1 infection (cold sores) an "acceptable" viral infection, whereas infection with HSV-2 is viewed as a "bad" infection. The social stigma and emotional perspective of genital herpes make it difficult to objectively compare it with an oral infection, labeled as "just a cold sore" and acceptable to most people. HSV types 1 and 2, nonetheless, both cause oral and genital herpes. People who have an outbreak of oral herpes should not touch their own or someone else's genitals after touching the oral cold sores. Doing so can lead to a herpes infection of the genitals (genital HSV-1 infection). Oral sex can also result in transmission of HSV from the lips to the genitals. *Thirty percent of all new cases of genital herpes result from HSV-1 infection.* A 2011 study showed that among college students, HSV-1 accounts for 78 percent of female and 85 percent of male genital herpes infections.[33] As with other health risk factors, prevention is the best medicine when it comes to STIs avoidance.

or sharing hypodermic needles. When a person becomes infected with HIV, the virus multiplies and attacks and destroys white blood cells. These cells are part of the immune system, whose function is to fight off infections and diseases in the body. As the number of white blood cells killed increases, the body's immune system breaks down gradually or may be destroyed totally. Without a functioning immune system, a person becomes susceptible to **opportunistic infections** or cancers ordinarily not seen in healthy people.

HIV is a progressive infection. At first, people who become infected with HIV might not know they are infected. An incubation period of weeks, months, or years may pass during which no symptoms appear. The virus may live in the body 10 years or longer before symptoms emerge. HIV infection can produce neurological abnormalities, leading to depression, memory loss, slower mental and physical response time, and sluggishness in limb movements that may progress to a severe disorder known as HIV dementia.

As the infection progresses to the point at which certain diseases develop, the person is said to have AIDS. HIV itself doesn't kill. Nor do people die from AIDS.

AIDS is the term used to define the final stage of HIV infection. Death is caused by a weakened immune system that is unable to fight off opportunistic diseases.

No one has to become infected with HIV. At present, once infected, with the exception of a handful of rare cases, a person cannot become uninfected. There is no second chance. Everyone must protect themselves

GLOSSARY

Sexually transmitted infections (STIs) Communicable infections spread through sexual contact.

Human immunodeficiency virus (HIV) Virus that leads to acquired immunodeficiency syndrome (AIDS).

Acquired immunodeficiency syndrome (AIDS) End stage of HIV infection, manifested by any of a number of diseases that arise when the body's immune system is compromised by HIV.

Opportunistic infections Diseases that arise in the absence of a healthy immune system that would fight them off in healthy people.

against this chronic infection. If people do not—and are so ignorant as to believe it cannot happen to them—they are putting themselves and their partners at risk.

HIV is transmitted by the exchange of cellular body fluids—blood, semen, vaginal secretions, and maternal milk. These fluids may be exchanged during sexual intercourse, by using hypodermic needles that infected individuals have used previously, between a pregnant woman and her developing fetus, in babies from infected mothers during childbirth, less frequently during breastfeeding, and, rarely, from a blood transfusion or an organ transplant.

People do not get HIV because of who they are but, rather, because of what they do. HIV and AIDS threaten anyone of any age or race. Nobody is immune to HIV.

You cannot tell if people are infected with HIV or have AIDS simply by looking at them or taking their word. Not you, not a nurse, not even a physician can tell without an HIV antibody test. Therefore, every time you engage in risky behavior, you run the risk of contracting HIV. The two most basic risky behaviors are (a) having unprotected vaginal, anal, or oral sex with an HIV-infected person and (b) sharing hypodermic needles or other drug paraphernalia with someone who is infected.

About 1.1 million people in the United States are infected with HIV and approximately 14 percent of them are unaware of the infection. One in every four newly reported cases is in youth ages 13 to 24, and because most don't know they are infected, they are not receiving treatment and have a high risk of passing the virus to others unknowingly. African Americans, Latinos, and gay and bisexual men of all races remain the most disproportionately affected by HIV. Although men who have sex with men (MSM) represent only 4 percent of American males, this group accounts for 78 percent of new HIV infections among males as well as 68 percent of new infections overall. Through the end of 2012, an estimated 658,500 people diagnosed with AIDS have died from diseases caused by HIV.

Antiretroviral drug therapy (ART) uses regular doses of drug combinations to delay the progress of HIV infection and even keep many people from developing AIDS. These drugs, commonly referred to as "AIDS cocktails," have turned HIV infection from an almost imminent predecessor of death to a lifelong chronic disease. Thanks to advances in the development of these drugs, many HIV-infected people can now look forward to decades of life. HIV-infected individuals, however, must take the drugs every day for the rest of their life. In most cases, failure to do so results in the virus coming back with full strength. The drugs don't eradicate HIV but rather suppress the virus and make it almost undetectable in the blood.

As with anyone who has a serious illness, AIDS patients deserve respect, understanding, and support. Rejection and discrimination are traits that come from immaturity, hate, and ignorance. Education, knowledge, and responsible behaviors are the best ways to minimize fear and discrimination.

Preventing STIs

With all the grim news about STIs, the good news is that you can do things to prevent their spread and take precautions to keep yourself from becoming a victim. The facts are in: The best preventive technique is a mutually monogamous sexual relationship—sex with only one person who has sexual relations only with you. That one behavior will remove you almost completely from any risk for developing an STI.

Unfortunately, in today's society, trust is an elusive concept. You may be led to believe you are in a monogamous relationship when your partner actually (a) may be cheating on you and gets infected, (b) ends up having a one-night stand with someone who is infected, (c) got the virus several years ago before the present relationship and still isn't aware of the infection, (d) may not be honest with you and chooses not to tell you about the infection, or (e) is injecting drugs and becomes infected. In any of these cases, HIV can be passed on to you.

Because your future and your life are at stake, and because you may never know if your partner is infected, you should give serious and careful consideration to postponing sex until you believe you have found a lifetime monogamous relationship. In doing so, you will not have to live with the fear of catching HIV or other STIs or deal with an unplanned pregnancy.

Many people postpone sexual activity until they are married. This is the best guarantee against STIs and HIV. Young people should understand that married life will provide plenty of time for fulfilling and rewarding sex. If you choose to delay sex, do not let peers pressure you into having sex. Manhood and womanhood are not proved during sexual intercourse but, instead, through mature, responsible, and healthy choices. Other people lead you to believe that love doesn't exist without sex. Sex in the early stages of a relationship is not the product of love but is simply the fulfillment of a physical, and often selfish, drive. A loving relationship develops over a long time with mutual respect for each other.

Teenagers are especially susceptible to peer pressure leading to premature sexual intercourse. As a result, about 270,000 girls under age 20 get pregnant each year in the United States. Too many young people wish they had postponed sex and silently admire those who do. Sex lasts only a few minutes. The consequences of irresponsible sex may last a lifetime, and in some cases they are fatal.

Sexual promiscuity never leads to a trusting, loving, and lasting relationship. Mature people respect others' choices. If someone does not respect your choice to wait, he or she certainly does not deserve your friendship or, for that matter, anything else. There is no greater sex than that between two loving and responsible individuals who mutually trust and admire each other. These relationships are possible when built upon unselfish attitudes and behaviors.

As you look around, you will find people who have these values. Seek them out and build your friendships and future around people who respect you for who you are and what you believe. You don't have to compromise your choices or values. In the end, you will reap the greater rewards of a fulfilling and lasting relationship, free of AIDS and other STIs.

Also, be prepared so that you will know your course of action before you get into an intimate situation. Look for common interests and work together toward them. Express your feelings openly: "I'm not ready for sex; I just want to have fun, and kissing is fine with me." If your friend does not accept your answer and is not willing to stop the advances, be prepared with a strong response. If statements such as "Please stop" or "Don't!" are ineffective, use a firm statement such as, "No, I'm not willing to have sex" or "I've already thought about this, and I'm not going to have sex." If this still doesn't work, inform them that their forceful behavior is considered rape and say,

"This is rape, and I'm going to call the police. "What about those who do not have—or do not desire—a monogamous relationship? The following are some risky behaviors that significantly increase the chances of contracting an STI, including HIV infection:

1. Multiple or anonymous sexual partners such as a pickup or prostitute
2. Anal sex with or without a condom
3. Vaginal or oral sex with someone who injects drugs or engages in anal sex
4. Sex with someone you know who has several sex partners
5. Unprotected sex (without a condom) with an infected person
6. Sexual contact of any kind with anyone who has symptoms of AIDS or who is a member of a group at high risk for AIDS
7. Sharing toothbrushes, razors, or other implements that could become contaminated with blood with anyone who is, or might be, infected with the HIV virus

Avoiding risky behaviors that destroy quality of life and life itself is a critical component of a healthy lifestyle. Learning the facts so you can make responsible choices can protect you and those around you from startling and unexpected conditions. Using alcohol moderately (or not at all), refraining from substance abuse, and preventing sexually transmitted infections are keys to averting both physical and psychological damage.

Assess Your Behavior

1. Is your diet fundamentally low in saturated fats, trans fats, and processed meats, and do you meet the daily suggested amounts of fruits, vegetables, and fiber?

2. Are you familiar with basic lifestyle guidelines to prevent cancer?

3. Is your life free of addictive behavior? If not, will you commit right now to seek professional help at your institution's counseling center? Addictive behavior destroys health and lives—don't let it end yours.

4. Do you believe in a mutually monogamous sexual relationship as the best way to prevent STIs? If not, do you always take precautions to practice safer sex?

Assess Your Knowledge

1. Coronary heart disease
   a. is the single leading cause of death in the United States.
   b. is the leading cause of sudden cardiac deaths.
   c. is a condition in which the arteries that supply the heart muscle with oxygen and nutrients are narrowed by fatty deposits.
   d. accounts for approximately 20 percent of all deaths.
   e. All are correct choices.

2. The risk of heart disease increases with
   a. high LDL-cholesterol.
   b. high HDL-cholesterol.
   c. lack of homocysteine.
   d. low levels of hs-CRP
   e. All are correct choices.

3. Type 2 diabetes is related closely to
   a. low BMI.
   b. obesity and lack of physical activity.
   c. genetically low homocysteine.
   d. increased insulin sensitivity.
   e. All are correct choices.

4. Metabolic syndrome is related to
   a. low HDL-cholesterol.
   b. high triglycerides.
   c. increased blood-clotting mechanism.
   d. an abnormal insulin response to carbohydrates.
   e. All are correct choices.

5. Cancer can be defined as
   a. a process whereby some cells invade and destroy the immune system.
   b. an uncontrolled growth and spread of abnormal cells.
   c. the spread of benign tumors throughout the body.
   d. the interference in normal body functions through blood flow disruption caused by angiogenesis.
   e. All are correct choices.

6. Cancer
   a. is primarily a preventable disease.
   b. is often related to tobacco use.
   c. has been linked to dietary habits.
   d. risk increases with obesity.
   e. All are correct choices.

7. A cancer prevention diet should include
   a. ample amounts of fruit and vegetables.
   b. cruciferous vegetables.
   c. phytonutrients.
   d. soy products.
   e. All are correct choices.

8. The biggest carcinogenic exposure in the workplace is
   a. asbestos fibers.
   b. cigarette smoke.
   c. biological agents.
   d. nitrosamines.
   e. pesticides.

9. Treatment of chemical dependency is
   a. primarily accomplished by the individual alone.
   b. most successful when there is peer pressure to stop.
   c. best achieved with the help of family members.
   d. seldom accomplished without professional guidance.
   e. usually done with the help of friends.

10. The best way to protect yourself against sexually transmitted infections is
   a. through the use of condoms with a spermicide.
   b. by knowing about the people who have previously had sex with your partner.
   c. through a mutually monogamous sexual relationship.
   d. by having sex only with an individual who has no symptoms of STIs.
   e. All of the above choices provide equal protection against STIs.

Correct answers can be found on page 307.

Activity 8.1   **Managing Cardiovascular Disease and Cancer Risks**

Name _____   Date _____

Course _____   Section _____

I. Cardiovascular Disease

	Yes	No
1. I accumulate between 30 and 60 minutes of physical activity at least five days per week.	☐	☐

Total number of daily steps: [＿＿＿＿]   Total minutes of daily physical activity: [＿＿＿＿]

	Yes	No
2. I exercise aerobically a minimum of three times a week in the appropriate target zone for at least 20 minutes per session.	☐	☐
3. I am at or slightly below the health fitness recommended percent body fat (see Chapter 2, Table 2.11, page 51), or my BMI is below 25.	☐	☐
4. My blood lipids are within normal range.	☐	☐
5. I consume whole-grain foods daily.	☐	☐
6. I get 25 (women) to 38 (men) grams of fiber in my daily diet.	☐	☐
7. I eat more than five servings of fruits and vegetables every day.	☐	☐
8. I limit saturated fat, trans fats, and cholesterol in my daily diet.	☐	☐
9. I limit the use of simple carbohydrates (including sugars), refined carbohydrates, and processed foods.	☐	☐
10. I eat primarily oily/cold-water fish at least twice per week.	☐	☐
11. I am not a diabetic.	☐	☐
12. I choose and prepare foods with little or no salt.	☐	☐
13. My blood pressure is normal.	☐	☐
14. I do not smoke cigarettes or use tobacco in any other form.	☐	☐
15. I manage stress adequately in daily life.	☐	☐
16. I do not have a personal or family history of heart disease.	☐	☐

Evaluation

A "no" answer to any of the above items increases your risk for cardiovascular disease. The greater the number of "no" responses, the higher the risk for developing cardiovascular disease.

Please indicate lifestyle changes you will implement or maintain to decrease your personal risk for cardiovascular disease.

_____

_____

_____

_____

Activity 8.1 Managing Cardiovascular Disease and Cancer Risks *(continued)*

14 Steps to a Healthier Life and Reduced Cancer Risk

	Yes	No

Scientists think most cancers may be related to lifestyle and environment—what you eat and drink, whether you smoke, and where you work and play. This means that you can help reduce your own cancer risk by taking control of actions in your daily life.

1. Are you eating more cruciferous vegetables?

   They include broccoli, cauliflower, Brussels sprouts, all cabbages, and kohlrabi. ☐ ☐

2. Are high-fiber foods included in your diet? ☐ ☐

3. Do you choose foods with vitamin A?

   Fresh foods with beta-carotene—including carrots, peaches, apricots, squash, and broccoli—are the best source, not vitamin pills. ☐ ☐

4. Is vitamin C included in your diet?

   You'll find it naturally in lots of fresh fruits and vegetables including grapefruit, cantaloupe, oranges, strawberries, red and green peppers, broccoli, and tomatoes. ☐ ☐

5. Do you eat sufficient selenium-bearing foods (fish, Brazil nuts, whole grains) so you obtain at least 100 mcg of selenium per day (but no more than 400 mcg per day)? ☐ ☐

6. Are you physically active for at least 30 minutes, and do you avoid excessive sitting on most days of the week? ☐ ☐

7. Do you maintain a healthy weight (a BMI between 18.5 and 25)? ☐ ☐

8. Do you limit salt-cured, smoked, and nitrite-cured foods?

   Choose bacon, ham, hot dogs, or salt-cured fish only occasionally if you like them a lot. ☐ ☐

9. Do you limit barbecuing and cooking meats at high temperatures to the point that they are "medium well" or "well done"? ☐ ☐

10. Do you smoke cigarettes or use tobacco in any other form? ☐ ☐

11. If you drink alcohol, are you moderate in your intake (no more than 2 drinks per day for men, 1 for women, or none at all for women with a family history of breast, esophagus, larynx, rectum, or liver cancers)? ☐ ☐

12. Do you get almost daily "safe sun" exposure (face, arms, and hands) and yet respect the sun's rays? "Safe sun" exposure means 10 to 20 minutes of unprotected sun exposure (without sunscreen) to the face, arms, and hands during peak daylight hours on most days of the week (10:00 a.m. to 4:00 p.m.), but yet you respect the sun's rays (your skin does not turn red, and you do not sunburn). If not, do you take a Vitamin D_3 supplement?

    Do you protect yourself with sunscreen (at least SPF 15) and wear long sleeves and a hat, especially during midday hours if you are going to be exposed to the sun for a prolonged period of time? ☐ ☐

13. Do you have a family history of any type of cancer?

    (If so, you should bring this to the attention of your personal physician.) ☐ ☐

14. Are you familiar with the seven warning signals for cancer? ☐ ☐

Evaluation

If you answered yes to most of these questions, congratulations. You are taking control of simple lifestyle factors that will help you feel better and reduce your risk for cancer.

Please indicate lifestyle changes you will implement or maintain to decrease your personal risk for cancer:

_____

_____

_____

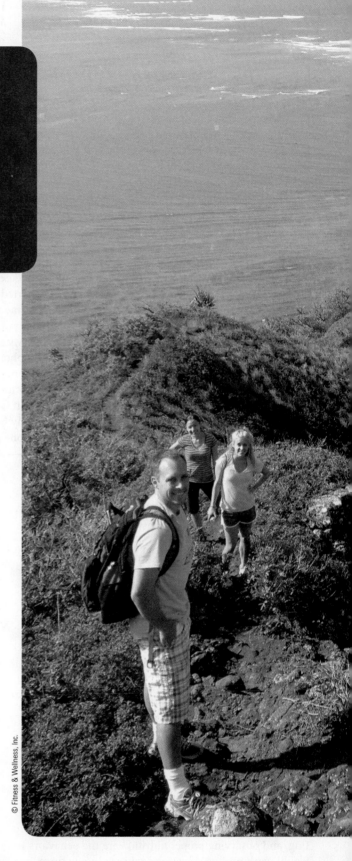

9

Relevant Fitness and Wellness Issues

The human body is extremely resilient during youth—not so during middle and older age. Thus, lifestyle choices you make and live today will affect your health, well-being, and quality of life tomorrow.

Objectives

> Dispel common misconceptions related to physical fitness and wellness.

> Give practical advice and tips regarding safety.

> Address some concerns specific to women.

> Clarify additional concepts regarding nutrition and weight control.

> Answer some questions regarding wellness and aging.

> Provide guidelines related to fitness/wellness consumer issues.

© Fitness & Wellness, Inc.

REAL LIFE STORY | Sonia's Recurrent Stress Fractures

I started gymnastics at a very young age. I participated in club gymnastics and competed extensively at an elite level until I graduated from high school. I earned a college scholarship and was looking forward to intercollegiate competition. Halfway through the fall semester my first year, I suffered a stress (bone) fracture in my lower left leg. The bone healed very slowly and kept me from competing that year. I was devastated because I wanted to compete so badly. At the end of the spring semester, I ran into an exercise science professor who had also been a gymnast. We talked about my injury, and during the conversation it came up that now at age 19, I had never menstruated. My percent body fat was

very low throughout all my teenage years and I didn't really drink that much milk. The professor strongly encouraged me to see my personal physician during the summer.

After seeing my doctor, I was placed on hormone replacement therapy and started to have regular menses. I also discovered that my bone density was quite low. My stress fracture recurred my sophomore and junior years and I was never able to compete. I took a Fit for Life course in my junior year. It was at that point I decided that my health would be my number one priority and I

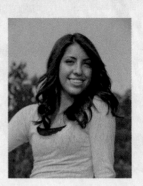

Laura Gangi Pond/Shutterstock.com

opted to end my gymnastics career. I gained a few pounds, more along a healthy weight guideline. I started to jog and lift weights for fitness. My menses stayed regular even after discontinuing hormone replacement therapy. I now know that I will need to maintain a lifetime physical activity program with some form of weight-bearing exercises, along with adequate daily calcium in my diet. I also need to monitor the regularity of my menstrual cycles and watch my bone density as recommended by my doctor.

This chapter addresses some of the most frequently asked questions about various facets of physical fitness and wellness. The answers will further clarify concepts discussed throughout the book, as well as put to rest several myths that misinform fitness and wellness participants. "Q" denotes the question, and "A" designates the answer.

9.1 *Wellness Behavior Modification Issues*

Q: If a person is going to do only one thing to improve health, what would it be?
A: This is a common question. It is a mistake to think, though, that you can modify just one factor and enjoy wellness. Wellness requires a constant and deliberate effort to change unhealthy behaviors and reinforce healthy behaviors. Although it is difficult to work on many lifestyle changes all at once, being involved in a regular physical activity program, avoiding excessive sitting, and observing proper nutrition are the behaviors I would work on first. If you use tobacco in any form, or you have any other form of chemical dependency, stop

today and seek professional counseling to overcome the addictive behavior. Other behavioral changes should follow, depending on your lifestyle.

Q: Why is it so hard to change?
A: Change is incredibly difficult for most people. Whether we are trying to increase physical activity, quit smoking, change unhealthy eating habits, or reverse heart disease, it is human nature to resist change even when we know that change will provide substantial benefits.

To understand human behavior, or why people do what they do, we need to understand values. Values are defined as the core beliefs and ideals that people have. Values govern behavior as people look to conduct themselves in a manner that is conducive to living and attaining goals consistent with their beliefs and what's important to them. A person's values reflect who they are.

Values are established through experience and learning, and their development is a lifelong process that influences all aspects of life. When making a choice between short-term urges and long-term desires, a person uses two different areas of their brain. One part of the brain is active as a response to immediate urges, and a completely different part of the brain is active when considering long held beliefs and lifetime goals. Personal values are first developed within family circles, schools, the media, and the culture where people grow up and live; according to what is acceptable or unacceptable, desirable or undesirable, good or bad, and rewarded or ignored/punished. Educational experiences, such as obtained in this course, play a key role in the establishment of values. Education is power: It provides people with knowledge to form opinions, allows them to better grasp future outcomes from today's choices, and forces them to question issues and take stands.

Furthermore, Dr. Richard Earle, managing director of the Canadian Institute of Stress and the Hans Selye Foundation, explains that people have a tendency toward pessimism. This tendency, commonly referred to as a "negativity bias," is hardwired into our biology. In every spoken language, there is a ratio of three pessimistic adjectives to one positive adjective. Thus, linguistically, psychologically, and emotionally, we focus on what can go wrong and we lose motivation before we even start.

Motivation for change comes from within. In most instances, neither pressure, nor reasoning, nor fear will inspire people to take action. Change in behavior is most likely to occur by addressing values and speaking to people's feelings. Most people start contemplating change when there is a change in core values that will make them feel uncomfortable with the present behavior(s) or lack thereof.

Core values change when feelings are addressed. The challenge is to find ways that will help people understand the problems and solutions in a manner that will influence emotions and not just the thought process. Once the problem behavior is understood and "felt," the person may become uncomfortable with the situation and will be more inclined to address the problem behavior or adoption of a healthy behavior. Discomfort is a great motivator. People tolerate any situation until it becomes too uncomfortable for them. At that point, they seek ways to make changes in their lives. It is then that the information presented in this book provides the tools to implement a successful plan for change.

Keep in mind that when lifestyle changes are addressed, relationships and friendships may also need to be addressed. You need to distance yourself from those individuals who share your bad habits (smoking, drinking, unhealthy eating, or sedentary lifestyle) and associate with people who practice healthy habits. Are you prepared to do so?

Q: Why is it so difficult to change dietary habits?
A: In most developed countries there is an overabundance of food and practically an unlimited number of food choices. With unlimited supply and choices, most people do not have the willpower, stemming from their core values, to avoid overconsumption.

Our bodies were not created to go hungry or to overeat. We are uncomfortable overeating and we feel even worse when we have to go hungry. Our health values, however, are not strong enough to prevent overconsumption. The end result: weight gain. Next, we restrict calories (go on a diet), we feel hungry, and we have a difficult time adhering to the diet. Stated quite simply, going hungry is an uncomfortable and unpleasant experience. And people do not like to feel this way.

To avoid this vicious cycle, our dietary habits—and most likely physical activity habits—must change. A question you need to ask yourself is: Do you value health and quality of life more than food overindulgence? If you do not, then the achievement and maintenance of recommended body weight and good health is a moot point. If you desire to avoid disease and increase quality of life, you have to value health more than food overconsumption. If you have spent the past 20 years tasting and "devouring" every food item in sight, it is now time to make healthy choices and consume only moderate amounts (portion control) of healthy food at a time. You do not have to taste and eat everything that is placed before your eyes. If you can make such a change in your eating habits, you may not have to worry about another diet throughout life.

9.2 *Safety of Exercise Participation and Injury Prevention*

Q: What amount of aerobic exercise is optimal to significantly decrease the risk for cardiovascular disease?
A: Physical inactivity by itself is a major risk factor for cardiovascular disease and often contributes to the development of other risk factors such as an increase in (a) body fat, (b) LDL-cholesterol, (c) triglycerides, (d) inflammation, (e) stress, (f) blood pressure, and (g) risk for diabetes, and studies have documented that these risk factors have multiple interrelations (see Figure 9.1).

Although a regular aerobic exercise program significantly decreases the risk for cardiovascular disease, the amount of exercise required to offset the risk cannot be pinpointed specifically because of the many individual differences (genetic and lifestyle) among people. Research, however, has shed some light on this subject.

One of the earlier studies published in the mid-1980s indicated that about 300 calories should be expended

Figure 9.1 Interrelationships among leading cardiovascular risk factors.

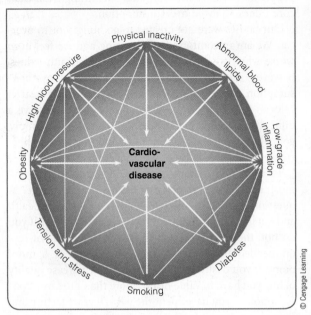

Physical inactivity · Abnormal blood lipids · High blood pressure · Low-grade inflammation · Obesity · **Cardio-vascular disease** · Tension and stress · Diabetes · Smoking

© Cengage Learning

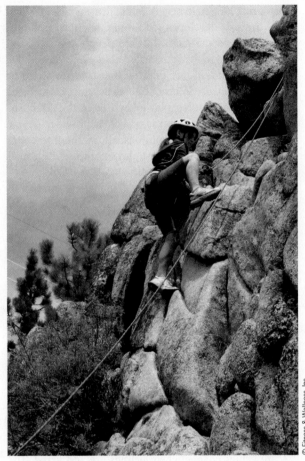

Individuals who initiate physical activity and exercise habits at a young age are more likely to participate throughout life.

© Fitness & Wellness, Inc.

daily through aerobic exercise to obtain a certain degree of protection against cardiovascular disease.[1] The work alluded to in Chapter 8 (see Figure 8.5, page 209) indicated that even moderate fitness levels—that is, a caloric expenditure of 150 to 200 calories 5 to 7 days per week—can reduce the incidence of cardiovascular problems substantially.[2] Greater protection, however, is achieved at higher energy expenditures and better fitness levels.

For individuals with or at risk for coronary heart disease, data suggest that more than 1,400 calories per week may have to be expended to improve cardiorespiratory fitness; more than 1,500 weekly calories to stop the progression of atherosclerotic lesions; and more than 2,200 calories per week, or the equivalent of 5 to 6 hours of weekly exercise, for regression of lesions.[3] Keep in mind that neither physical activity nor exercise by itself provides an absolutely risk-free guarantee against cardiovascular disease. Overall risk factor management is the best approach to disease risk reduction.

Q: At what age should I start concerning myself with cardiovascular disease?
A: The disease process for cardiovascular disease, as well as cancer, starts early in life as a result of poor lifestyle habits. Studies have shown beginning stages of atherosclerosis and elevated blood lipids in children as young as 10 years old.

Many positive habits can be established early in life. If at a young age you learn to avoid excessive calories, saturated and trans fats, sweets, salt, and alcohol; to not use

tobacco; and to participate in physical activity, your chances of leading a healthier life are much greater than is true with the present generation.

Q: What is more important for good health—aerobic fitness or muscular fitness (good muscular strength)?
A: They are both important. During the initial fitness boom in the 1970s and 1980s, the emphasis was placed almost exclusively on aerobic fitness. We now know that they both contribute to health, fitness, work capacity, and overall quality of life. Among others, aerobic fitness is particularly important for the prevention of cardiovascular diseases, diabetes, and some types of cancer; whereas muscular fitness builds strong muscles and bones, helps prevent osteoporosis, decreases the risk for low back pain and musculoskeletal injuries, improves overall functional capacity, and to a lesser extent also contributes to the prevention of cardiovascular disease and diabetes.

Q: Should I do aerobic exercise or strength training first?
A: Ideally, allow some recovery hours between the two types of training. There is really no consensus as to which sequence is most beneficial. If you can't afford the time, the training order should be based on your fitness goals and preferences.

Aerobic training first can help improve running performance and VO_{2max} to a larger extent than following the strength training segment of exercise. Aerobic exercise followed by strength training also has been shown to enhance post exercise energy expenditure (calories burned during recovery from exercise). If you are trying to develop the cardiorespiratory system or enhance caloric expenditure for weight-loss purposes, heavy lower body lifting will make it very difficult to sustain a good cardio workout thereafter.

Resistance training first is more effective for developing strength, power, and muscular hypertrophy. In adults over the age of 65, strength training first seems more effective in enhancing aerobic power because in older adults VO_{2max} is somewhat limited due to age-related loss of muscle and strength. If strength development is the primary objective, unless exhausting, aerobic exercise provides a sound warm-up prior to resistance training. Excessive fatigue from vigorous aerobic exercise, however, can lead to bad form while lifting and may result in injury. Thus, you need to evaluate your goals and select the training order accordingly.

Q: Do big muscles turn into fat when the person stops training?
A: Muscle and fat tissue are two completely different types of tissue. Just as an apple will not turn into an orange, muscle tissue cannot turn into fat or vice versa. Muscle cells increase and decrease in size according to your training program. If you train quite hard, muscle cells increase in size. This increase is limited in women due to hormonal differences compared with men. When one stops training, muscle cells again decrease in size. If the person maintains a high caloric intake without physical training, however, fat cells will increase in size as weight (fat) is gained.

Q: What strength-training exercises are best to get an abdominal "six-pack"?
A: Most men tend to store body fat around the waist, while women do so around the hips. There are, however, no "miracle" exercises to spot-reduce. Multiple sets of abdominal curl-ups, crunches, reverse crunches, or sit-ups performed three to five times per week will strengthen the abdominal musculature but will not be sufficient to allow the muscles to appear through the layer of fat between the skin and the muscles. The total energy (caloric) expenditure of a few sets of abdominal exercises will not be sufficient to lose a significant amount of weight (fat). If you want to get a "washboard stomach" (or, for women, achieve shapely hips), you need to engage in a moderate to vigorous aerobic and strength-training program combined with a moderate reduction in daily caloric intake (diet).

Q: Can too much exercise be detrimental to health?
A: Moderate exercise training provides many health benefits and strengthens immune function. Prolonged, intense, and exhaustive exercise, however, can negatively affect immune function and result in increased susceptibility to upper respiratory tract infections (common cold and influenza) and viral infections. The primary concern in this area is with elite endurance athletes who train for lengthy periods of time each day. These athletes are more susceptible to infections during intense training and competition.

From a health fitness point of view, if you overdo your exercise session, your body will let you know by becoming excessively sore and fatigued. You may now have to skip your exercise session for a day or two to recover from the overexertion, thus defeating the purpose of having trained so hard. The best guide is to be "comfortably sore" following a day of hard training. You should never be so sore that you cannot exercise at all or are too uncomfortable doing so. Remember to use a progressive approach to increase your exercise volume and each hard day of training (being just "comfortably sore") should be followed by a lighter exercise day. With few exceptions in athletic instances, back to back hard days of training are not recommended to improve fitness.

> **!**
> **Critical Thinking**
> What role do physical activity and exercise play in your life? • What impact do these have on your emotional well-being?

Q: Should I exercise when I have a cold or the flu?
A: The most important consideration is to use common sense and pay attention to your symptoms. Usually you may continue exercise if your symptoms are a runny nose, sneezing, or a scratchy throat. But if you have a fever or achy muscles, if you are vomiting, have diarrhea, or have a hacking cough, you should avoid exercise. Following an illness, be sure to ease back gradually into your program. Do not attempt to return at the same intensity and duration that you were used to prior to your illness.

Q: How fast does a person lose the benefits of exercise after stopping an exercise program?

A: How quickly the benefits of exercise are lost differs among the various components of physical fitness and also depends on the condition the person achieves before discontinuing the exercise. Specifically with regard to cardiorespiratory endurance, it has been estimated that four weeks of aerobic training are completely reversed in two consecutive weeks of physical inactivity.

If you have been exercising regularly for months or years, two weeks of inactivity (due to illness and hopefully not a lack of desire to be active), will not hurt you as much as it will someone who has exercised only a few weeks. Generally speaking, within two to three days of aerobic inactivity, the cardiorespiratory system starts to lose some of its capacity. Flexibility can be maintained with two or three stretching sessions per week, and strength is maintained with just one maximal training session per week.

You should maintain a regular fitness program even during traveling and vacation periods. When traveling, plan ahead and examine your options before you leave home. Many hotels provide in-house fitness facilities. Although the equipment often is limited, it's generally sufficient for an adequate cardiorespiratory and strength workout. Frequent travelers would benefit from joining a nationally franchised health club or a YMCA. In this manner, you can continue the same exercise program while visiting different cities.

Activities that require a minimum of equipment and no facilities, such as walking, jogging, and rope jumping, are excellent alternatives for the road. If you are going to venture out in a new city, always ask for safe places to walk and jog. Do not venture into an area, even though it looks safe, without inquiring about the area first. Nearby parks or a high school track are usually safe (but inquire first) and help you stay away from traffic and stoplights. The strength-training (without equipment) and flexibility exercises provided in Appendix A and Appendix B, pages 272–283, can be used to maintain your strength and flexibility.

Q: What type of clothing should I wear when I exercise?

A: The type of clothing you wear during exercise is important. In general, clothing should fit comfortably and allow free movement of the various body parts. Select clothing according to expected air temperature, humidity, and exercise intensity. Avoid nylon and rubberized materials and tight clothes that interfere with the body's cooling mechanism or obstruct normal blood flow. Cotton is not an ideal choice either. While it may feel comfortable at the beginning of your workout, 100 percent cotton will absorb and hold moisture throughout your workout (think of the weight of a pair of wet jeans). A cotton-synthetic blend will perform better. Fabrics made from Capilene, Thermax, or any synthetic that draws (wicks) moisture away from the skin will work. The fibers of these synthetic fabrics are nonabsorbent. The moisture moves along the fibers to disperse and evaporate, enhancing cooling of the body. Polypropylene is another moisture-wicking synthetic, but it requires special care to remove odors. Exercise intensity also is important in determining the clothing you wear because the harder you exercise, the more heat your body produces.

When exercising in the heat, avoid the hottest time of the day, between 11:00 a.m. and 5:00 p.m. Avoid surfaces such as asphalt, concrete, and artificial turfs because they absorb heat, which then radiates to the body. (Also see the discussion on exercise in hot and humid conditions on pages 247–248).

Only minimal clothing is necessary during exercise in the heat, to allow for maximal evaporation. Clothing should be lightweight, light-colored, loose-fitting, airy, and absorbent. Examples of commercially available products that can be used during exercise in the heat are Asci's Perma Plus, Coolmax, and Nike's Dri-FIT. Double-layer acrylic socks are preferable to cotton and help prevent blistering and chafing of the feet. A straw-type hat can be worn to protect the eyes and head from the sun. Clothing for exercise in the cold is discussed on pages 249–250.

For decades, a good pair of shoes has been recommended by most professionals to prevent injuries to lower limbs. Shoes manufactured specifically for the choice of activity have been encouraged. Shoes should have good stability and motion control and comfortable fit. Purchase shoes in the middle of or later in the day when feet have expanded and might be one half size larger. For increased breathability, shoes with nylon or mesh uppers are recommended. Salespeople at reputable athletic shoe stores can help you select a good shoe that fits your needs.

More recently, a trend has emerged toward barefoot running. For most of human history, people ran either barefoot or with minimal shoes. As in walking, the modern running shoe with its bulky padded heel cushion allows runners to land on the heel and roll forward toward the ball of the foot. The impact-collision force while running is often more than three times the person's body weight. Researchers have observed that joggers/runners who don't wear shoes, or use minimal footwear, land on the front (ball) or middle of the foot. This motion induces them to flex the ankle as contact is made with the ground, resulting in smaller impact forces than ankle strikers. Such running mechanics are thought to decrease impact-related repetitive stress injuries.

Some experts believe that the spring in the arch of the foot and the Achilles tendon diminish ground impact forces. A good illustration is to compare the impact forces generated by landing a jump on the heels versus the toes.

Shoeless-running proponents believe that wearing cushioned shoes with arch supports alters natural foot-landing actions, weakening muscles and ligaments and rendering feet, ankles, and knees more susceptible to injuries. They recommend wearing a flexible shoe without a heel cushion or arch support. This recommendation has led to the development of "barefoot running shoes." These "shoes" feature a thin, abrasion-resistant stretch nylon with breathable mesh upper material that wraps around the entire foot to keep rocks and dirt out. At present, the verdict is still out. Data are insufficient to support either recommendation (shod vs. shoeless running). Research is now being conducted to determine the best type of footwear to use with repetitive-impact activities.

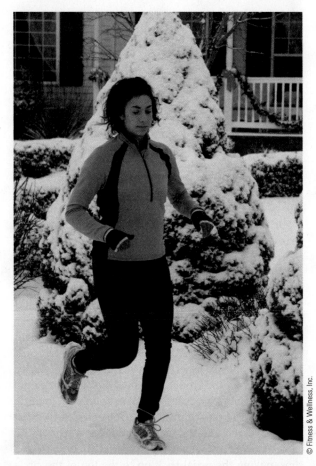

Several layers of heat-conserving, lightweight clothing are recommended when exercising outdoors during the winter months.

© Fitness & Wellness, Inc.

Q: What time of the day is best for exercise?
A: A person can exercise at almost any time of the day except about two hours following a large meal, or the noon and early afternoon hours on hot and humid days. Many people enjoy exercising early in the morning because it gives them a good boost to start the day. If you have a difficult time sticking to an exercise program, early morning exercise is best because the chances of some other activity or conflict interfering with your exercise time are minimal. Some people prefer the lunch hour for weight control reasons. By exercising at noon, they do not eat as big a lunch, which helps keep down daily caloric intake. Highly stressed people seem to like the evening hours because of the relaxing effects of exercise.

Q: How should acute sports injuries be treated?
A: The best treatment always has been prevention. If an activity causes unusual discomfort or chronic irritation, you need to treat the cause by decreasing the intensity, switching activities, substituting equipment, or upgrading clothing, such as buying properly fitted shoes.

In cases of acute injury, the standard treatment is rest, cold application, compression or splinting (or both), and elevation of the affected body part. The applicable acronym is RICE:

> R = rest
> I = ice application
> C = compression
> E = elevation

Cold should be applied 3 to 5 times a day for 15 minutes at a time during the first 36 to 48 hours, by submerging the injured area in cold water, using an ice bag, or applying ice massage to the affected part. An elastic bandage or wrap can be used for compression. Elevating the body part decreases blood flow to it. The purpose of these treatment modalities is to minimize swelling in the area, which hastens recovery time.

After the first 36 to 48 hours, heat can be used if the injury shows no further swelling or inflammation. If you have doubts regarding the nature or seriousness of the injury (such as suspected fracture), you should seek a medical evaluation.

Obvious deformities (such as in fractures, dislocations, or partial dislocations) call for splinting, cold application with an ice bag, and medical attention. Never try to reset any of these conditions by yourself, as muscles, ligaments, and nerves could be damaged further. These injuries should be treated by specialized medical personnel. A quick reference guide for the signs or symptoms and treatment of exercise-related problems is provided in Table 9.1.

Table 9.1 Reference Guide for Exercise-Related Problems

Injury	Signs/Symptoms	Treatment*
Bruise (contusion)	Pain, swelling, discoloration	Cold application, compression, rest
Dislocations/ fractures	Pain, swelling, deformity	Splinting, cold application, seek medical attention
Heat cramps	Cramps, spasms, and muscle twitching in the legs, arms, and abdomen	Stop activity, get out of the heat, stretch, massage the painful area, drink plenty of fluids
Heat exhaustion	Fainting, profuse sweating, cold/clammy skin, weak/rapid pulse, weakness, headache	Stop activity, rest in a cool place, loosen clothing, rub body with cool/wet towel, drink plenty of fluids, stay out of heat for 2–3 days
Heatstroke	Hot/dry skin, no sweating, serious disorientation, rapid/full pulse, vomiting, diarrhea, unconsciousness, high body temperature	Seek immediate medical attention, request help and get out of the sun, bathe in cold water/spray with cold water/rub body with cold towels, drink plenty of cold fluids
Joint sprains	Pain, tenderness, swelling, loss of use, discoloration	Cold application, compression, elevation, rest, heat after 36 to 48 hours (if no further swelling)
Muscle cramps	Pain, spasm	Stretch muscle(s), use mild exercises for involved area
Muscle soreness and stiffness	Tenderness, pain	Mild stretching, low-intensity exercise, warm bath
Muscle strains	Pain, tenderness, swelling, loss of use	Cold application, compression, elevation, rest, heat after 36 to 48 hours (if no further swelling)
Shin splints	Pain, tenderness	Cold application prior to and following any physical activity, rest, heat (if no activity is carried out)
Side stitch	Pain on the side of the abdomen below the rib cage	Decrease level of physical activity or stop altogether, gradually increase level of fitness
Tendinitis	Pain, tenderness, loss of use	Rest, cold application, heat after 48 hours

*Cold should be applied three to four times a day for 15 minutes. Heat can be applied three times a day for 15 to 20 minutes.

© Cengage Learning

Q: What causes muscle soreness and stiffness?

A: Muscle soreness and stiffness are common in individuals who (a) begin an exercise program or participate after a long layoff from exercise, (b) exercise beyond their customary intensity and duration, and (c) perform eccentric training. The acute soreness that sets in during the first few hours after exercise is related to general fatigue caused by chemical waste products that build up in the exercised muscles.

The delayed-onset muscle soreness (DOMS) that appears several hours after exercise (usually 12 hours or so later) and lasts two to four days may be related to microtears in muscle tissue, muscle spasms that increase fluid retention and thereby stimulate the pain nerve endings, and overstretching or tearing of connective tissue in and around muscles and joints.

Two types of contraction accompany muscular activity with movement (also see the Chapter 3 discussion on mode of training—concentric muscle contraction and eccentric muscle contraction—page 71). **Concentric muscle contraction** is a dynamic contraction in which the muscle shortens as it develops tension. **Eccentric muscle contraction** is a dynamic contraction in which the muscle fibers lengthen while developing tension.

For example, during the arm-curl exercise, the elbow flexor muscles (biceps, brachioradialis, and brachialis) shorten as the weight is brought toward the shoulder (concentric contraction). On the way down, the muscles contract eccentrically as they lengthen while the person lowers the weight slowly to the starting position.

As you place your foot on the ground when running, the muscles contract eccentrically to absorb the weight of the body as you strike the ground. This eccentric contraction is followed by a concentric contraction of the leg as you push off the ground to propel the body forward.

Unlike running, cycling requires only concentric contractions of the leg muscles as you pedal the bicycle. Pushing down on the pedal produces a concentric contraction of the quadriceps muscles. If you use toe clips, pulling the pedal back up to the top of the circle produces a concentric contraction of the hamstring muscles.

Eccentric training has been shown to produce more muscle soreness than concentric training does. A hard running workout, therefore, produces greater muscle soreness than a hard cycling workout of similar intensity and duration.

To prevent soreness and stiffness, the recommended approach is to warm up gradually before physical activity and to stretch adequately after exercise. Do not attempt to do too much too quickly. If you become sore and stiff, you have overdone your workout. In these cases, mild stretching, low-intensity exercise to stimulate blood flow, and a warm bath can bring relief.

Stretching may be of greatest significance following exercise. Tired muscles tend to contract to a length that is shorter than normal. By-products of exercise metabolism also may cause muscle spasms. Post-exercise stretching thus can help return a muscle to its normal length.

Q: What causes muscle cramps, and what should be done when they occur?
A: Muscle cramps are caused by the body's depletion of essential electrolytes or a breakdown in coordination between opposing muscle groups. If you have a muscle cramp, first attempt to stretch the muscle(s) involved. In the case of the calf muscle, for example, pull your toes up toward the knees. After stretching the affected muscles, rub them down gently, and finally do some mild exercises requiring the use of those specific muscles.

In pregnant and lactating women and people who get very little calcium in the diet, muscle cramps often are caused by a lack of this nutrient. Calcium supplements are recommended in these cases and usually relieve the problem. Tight clothing also can cause cramps because it restricts blood flow to active muscle tissue.

Q: Why is exercising in hot and humid conditions unsafe?
A: When a person exercises, only 30 percent to 40 percent of the energy the body produces is used for mechanical work or movement. The rest of the energy (60 percent to 70 percent) is converted into heat. If this heat cannot be dissipated properly because the weather is too hot or the relative humidity is too high, body temperature increases and, in extreme cases, can result in death.

The specific heat of body tissue (the heat required to raise the temperature of the body by 1°C) is .38 calories per pound of body weight per 1°C (.38 cal/lb/°C). This indicates that if no body heat is dissipated, a 150-pound person has to burn only 57 calories (150 × .38) to increase total body temperature by 1°C. If this person were to engage in an exercise session requiring 300 calories (about 3 miles running) without dissipating any heat, the inner body temperature would increase by 5.3°C, the equivalent of going from 98.6°F to 108.1°F.

This example clearly illustrates the need for caution when exercising in hot or humid weather. If the weather is too hot or the relative humidity is too high, body heat cannot be lost through evaporation because the atmosphere already is saturated with water vapor. In one instance, a football casualty occurred when the outdoor temperature was only 64°F but the relative humidity was 100 percent. As a general rule, a person must take care when air temperature is above 90°F and relative humidity is above 60 percent.

Following are symptoms of and first-aid measures for the three major signs of trouble when exercising in the heat:

1. Heat cramps. Symptoms include cramps and spasms and muscle twitching in the legs, arms, and abdomen. To relieve heat cramps, stop exercising, get out of the heat, stretch slowly, massage the painful area, and drink plenty of fluids (water, fruit drinks, or electrolyte beverages).

2. Heat exhaustion. Symptoms include fainting; dizziness; profuse sweating; cold, clammy skin; weakness; headache; and a rapid, weak pulse. If you develop any of these symptoms, stop and find a cool place to rest. Drink cool water only if conscious. Loosen or remove clothing, and rub your body with a cool/wet towel or ice packs. Place yourself in a supine position with legs elevated 8 to 12 inches. If you are not fully recovered in 30 minutes, seek immediate medical attention.

3. Heatstroke. Symptoms include serious disorientation; warm, dry skin; no sweating; rapid, full pulse; vomiting; diarrhea; unconsciousness; and high body temperature. As the body temperature climbs, unexplained anxiety sets in. When the body temperature reaches 104°F to 105°F, the individual may feel a cold sensation in the trunk of the body, goose bumps, nausea, throbbing in the temples, and numbness in the extremities. Most people become incoherent after this stage. When body temperature reaches 105°F to 106°F, disorientation, loss of fine motor control,

---

GLOSSARY

Concentric muscle contraction A dynamic contraction in which the muscle shortens as it develops tension.

Eccentric muscle contraction A dynamic contraction in which the muscle lengthens as it develops tension.

and muscular weakness set in. If the temperature exceeds 106°F, serious neurologic injury and death may be imminent.

Heatstroke requires immediate emergency medical attention. Request help and get out of the sun and into a cool, humidity-controlled environment. While you're waiting to be taken to the hospital's emergency room, you should be placed in a semiseated position, and your body should be sprayed with cool water and rubbed with cool towels. If possible, cold packs should be placed in areas with abundant blood supply, such as the head, neck, armpits, and groin. Fluids should not be given if you are unconscious.

In any case of heat-related illness, if the person refuses water, vomits, or starts to lose consciousness, call for an ambulance immediately. Proper initial treatment of heatstroke is critical.

Q: What are the recommended guidelines for fluid replacement during prolonged aerobic exercise?
A: Especially for prolonged aerobic exercise, make sure you are well-hydrated before you begin. Thirst is not an adequate indicator of hydration, as feelings of thirst indicate that dehydration has already begun. Exercise performance is impaired when an individual is dehydrated by as little as 2 percent of body weight. Dehydration at 5 percent of body weight decreases performance by about 30 percent. During prolonged aerobic exercise, the main objective of fluid replacement is to maintain the blood volume so circulation and sweating can continue at normal levels. Adequate water replacement is the most important factor in preventing heat disorders. Drinking about 6 to 8 ounces of cool water every 15 to 20 minutes during exercise seems to be ideal to prevent dehydration. Cold fluids are absorbed more rapidly from the stomach.

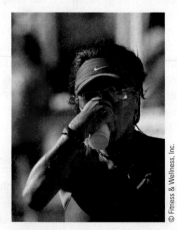

Fluid and carbohydrate replacement is essential during prolonged exercise.

Commercial fluid-replacement solutions (e.g., Powerade, All-Sport, and Gatorade) contain about 6 percent to 8 percent glucose, which seems to be optimal for fluid absorption and performance in most cases. Commercially prepared sports drinks are recommended especially when exercise will be strenuous and carried out for more than an hour. For exercise lasting less than an hour, water is sufficient to replace fluid loss. The sports drinks you select should be based on your personal preference. Try different drinks at 6 percent to 8 percent glucose concentration to see which drink you tolerate best and suits your taste as well. The sugar in these products does not become available to the muscles until about 30 minutes after drinking a glucose solution.

Drinks high in fructose or with a glucose concentration above 8 percent will actually slow water absorption when you exercise in the heat. Most soft drinks (cola, noncola) contain between 10 percent and 12 percent glucose, an amount that is too high for proper rehydration in these circumstances.

For long-distance events, researchers recommend that 30 to 60 grams of carbohydrates (120 to 240 calories) be consumed every hour. This is best accomplished by drinking 8 ounces of a 6 percent to 8 percent carbohydrate sports drink every 15 minutes. The percentage of the carbohydrate drink is determined by dividing the amount of carbohydrates (in grams) by the amount of fluid (in milliliters) and multiplying by 100. For example, 18 grams of carbohydrates in 240 mL (8 oz) of fluid yields a drink at 7.5 percent (18 ÷ 240 × 100).

Q: Do energy drinks enhance work capacity?
A: People tend to associate energy with work. If an energy drink can enhance work capacity, the benefits of such drinks would surpass plain thirst-quenching drinks. Unlike sports drinks, energy drinks typically contain sugar, herbal extracts, large amounts of caffeine, and water-soluble vitamins. Consumers are led to believe that these ingredients increase energy metabolism, provide an energy boost, improve endurance, and aid in weight loss. These purported benefits have yet to be proven through scientific research.

The energy content of many of these drinks is around 60 grams of sugar and 240 calories in a 16-ounce drink (a 12.5 percent glucose concentration), with little additional nutritive value. If you are going to participate in an intense and lengthy workout, the carbohydrate content can boost performance and help you get through the workout. If, however, you are concerned with weight management, 240 calories is an extraordinarily large amount of calories in a 2-cup drink. Weight gain may be the end result if you drink a few of these throughout the day to give you a boost while studying or while at work. Sugar-free energy drinks, available for the weight-conscious consumer, provide little or no energy (calories), although they are packed with nervous system stimulants.

The high caffeine content can also have adverse health effects. Caffeine intake greater than 400 mg can precipitate cardiac arrhythmias, nervousness, irritability, and gastrointestinal discomfort. Many of the popular energy drinks (Red Bull, Sobe Adrenaline Rush, Full Throttle, and Rip It Energy Fuel) contain about 80 mg of caffeine per 8-ounce cup. If you drink two 16-ounce cans, you'll end up with upward of 300 mg of caffeine through these drinks alone. You may also have to consider additional caffeine intake from other beverages that you routinely consume during the day (coffee, tea, or sodas).

Consumption of energy drinks has been linked with many a rapid heart rate (palpitations and tachycardia), ischemia (lack of blood flow to the heart muscle), chest pain, increased blood pressure, tremors, jitters, convulsions, agitation, restlessness, gastrointestinal disturbance, increased urination, nausea, dizziness, irritability, nervousness, syncope (loss of consciousness), paraesthesia (tingling or numbing of the skin), insomnia, respiratory distress, headaches; and most seriously, based on circumstantial evidence, myocardial infarctions and sudden cardiac deaths. At least one sudden cardiac death has been reported in a 28-year-old man who consumed eight cans of an energy drink containing 80 mg of caffeine each over a seven-hour span of time. Between 2008 and 2012, the Food and Drug Administration (FDA) received reports of 13 deaths possibly linked to the highly caffeinated drink 5-Hour Energy (215 milligrams of caffeine per drink—about two cups of coffee) and more than 90 filings of adverse effects, including more than 30 citing life-threatening complications.

Furthermore, because of the high acid content, both sports and energy drinks are extremely erosive to tooth enamel, with energy drinks being twice as erosive as sports drinks. If you ever consume these drinks, to decrease the damage, rinse your mouth with water immediately thereafter and do not brush within an hour as such can actually exacerbate the damage on the enamel caused by the acids. The same can be said about soft drinks and fruit drinks, but to a lesser damaging extent.

Energy drink manufacturers state that the products are safe when used as directed. The potential for excessive use or abuse, however, is real because the FDA does not regulate the products. As with most addictive substances, invariably a sugar and caffeine rush is likely to end up in a physiological crash, requiring a subsequent larger intake to obtain a similar "physical high," thus augmenting the risk for adverse and life-threatening effects.

Q: What precautions must a person take when exercising in the cold?

A: The two factors to consider when you exercise in the cold are frostbite and hypothermia. In contrast to hot and humid conditions, exercising in the cold usually is not health threatening because clothing for heat conservation can be selected and exercise itself increases the production of body heat.

Most people actually overdress for exercise in the cold. Because exercise increases body temperature, a moderate workout on a cold day makes you feel that it is 20° to 30° warmer than the actual temperature. Overdressing for exercise can make the clothes damp from excessive perspiration. The risk for **hypothermia** increases when a person is wet or not moving around sufficiently to increase body heat. Initial warning signs of hypothermia include shivering, loss of coordination, and difficulty in speaking. With a continued drop in body temperature, shivering stops, the muscles weaken and stiffen, and the person feels elated or intoxicated and eventually loses consciousness. To prevent hypothermia, use common sense, dress properly, and be aware of environmental conditions.

The popular belief that exercising in cold temperatures (32°F and lower) freezes the lungs is false because the air is warmed properly in the air passages before it reaches the lungs. The threat is not the cold; it's the wind velocity—which affects the chill factor greatly.

For example, exercising at a temperature of 25°F with adequate clothing is not too cold, but if the wind is blowing at 25 miles per hour, the chill factor lowers the actual temperature to 15°F. This effect is even worse if a person is wet and exhausted. On windy days, exercise (jog or cycle) against the wind on the way out and with the wind when you return.

Even though the lungs are not at risk when you exercise in the cold, your face, head, hands, and feet should be protected because they are subject to frostbite. Watch for numbness and discoloration—signs of frostbite. In cold temperatures, as much as 50 percent of the body's heat can be lost through an unprotected head and neck. A wool or synthetic cap, hood, or hat will help to hold in body heat. Mittens are better than gloves because they keep the fingers together so the surface area from which to lose heat is less. Inner linings of synthetic material are recommended because they wick moisture away from the skin. Avoid cotton next to the skin because, once it gets wet—whether from perspiration, rain, or snow—cotton loses its insulating properties.

GLOSSARY

Hypothermia A breakdown in the body's ability to generate heat, resulting in body temperature below 95°F.

Wearing several layers of lightweight clothing is preferable to wearing one single, thick layer because warm air is trapped between layers of clothes, enabling greater heat conservation. As body temperature increases, you can remove layers as necessary. For prolonged or long-distance workouts (cross-country skiing or long runs), take a small backpack to carry any clothing you remove. You also can carry extra warm and dry clothes in case you stop exercising away from shelter. If you remain outdoors following exercise, added clothing and continuous body movement are essential.

The first layer of clothes should wick moisture away from the skin. Polypropylene, Capilene, and Thermax are recommended. Next, a layer of wool, Dacron, or polyester fleece insulates well even when wet. Lycra tights or sweatpants help to protect the legs. The outer layer should be waterproof, wind-resistant, and breathable. A synthetic material such as Gore-Tex is best so moisture still can escape from the body. A ski mask or face mask helps to protect the face. In extremely cold conditions, petroleum jelly can be used to protect exposed skin such as the nose, cheeks, or around the eyes.

9.3 *Considerations for Women*

Q: What are the physiological differences between men and women as related to exercise?
A: Men and women have several basic differences that affect their physical performance. On average, men are about 3 to 4 inches taller and 25 to 30 pounds heavier than women. The average body fat in college males is about 12 percent to 16 percent, whereas in college females it is 22 percent to 26 percent.

Maximal oxygen uptake (aerobic capacity) is about 15 percent to 30 percent greater in men, caused primarily by their lower body fat content (essential fat), higher **hemoglobin** concentration, and larger heart size. The higher hemoglobin concentration allows men to carry more oxygen during exercise, which is advantageous during aerobic events. A larger heart pumps more blood with each stroke, thereby increasing the amount of oxygenated blood available to the working muscles.

The quality of muscle in men and women is the same. Men, however, are stronger because they have more muscle mass and a greater capacity for muscle hypertrophy, the muscle's ability to increase in size. The larger capacity for muscle hypertrophy is related to sex-specific hormones. Strength differences are significantly less, though, when taking into consideration body size and composition.

Men also have wider shoulders, longer extremities, and a 10 percent greater bone width, except for pelvic width. Notwithstanding all these gender differences in physiological characteristics, the two sexes respond to training in a similar way.

Q: Does participation in exercise hinder menstruation?
A: In some instances highly trained athletes develop **oligomenorrhea** or **amenorrhea** during training and competition. These conditions are often seen in extremely lean women with disordered eating behaviors who engage in strenuous physical training over a sustained time. Amenorrhea is often associated with lower estrogen levels. Lack of estrogen leads to bone loss and a subsequent increase in risk for osteoporosis (also see question on osteoporosis on pages 252–254).

Primary amenorrhea exists when a girl has reached the age of 16 without menstruating or she has gone 2 years following the development of secondary sex characteristics without the onset of menses. Secondary amenorrhea is defined as cessation of menses following normal menstrual cycles.

At present we do not know whether the disorders are caused by physical stress or emotional stress related to high-intensity training, excessively low body fat, or other factors. Intense training and decreased caloric intake (often seen in athletes in an attempt to improve performance) appears to hinder the release of hormones needed for normal menses.

The combination of disordered eating, secondary amenorrhea, and bone mineral disorders is known as the **female athlete triad** (see Figure 9.2). The triad is seen most often in highly trained young women who participate in sports. It is also referred to as the female triad because it is seen in some nonathlete women who are very lean and extremely active. A woman can have one, two, or all three parts of the triad.

The American College of Sports Medicine has issued a position statement on the female athlete triad indicating that these disorders can lead to decreased physical

Figure 9.2 The female athlete triad.

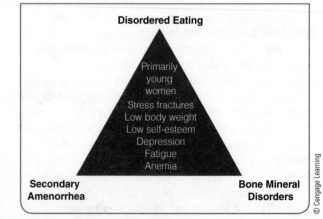

Disordered Eating

Primarily young women
Stress fractures
Low body weight
Low self-esteem
Depression
Fatigue
Anemia

Secondary Amenorrhea

Bone Mineral Disorders

© Cengage Learning

capacity, illness, and premature death.[4] These conditions are by no means irreversible. Women who stop menstruating because of heavy exercise training should seek the advice of a physician. A gradual increase in daily caloric intake, slight weight gain, decreased exercise training, maintenance of adequate calcium intake, and possible estrogen replacement therapy are all recommended to treat the female athlete triad.

Q: Does exercise help relieve dysmenorrhea?
A: Although exercise has not been shown to either cure or aggravate **dysmenorrhea**, it has been shown to help relieve menstrual cramps because it improves circulation to the uterus. Particularly, stretching exercises of the muscles in the pelvic region seem to reduce and prevent painful menstruation that is not the result of a disease.

Q: Is exercising safe during pregnancy?
A: Exercise is beneficial during pregnancy. According to the American College of Obstetricians and Gynecologists (ACOG), in the absence of contraindications, healthy pregnant women are encouraged to participate in regular moderate-intensity physical activities to continue to derive health benefits during pregnancy.[5] Pregnant women, however, should consult with their physicians to ensure there are no contraindications to exercise during pregnancy (see box on the next page).

As a general rule, healthy pregnant women can also accumulate 30 minutes of moderate-intensity physical activity on most, if not all, days of the week (a minimum of 150 minutes per week). Physical activity strengthens the body and helps prepare it for the challenges of labor and childbirth.

The average labor and delivery lasts 10 to 12 hours. In most cases, labor and delivery are highly intense, with repeated muscular contractions interspersed with short rest periods. Proper conditioning will better prepare the body for childbirth. Moderate exercise during pregnancy also helps to prevent back pain and excessive weight gain, and it speeds up recovery following childbirth.

The most common recommendations for exercise during pregnancy for healthy pregnant women with no additional risk factors are as follows:

1. Do not start a new or more rigorous exercise program without proper medical clearance.
2. Accumulate 30 minutes of moderate-intensity physical activities on most days of the week.
3. Instead of using heart rate to monitor intensity, exercise at an intensity level that is perceived between "light" and "somewhat hard." An exertion above "somewhat hard" is not recommended during pregnancy.
4. Gradually switch from weight-bearing and high-impact activities such as jogging and aerobics, to non-weight-bearing/lower-impact activities such as walking, stationary cycling, swimming, and water aerobics. The latter activities minimize the risk of injury and may allow exercise to continue throughout pregnancy.
5. Avoid exercising at an altitude above 6,000 feet (1,800 meters) or scuba diving because these may compromise availability of oxygen to the fetus.
6. Women who are accustomed to strenuous exercise may continue in the early stages of pregnancy but should gradually decrease the amount, intensity, and exercise mode as pregnancy advances (most healthy pregnant women, however, slow down during the first few weeks of pregnancy because of morning sickness and fatigue).
7. Pay attention to the body's signals of discomfort and distress and never exercise to exhaustion. When fatigued, slow down or take a day off. Do not stop exercising altogether unless you experience any of the contraindications for exercise listed in the box on the next page.

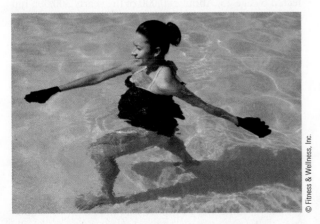

Light- to moderate-intensity exercise is recommended throughout pregnancy.

© Fitness & Wellness, Inc.

GLOSSARY

Hemoglobin Protein-iron compound in red blood cells that transports oxygen in the blood.

Oligomenorrhea Irregular menstrual cycles.

Amenorrhea Absence (primary amenorrhea) or cessation (secondary amenorrhea) of normal menstrual function.

Female athlete triad Three interrelated disorders—disordered eating, amenorrhea, and bone mineral disorders— seen in some highly trained female athletes.

Dysmenorrhea Painful menstruation.

8. To prevent fetal injury, avoid activities that involve potential contact or loss of balance or could cause even mild trauma to the abdomen. Examples of these activities are basketball, soccer, volleyball, Nordic or water skiing, ice skating, road cycling, horseback riding, and motorcycle riding.

9. During pregnancy, do not exercise for weight loss purposes.

10. Get proper nourishment (pregnancy requires between 150 and 300 extra calories per day), and eat a small snack or drink some juice 20 to 30 minutes prior to exercise.

11. Prevent dehydration by drinking a cup of fluids 20 to 30 minutes before exercise and drink 1 cup of liquid every 15 to 20 minutes during exercise.

12. During the first three months in particular, do not exercise in the heat. Wear clothing that allows for proper dissipation of heat. A body temperature above 102.6°F (39.2°C) can harm the fetus.

13. After the first trimester, avoid exercises that require lying on the back. This position can block blood flow to the uterus and the baby.

14. Perform stretching exercises gently because hormonal changes during pregnancy increase the laxity of muscles and connective tissue. Although these changes facilitate delivery, they also make women more susceptible to injuries during exercise.

Contraindications to Exercise During Pregnancy

Stop exercise and seek medical advice if you experience any of the following symptoms:

- Unusual pain or discomfort, especially in the chest or abdominal area
- Cramping, primarily in the pelvic or lower back areas
- Muscle weakness, excessive fatigue, or shortness of breath
- Abnormally high heart rate or a pounding (palpitations) heart rate
- Decreased fetal movement
- Insufficient weight gain
- Amniotic fluid leakage
- Nausea, dizziness, or headaches
- Persistent uterine contractions
- Vaginal bleeding or rupture of the membranes
- Swelling of ankles, calves, hands, or face

© Cengage Learning

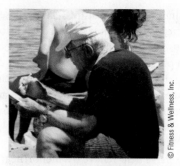
© Fitness & Wellness, Inc.

Osteoporosis is a major cause of functional loss and premature morbidity in older adults.

Q: Can osteoporosis be prevented?

A: Osteoporosis, literally meaning "porous bones," is a condition in which bones lack the minerals required to keep them strong. In osteoporosis, bones—primarily of the hip, wrist, and spine—become so weak and brittle that they fracture readily. The process begins slowly in the third and fourth decades of life. Women are especially susceptible after menopause because of the accompanying loss of **estrogen,** which increases the rate at which bone mass is broken down.

Osteoporosis is the leading cause of serious morbidity and functional loss in the elderly population. One of every two women and one in eight men over age 50 will have an osteoporotic-related fracture at some point in their lives. Up to 20 percent of people who have a hip fracture die within a year because of complications related to the fracture. As alarming as these figures are, they do not convey the pain and loss of quality of life in people who suffer the crippling effects of osteoporotic fractures.

Although osteoporosis is viewed primarily as a women's disease, more than 30 percent of all men will be affected by age 75. About 100,000 of the yearly 300,000 hip fractures in the United States occur in men.

Despite the strong genetic component, osteoporosis is preventable. Maximizing bone density at a young age and subsequently decreasing the rate of bone loss later in life are critical to preventing osteoporosis.

Normal hormone levels prior to menopause and adequate calcium intake and physical activity throughout life cannot be overemphasized. These factors are all crucial to prevent osteoporosis. The absence of any one of these three factors leads to bone loss for which the other two factors never completely compensate. Smoking, excessive use of alcohol, and corticosteroid drugs also accelerate the rate of bone loss in women and men alike. Osteoporosis is also more common in whites, Asians, and small-frame people. Figure 9.3 depicts these variables.

Figure 9.3 Factors that diminish bone health (osteoporosis).

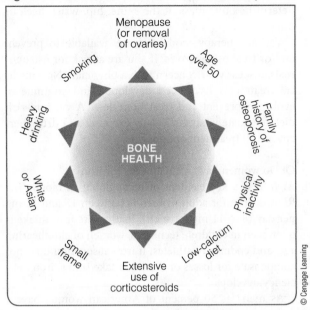

© Cengage Learning

Table 9.3 Calcium-Rich Foods

Food	Amount	Calcium (mg)	Calories
Beans, red kidney, cooked	1 cup	70	218
Beet, greens, cooked	½ cup	82	19
Bok choy (Chinese cabbage)	1 cup	158	20
Broccoli, cooked, drained	1 cup	72	44
Burrito, bean (no cheese)	1	57	225
Cottage cheese, 2% low-fat	½ cup	78	103
Ice milk (vanilla)	½ cup	102	100
Instant breakfast, nonfat milk	1 cup	407	216
Kale, cooked, drained	1 cup	94	36
Milk, nonfat, powdered	1 tbs	52	15
Milk, skim	1 cup	296	88
Oatmeal, instant, fortified, plain	½ cup	109	70
Okra, cooked, drained	½ cup	74	23
Orange juice, fortified	1 cup	300	110
Soy milk, fortified, fat free	1 cup	400	110
Spinach, raw	1 cup	56	12
Turnip greens, cooked	1 cup	197	29
Tofu (some types)	½ cup	138	76
Yogurt, fruit	1 cup	372	250
Yogurt, low-fat, plain	1 cup	448	155

© Cengage Learning

Bone health begins at a young age. Some experts have called osteoporosis a "pediatric disease." Bone density can be promoted early in life by making sure the diet has sufficient calcium and participating in weight-bearing activities. Adequate calcium intake in both women and men is also associated with a reduced risk for colon cancer. The RDA for calcium is between 1,000 and 1,300 mg per day (see Table 9.2).

To obtain your daily calcium requirement, get as much calcium as possible from calcium-rich foods, including calcium-fortified foods. If you don't get enough, you need to make a conscious and deliberate effort to reach the RDA. Calcium supplements are no longer recommended because they may cause more harm than good, including a higher risk of heart attack, kidney stones in both men and women, and possibly increased risk of prostate cancer in men. Calcium obtained from food has not been linked to these negative health risks. Supplements are only warranted in extreme cases, when dietary intake from food absolutely does not supply the need.

Table 9.3 provides a list of selected foods and their calcium content. Along with adequate calcium intake, taking 400 to 800 IU of vitamin D daily is the recommendation for optimal calcium absorption (for overall health benefits, 1,000 to 2,000 IU of vitamin D is preferable). Close to half of people over 50 are vitamin D deficient. Without vitamin D, it is practically impossible for the body to absorb sufficient calcium to protect the bones.

Vitamin B_{12} may also be a key nutrient in the prevention of osteoporosis. Several reports have shown an association between low vitamin B_{12} and lower bone mineral density in both men and women. Vitamin B_{12} is found primarily in dairy products, meats,

Table 9.2 Recommended Daily Calcium Intake

Age	Amount (gr)
9–18	1,300
19–50	1,000
51–70 Men	1,000
51–70 Women	1,200
>70	1,200

© Cengage Learning

GLOSSARY

Osteoporosis Softening, deterioration, or loss of bone.

Estrogen Female sex hormone; essential for bone

formation and conservation of bone density.

poultry, fish, and some fortified cereals. Other nutrients vital for bone health are potassium (also neutralizes acid), vitamin K (works with bone-building proteins), and magnesium (also keeps bone from becoming too brittle).

Soft drinks, coffee, and alcoholic beverages can also contribute to a loss in bone density if consumed in large quantities. The damage may not be caused directly by these food items but, rather, because they take the place of dairy products in the diet.

Exercise plays a key role in preventing osteoporosis by decreasing the rate of bone loss following menopause. Active people are able to maintain bone density much more effectively than their inactive counterparts. A combination of weight-bearing exercises, such as walking or jogging and strength training, is especially helpful.

The benefits of exercise go beyond maintaining bone density. Exercise strengthens muscles, ligaments, and tendons—all of which provide support to the bones (skeleton). Exercise also improves balance and coordination, which can help prevent falls and injuries.

Current studies indicate that, on average, people who are active have denser bone mineral than inactive people do. Similar to other benefits of participating in exercise, there is no such thing as "bone in the bank." To have good bone health, people need to participate in a lifetime exercise program

Prevailing research also tells us that estrogen is the most important factor in preventing bone loss. Lumbar bone density in women who have always had regular menstrual cycles exceeds that of women with a history of oligomenorrhea and amenorrhea interspersed with regular cycles. Furthermore, the lumbar density of these two groups of women is higher than that of women who have never had regular menstrual cycles.

For instance, athletes with amenorrhea (who have lower estrogen levels) have lower bone mineral density than even nonathletes with normal estrogen levels. Studies have shown that amenorrheic athletes at age 25 have the bones of women older than 50. It has become clear that sedentary women with normal estrogen levels have better bone mineral density than active amenorrheic athletes. Many experts believe the best predictor of bone mineral content is the history of menstrual regularity.

As a baseline, women age 65 and older should have a bone density test to establish the risk for osteoporosis. Younger women who are at risk for osteoporosis should discuss a bone density test with their physician at menopause. The test also can be used to monitor changes in bone mass over time and to predict the risk of future fractures. The bone density test is a painless scan requiring only a small amount of radiation to determine bone mass of the spine, hip, wrist, heel, or fingers.

Various therapy modalities are available to prevent and/or treat osteoporosis. If you are at risk for osteoporosis, discuss your concern with a physician. New medical treatments have been developed and continue to evolve to prevent and treat bone loss. A calcium-rich diet, adequate vitamin D, daily exercise, and drug therapy are all treatment options.

Q: Do women have special needs for iron?

A: Iron is a key element of hemoglobin in blood. The RDA of iron for adult women is between 15 and 18 mg per day (8 to 11 mg for men). Inadequate iron intake is often seen in children, teenagers, women of childbearing age, and endurance athletes. If iron absorption does not compensate for losses or dietary intake is low, iron deficiency develops.

As many as 50 percent of American women have a deficiency of iron. Over time, excessive depletion of iron stores in the body leads to iron-deficiency anemia, a condition in which the concentration of hemoglobin in the red blood cells is lower than it should be; this leads to fatigue and headaches, among other symptoms.

Physically active individuals, women in particular, have a greater-than-average need for iron. Heavy training creates a demand for iron that is higher than the recommended intake because small amounts of iron are lost through sweat, urine, and stools. Mechanical trauma, caused by the pounding of the feet on the pavement during extensive jogging, may also lead to destruction of iron-containing red blood cells.

A large percentage of female endurance athletes are reported to have iron deficiency. The blood **ferritin** levels of women who participate in intense physical training should be checked frequently.

The rates of iron absorption and iron loss vary from person to person. In most cases, though, people can get enough iron by eating more iron-rich foods such as beans, peas, green leafy vegetables, enriched grain products, egg yolk, fish, and lean meats. A list of foods high in iron is given in Table 9.4.

9.4 *Nutrition and Weight Control*

Q: What is the difference between a calorie and a kilocalorie (kcal)?

A: A calorie is the unit of measure indicating the energy value of food to the person who consumes it. It is also used to express the amount of energy a person expends

Table 9.4 Iron-Rich Foods

Food	Amount	Iron (mg)	Calories
Beans, red kidney, cooked	1 cup	4.4	218
Beef, ground lean	3 oz	3.0	186
Beef, sirloin	3 oz	2.5	329
Beef, liver, fried	3 oz	7.5	195
Beet greens, cooked	½ cup	1.4	13
Broccoli, cooked, drained	1 sm stalk	1.1	36
Burrito, bean	1	2.4	307
Egg, hard-cooked	1	1.0	72
Farina (Cream of Wheat), cooked	½ cup	6.0	51
Instant breakfast, whole milk	1 cup	8.0	280
Peas, frozen, cooked, drained	½ cup	1.5	55
Shrimp, boiled	3 oz	2.7	99
Spinach, raw	1 cup	1.7	14
Vegetables, mixed, cooked	1 cup	2.4	116

© Cengage Learning

in physical activity. Technically, a kilocalorie (kcal), or large calorie, is the amount of heat necessary to raise the temperature of 1 kilogram of water 1° Celsius. For simplicity, people call it a calorie rather than a kcal. For example, if the caloric value of a food is 100 calories (that is, 100 kcal), the energy in this food would raise the temperature of 100 kilograms of water 1° Celsius. Similarly, walking 1 mile would burn about 100 calories (again, 100 kcal).

Q: What constitutes ideal body weight?
A: There is no such thing as "ideal" body weight. Health/fitness professionals prefer to use the terms "recommended" or "healthy" body weight. Let's examine the question in more detail. For instance, 25 percent body fat is the recommended health fitness standard for a 40-year-old man. For the average "apparently healthy" individual, this body fat percentage does not constitute a threat to good health. Due to genetic and lifestyle conditions, however, if a person this same age at 25 percent body fat is pre-diabetic, pre-hypertensive, and with abnormal blood lipids (cholesterol and triglycerides—see Chapter 8), weight (fat) loss and a lower percent body fat may be recommended. Thus, what will work as recommended weight for most individuals may not be the best standard for individuals with disease risk factors. The current recommended or healthy weight standards (based on percent body fat or BMI) are established at the point where there appears to be a lower incidence for overweight-related conditions for most people. Individual differences

have to be taken into consideration when making a final recommendation, especially in people with risk factors or a personal and family history of chronic conditions.

Q: What is more important for weight loss—a negative caloric balance (diet) or an increase in physical activity?
A: Most of the research shows that weight loss is more effective when cutting back on calories (dieting) as opposed to only increasing physical activity or exercise. Weight loss is accelerated, nonetheless, when physical activity is added to dieting, as long as the person doesn't compensate with extra food intake following physical activity (a common occurrence among people who exercise, as they feel justified in doing so because they exercised).

There is a fair amount of media distortion stating that "exercise makes a person fat," "why most of us believe that exercise makes us thinner—and why we are wrong," and "the myth about exercise: of course it's good for you, but it won't make you lose weight." There is ample scientific evidence that exercise is an important component of a successful weight loss program. The problem is that following exercise, many people eat more (particularly more junk food).

When attempting to lose weight, initial lengthy exercise sessions (longer than 60 minutes) by unfit people may not be the best approach to weight loss—unless they carefully monitor daily caloric intake and avoid caloric compensation for the energy expended during exercise. In active or fit individuals, lengthy exercise sessions are not counterproductive.

Body composition changes are also more effective when dieting and exercise are combined while attempting to lose body weight. Most weight loss when dieting with exercise comes in the form of body fat and not lean body tissue, a desirable outcome. Weight loss maintenance, however, in most cases is possible only with 60 to 90 minutes of sustained daily physical activity and exercise. If you are still not convinced that exercise is the best approach to weight management, take a look around the gym or the jogging trail. If this were the case, wouldn't those who regularly exercise be the fattest?

Q: Are some diet plans more effective than others?
A: The term "diet" implies a negative caloric balance. A negative caloric balance means that you are consuming

---

GLOSSARY

Ferritin Iron stored in the body.

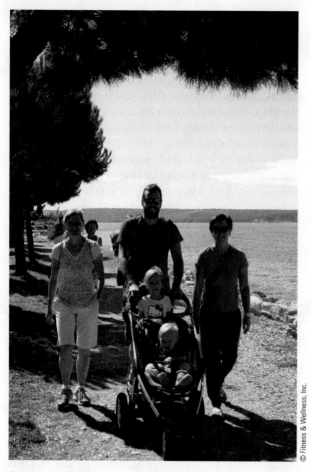

A wellness lifestyle provides the freedom to live life to its fullest without functional limitations.

energy comes from fat when doing absolutely nothing (resting/sleeping). And when one does nothing, as in a sedentary lifestyle, one doesn't burn many calories.

Let's examine this issue. During resting conditions, the human body is a very efficient "fat-burning machine." That is, most of the energy, approximately 70 percent, is derived from fat and only 30 percent from carbohydrates. But we burn few calories at rest, about 1.5 calories per minute compared to 3 to 4 calories during light-intensity exercise and 8 to 10 calories per minute during vigorous-intensity exercise. As we begin to exercise, and subsequently increase the intensity of exercise, we progressively rely more on carbohydrates and less on fat for energy, until we reach maximal intensity when 100 percent of the energy is derived from carbohydrates. Even though a lower percentage of the energy is derived from fat during vigorous-intensity exercise, the total caloric expenditure is so much greater (twice as high or more), that overall the total fat burned is still higher than during moderate intensity.

A word of caution, nonetheless: Do not start vigorous-intensity exercise without several weeks of proper and gradual conditioning. This advice particularly applies if such exercise is a high-impact activity. If you participate in high-impact activities from the outset, you increase the risk of injury and may have to stop exercising altogether.

Q: Do fasting or detox diets "cleanse" the body and rid it of toxins and poisons?
A: Popular cleansing, fasting, liquid, and detox diets on the market today lead consumers to believe that they aid the body in removing toxins and chemicals. It may sound like a good concept, but the claims are unsubstantiated with no scientific proof to this effect. The notion behind these claims is that the body holds onto harmful substances in the gastrointestinal tract and the lymph system. The digestive system, liver, kidneys, and lungs, however, are very effective at cleansing the body and you do not need to stop eating to help the process. If you are concerned about your diet and the environment in which you live (excess alcohol and caffeine, tobacco use, drugs, pesticides, smog, chemicals to grow and prepare food, sugar, artificial sweeteners, or unhealthy water), you need to make healthy changes in your lifestyle, but you do not need cleansing.

Weight loss as a result of one to three days of near fasting is primarily due to water loss and not fat loss. Your health may improve with a detox diet because these diets are highly restrictive in food choices. You can accomplish the same results by eating more fruits and vegetables, and

fewer calories than those required to maintain your current weight. When energy output surpasses energy intake, weight loss will occur. Popular diets differ widely in the food choices you are allowed to have. The more limited the choices, the lower the chances to overeat, and thus you will have a lower caloric intake. And the fewer the calories that you consume, the greater the weight loss. *For health reasons,* to obtain the variety of nutrients the body needs, even during weight loss periods, most people should not consume fewer than 1,500 calories per day. These calories should be distributed over a wide range of foods, emphasizing grains, fruits, vegetables, and small amounts of low-fat animal products or fish.

Q: Is light-intensity aerobic exercise more effective in burning fat for weight loss purposes?
A: Without a question, vigorous-intensity aerobic exercise is more effective. True, during light-intensity exercise a greater percentage of the energy is derived from fat. It is also true that an even greater percentage of the

fewer calories, refined/processed foods, and high fat/saturated/trans fat foods.

Q: Are organic foods better than conventional foods?
A: Concerns over pesticides in foods have led many people to turn to organic foods. Currently, less than 2 percent of imported food products are inspected by the FDA and domestic food is seldom inspected at all. Health risks from pesticide exposure from foods are relatively small for healthy adults. The health benefits of produce far outweigh the risks. Children, older adults, pregnant and lactating women, and people with a weak immune system, however, may be vulnerable to some types of pesticides.

Organic crops have to be grown without the use of conventional pesticides, artificial fertilizers, human waste, or sewage sludge and have been processed without ionizing radiation or food additives. Organic livestock is raised under certain grazing conditions, using organic feed, and without the use of antibiotics and growth hormones.

While pesticide residues in organic foods are substantially lower than in conventionally grown foods, organic foods can also be contaminated with bacteria, pathogens, and heavy metals that pose major health risks. The soil itself may become contaminated, or if the produce comes in contact with the feces of grazing cattle, wild animals or birds, farmworkers, or any other source, potentially harmful microorganisms can contaminate the produce.

Regardless of the type of produce you purchase, be sure to wash it. If you choose to take extra precaution, you may choose a trusted low-pesticide source for purchasing produce items likely to be heavily treated (apples, bell peppers, blueberries, celery, cherries, cherry tomatoes, collard greens, cucumbers, grapes, kale, nectarines, peaches, potatoes, snap peas, spinach, and strawberries). Pre-washed produce (indicated on the package) do not have to be washed again.

Q: Are "natural" supplements to boost metabolism safe?
A: Supplements to boost metabolism contain stimulants that are harmful to individuals sensitive to such substances. These stimulants can also cause damage to people with metabolic disorders, heart disease, and high blood pressure. A physician or registered dietitian should be consulted prior to taking such supplements.

Q: Do athletes or individuals who train for long periods need a special diet?
A: In general, athletes do not require special supplementation or any other special type of diet. Unless the diet is deficient in basic nutrients, no special, secret, or magic diet will help people perform better or develop faster as a result of what they eat. As long as the diet is balanced, based on a large variety of nutrients from the basic food groups, and with sufficient daily protein intake (see section on Proteins in Chapter 5, pages 130–131, and Chapter 3, page 78), athletes do not require additional supplements. Even in strength training and body building, protein in excess of 20 percent of total daily caloric intake is not necessary.

The main difference between a sedentary person and a highly active individual is in the total number of calories required daily and the amount of carbohydrate intake during bouts of prolonged physical activity. During training, people consume more calories because of the greater energy expenditure required as a result of intense physical training.

A regular diet should be altered to include about 70 percent carbohydrates (carbohydrate loading) during several days of heavy aerobic training or when a person is going to participate in a long-distance event of more than 90 minutes (marathons, triathlons, road cycling races). For events shorter than 90 minutes, carbohydrate loading does not seem to enhance performance.

Q: What is gluten sensitivity?
A: Gluten sensitivity falls under an umbrella of adverse effects on the body caused by gluten, a protein found in wheat, barley, rye, malts, and triticale. Gluten is also used as an additive for flavoring and stabilizing food or as a thickening agent.

About 1 percent of Americans suffer from celiac disease, an autoimmune disorder in genetically predisposed people of all ages that damages the lining of the small intestine and the ability to absorb nutrients. The disease is caused by a reaction to gluten, leading to an inflammatory reaction that induces a series of symptoms, including vomiting, severe abdominal pain, diarrhea, and fatigue. A gluten-free diet is the accepted treatment for individuals with celiac disease.

Many people test negative for celiac disease but appear to be gluten sensitive. They indicate that they feel better when they eliminate gluten from the diet. A gluten-free diet, however, is not completely free of gluten; rather, it contains a low, harmless level. Switching to a healthy diet often helps gluten-sensitive individuals because processed and junk foods tend to have high amounts of gluten. Some gluten in the diet may not affect these people much.

Q: Do I have to follow a diet 24/7 to derive health benefits?
A: A sound diet is vital for good health and wellness. An extreme approach, however, is not the best advice when

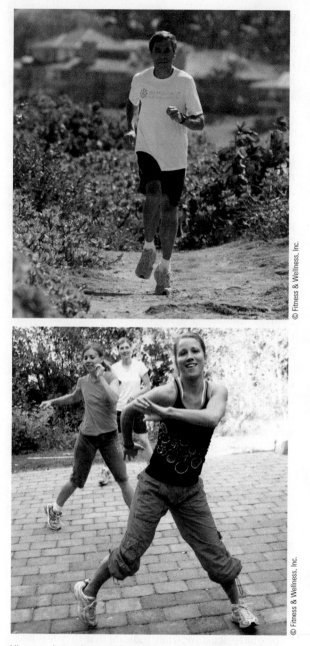

© Fitness & Wellness, Inc.

© Fitness & Wellness, Inc.

Vigorous-intensity exercise is by far more effective in producing weight (fat) loss, as long as the individual does not compensate by eating additional calories following exercise.

it comes to proper nutrition. Health experts believe that such an approach may lead to "orthorexia nervosa," a new category of eating disorder characterized by an unhealthy compulsion over food choices. Moderation and common sense in all things is solid advice when it comes to healthy diet and nutrition. Healthy eating patterns that can be maintained for a lifetime include small and occasional treats from time to time.

Q: Should I be concerned about antibiotics in meat?

A: The use of antibiotics in animals in the United States is a common practice to increase animal growth and prevent chronic livestock illness in overcrowded farms with unsanitary living conditions. Most mass-produced meat in the United States has been injected with antibiotics and hormones. The concern is that overuse may lead to antibiotic resistance in humans, a condition responsible for about two million illnesses and 23,000 deaths in the United States each year. The World Health Organization, the American Medical Association, and the National Resources Defense Council consider non-therapeutic antibiotic use in livestock as a significant public health risk. As a consumer you are encouraged to minimize the use of meats anyway, for overall health reasons (see Proteins in Chapter 5, pages 130–131), and when you do use them, search for products from companies that certify antibiotic use in animals for therapeutic purposes only. Imports of United States meats are banned by the European Union, Canada, Japan, Australia, Russia, and Taiwan.

Q: Should I worry about sugar in my diet?

A: Until recently, the most significant health concerns regarding excessive sugar intake included increased caloric intake, weight gain, obesity, tooth decay, and lower nutrient intake (empty calories with no nutritional benefit whatsoever). Consumption of one or two sugar-sweetened beverages per day has been found to increase coronary heart disease risk by up to 35 percent and regular soft drink consumers have about an 80 percent greater risk for developing type 2 diabetes. Excessive body weight increases the risk for metabolic syndrome and heart disease. People who consume a sugar-heavy diet also run a greater risk for pancreatic cancer. And most recently, in an article published in the *American Journal of Public Health* in December 2014, scientists established that regardless of weight gain, drinking an 8-ounce daily serving of soda is linked to 1.9 years of additional biological aging and drinking 20 ounces of soda daily is associated with 4.6 years of additional aging.

Data indicates that the typical American consumes about 13 percent of the daily calories from added sugar, or about 268 calories, the equivalent of 18 teaspoons per day. The American Heart Association recommends no more than six (100 calories) and nine (150 calories) daily teaspoons of added sugar for women and men, respectively.

Most people simply cannot afford all those extra daily empty calories. Data indicate that liquid calories (soft drinks) do not result in less food consumption during a meal. Liquid calories are not recognized by the body as are solid food calories and do little to suppress the body's hunger-stimulating hormone ghrelin, thus most often they lead to greater caloric consumption per meal. Adults who drink one or more sodas per day are 27 percent more likely to be overweight or obese. Not taking into account the greater caloric intake with meals, even just the one can (12 oz.) of soda per day can add 16.5 pounds of body weight per year (160 calories per can × 365 days ÷ 3,500—the equivalent of one pound of fat). Thus, for good health and proper weight management, steer clear of liquid calories and hydrate with plain water instead.

Q: Fish is known to be heart healthy, but should we have concerns about mercury toxicity?
A: Fish and shellfish contain high-quality protein, omega-3 fatty acids, and other essential nutrients. As little as six ounces of fatty fish per week can reduce the risk of premature death from heart disease by one-third and overall death rates by about one-sixth. Fish also appears to have anti-inflammatory properties that can help treat chronic inflammatory kidney disease, osteoarthritis, rheumatoid arthritis, Crohn's disease, and autoimmune disorders like asthma and lupus. Thus, fish is one of the healthiest foods we can consume.

Mercury in fish has created concerns among some people. Mercury cannot be removed from food. As it accumulates in the body, it harms the brain and nervous system. Mercury is a naturally occurring trace mineral that can be released into the air from industrial pollution. As mercury falls into streams and oceans, it accumulates in the aquatic food chain. Larger fish accumulate larger amounts of mercury because they eat medium- and small-size fish. Of particular concern are shark, swordfish, king mackerel, pike, bass, and tilefish, which have higher levels. Farm-raised salmon also have slightly higher levels of polychlorinated biphenyls (PCBs), which the U.S. Environmental Protection Agency lists as a "probable human carcinogen."

The risk for adverse effects from eating fish is extremely low and primarily theoretical in nature. For most people, eating two servings (up to six ounces) of fish per week poses no health threat. Pregnant and nursing women and young children, however, should avoid mercury in fish. The best recommendation is to balance the risks against the benefits. If you are still concerned, consume no more than 12 ounces per week of a variety of fish and shellfish that are lower in mercury, including canned light tuna, wild salmon, shrimp, pollock, catfish, and scallops. And check local advisories about the safety of fish caught by family and friends in local streams, rivers, lakes, and coastal areas. Some preventive medicine experts now believe that fish is most likely the single most important food an individual can consume for good health.

Q: Are there specific nutrient requirements for optimal development and recovery following exercise?
A: Carbohydrates with some protein appear to be best. Protein is recommended prior to and immediately following high-intensity aerobic or strength-training exercise. Intense exercise causes micro-tears in muscle tissue, and the presence of amino acids (the building blocks of proteins) in the blood contributes to the healing process and subsequent development and strengthening of the muscle fibers. Protein consumption along with carbohydrates also accelerates glycogen replenishment in the body after intense or prolonged exercise. Thus, carbohydrates provide energy for exercise and replenishment of glycogen stores after exercise, while protein optimizes muscle repair, growth, glycogen replenishment, and recovery following exercise. Aim for a ratio of 4-to-1 grams of carbohydrates to protein. For example, you may consume a snack that contains 40 grams of carbohydrates (160 calories) and 10 grams of protein (40 calories). Examples of good recovery foods include milk and cereal, a tuna fish sandwich, a peanut butter and jelly sandwich, or pasta with turkey meat sauce.

Q: What do the terms "glycemic index" and "glycemic load" mean?
A: The glycemic index (GI) provides a numeric value that measures the blood glucose (sugar) response following ingestion of individual carbohydrate foods. Carbohydrates that are quickly absorbed and cause a rapid rise in blood glucose are said to have a high GI. Those that break down slowly and gradually release glucose into the blood have a low GI. Consumption of high glycemic foods in combination with some fat and protein, nonetheless, brings down the average index. The glycemic load (GL) is calculated by multiplying the GI of a particular food by its carbohydrate content in grams and dividing by 100. The usefulness of the glycemic load is based on the theory that a high-glycemic-index food eaten in small quantities provides a similar effect in blood sugar rise as consumption of a larger quantity of a low-glycemic food. The most accurate source of the GI and GL of 750 foods has been published in the *Journal of Clinical Nutrition* at http://www.ajcn.org/content/ 76/ 1/5.full.pdf ++html.

Q: What is the difference between antioxidants and phytonutrients?
A: Antioxidants, comprising vitamins, minerals, and phytonutrients, help prevent damage to cells from highly reactive and unstable molecules known as oxygen free radicals (see page 140). Antioxidants are found in both plant and animal foods, whereas phytonutrients are

found in plant foods only, including fruits, vegetables, beans, nuts, and seeds. The actions of phytonutrients, however, go beyond those of most antioxidants. In particular, they appear to have powerful anticancer properties. For example, at almost every stage of cancer, phytonutrients can block, disrupt, slow, or even reverse the process. In terms of heart disease, they may reduce inflammation, inhibit blood clots, or prevent the oxidation of low-density lipoprotein cholesterol. People should consume ample amounts of plant-based foods to obtain a healthy supply of antioxidants, including a wide array of phytonutrients.

9.5 *Exercise and Aging*

Q: What is the difference between chronological and physiological age?

A: Chronological age is your actual age—that is, how old you are. Physiological age is used in reference to your functional capacity to perform physical work at any stage of your life. Data on individuals who have taken part in systematic physical activity throughout life indicate that these people maintain a higher level of functional capacity and do not experience the declines typical in later years. From a functional point of view, typical sedentary people in the United States are about 25 years older than their chronological age indicates. Thus, a sedentary 20-year-old college student can easily have the physical capacity of a 45-year-old active individual. Likewise, a 60-year-old individual can easily have a similar physical capacity to that of an inactive 35-year-old person.

Q: What is the relationship between aging and physical work capacity?

A: The elderly constitute the fastest-growing segment of the population. The number of Americans ages 65 and older increased from 3.1 million in 1900 (4.1 percent of the population) to about 40 million (13 percent) in 2010. By the year 2030, more than 72 million people, or 20 percent of the United States population, are expected to be older than 65.

The main objective of fitness programs for older adults is to help them improve their **functional fitness** and contribute to healthy aging. This implies the ability to maintain **functional independence** and to avoid disability. Older adults are encouraged to participate in programs that will help develop cardiorespiratory endurance, muscular strength and endurance, muscular flexibility, agility and balance, and motor coordination. A fitness program delivers results with gains in physical and mental capacity—even small efforts bring measurable rewards.

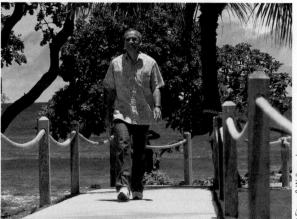

Regular physical activity enhances quality of life and longevity.

The physical and psychological benefits of regular physical activity for older adults make an impressive list. Physical activity decreases the risk for cardiovascular disease, stroke, hypertension, type 2 diabetes, osteoporosis, obesity, colon cancer, breast cancer, cognitive impairment, anxiety, and depression, and even dementia and Alzheimer's. Physical activity also improves self-confidence and self-esteem. Furthermore, both cardiorespiratory endurance and strength training help to increase functional capacity, improve overall health status, improve memory and mental acumen, and increase life expectancy. Strength training also decreases the rate at which strength and muscle mass are lost.

Unhealthy behaviors precipitate premature aging. For sedentary people, productive life ends at about age 60. Most of these people hope to live to be 65 or 70 and often must cope with serious physical ailments. These people stop living at age 60 but choose to be buried at age 70! (See the theoretical model in Figure 9.4.)

A healthy lifestyle allows people to live a vibrant life—a physically, intellectually, emotionally, socially active, and functionally independent existence—to age 95. When death comes to active people, it usually is rather quick and not as a result of prolonged illness (see Figure 9.4). Such are the rewards of a wellness way of life.

> **!** **Critical Thinking**
>
> Have you ever considered how you would like to feel and what type of activities you would like to carry on after age 65? • What will it take for you to accomplish your goals?

Figure 9.4 Relationships among physical work capacity, aging, and lifestyle habits.

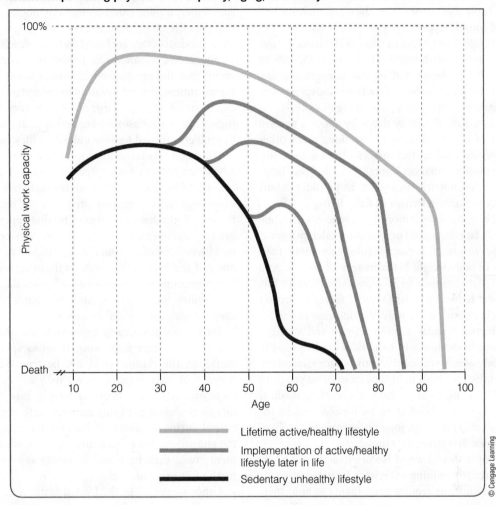

Lifetime active/healthy lifestyle

Implementation of active/healthy lifestyle later in life

Sedentary unhealthy lifestyle

© Cengage Learning

Q: Do older adults respond to physical training?

A: The trainability of older men and women alike and the effectiveness of physical activity in enhancing health have been demonstrated in prior research. Older adults who increase their physical activity experience significant changes in cardiorespiratory endurance, strength, and flexibility. The extent of the changes depends on their initial fitness level and the types of activities they select for their training (walking, cycling, strength training, and so on).

Improvements in maximal oxygen uptake in older adults are similar to those of younger people, although older people seem to require a longer training period to achieve these changes. Declines in maximal oxygen uptake average about 1 percent per year between ages 25 and 75. A slower rate of decline is seen in people who maintain a lifetime aerobic exercise program. Data show that the maximal oxygen uptake of older adults who regularly exercise is almost twice that of the nonexercisers.[6] Only about one-third of the loss in maximal oxygen

uptake results from aging and two-thirds of the loss comes from inactivity.

Blood pressure, heart rate, and body weight also were remarkably better in the exercising group. Furthermore, aerobic training seems to decrease high blood pressure in the older participants at the same rate as in young, hypertensive people.

Muscle strength declines by 10 percent to 20 percent between the ages of 20 and 50, but between ages 50 and 70 it drops by another 25 percent to 30 percent. Through

GLOSSARY

Functional fitness The physical capacity of the individual to meet ordinary and unexpected demands of daily life safely and effectively.

Functional independence Ability to carry out activities of daily living without assistance from other individuals.

strength training, frail adults in their 80s or 90s can double or triple their strength in just a few months. The amount of muscle hypertrophy achieved, however, decreases with age. Strength gains close to 200 percent have been found in previously inactive adults older than 90. In fact, research has shown that regular strength training improves balance, gait, speed, functional independence, morale, depression symptoms, and energy intake.[7]

Although muscle flexibility drops by about 5 percent per decade of life, 10 minutes of stretching every other day can prevent most of this loss as a person ages. Improved flexibility enhances mobility skills. The latter promotes independence because it helps older adults successfully perform **activities of daily living**.

In terms of body composition, inactive adults continue to gain body fat after age 60 despite the tendency toward lower body weight. Sedentary adults gain more than 30 pounds of body weight between ages 18 and 55. As a result, body fat continues to increase through adult life, with a greater tendency toward visceral fat accumulation (especially in men), leading to further increase in risk for chronic disease. Regular aerobic activity and strength training have been shown to help older adults properly manage body weight and significantly reduce visceral fat.

Older adults who wish to initiate an exercise program are strongly encouraged to have a complete medical evaluation. Recommended activities for older adults include calisthenics, walking, jogging, swimming, cycling, water aerobics, and strength training.

Older people should avoid isometric and very high-intensity strength-training exercises. Activities that require all-out effort or require participants to hold their breath (Valsalva maneuver) tend to lessen blood flow to the heart and cause a significant increase in blood pressure and the load placed on the heart. Older adults should participate in activities that require continuous and rhythmic muscular activity (about 40 percent to 60 percent of functional capacity). These activities do not cause large increases in blood pressure or place an intense overload on the heart.

9.6 *Fitness/Wellness Consumer Issues*

Q: How do I protect myself from quackery and fraud in the fitness/wellness industry?
A: The rapid growth in fitness and wellness programs during the past three decades has spurred **quackery** and **fraud**. The promotion of fraudulent products has deceived consumers into adopting "miraculous," quick, and easy ways toward total well-being.

Today's market is saturated with "special" foods, diets, supplements, pills, cures, equipment, books, and videos that promise quick, dramatic results. Advertisements for these products often are based on testimonials, unproven claims, secret research, half-truths, and quick-fix statements that the uneducated consumer wants to hear. In the meantime, the organization or enterprise making the claims stands to reap a large profit from consumers' willingness to pay for astonishing and spectacular solutions to problems related to their unhealthy lifestyle.

Television, social media, magazine, and newspaper advertisements are not necessarily reliable. For instance, one piece of equipment sold through television and newspaper advertisements promised to "bust the gut" through 5 minutes of daily exercise that appeared to target the abdominal muscle group. This piece of equipment consisted of a metal spring attached to the feet on one end and held in the hands on the other end. According to handling and shipping distributors, the equipment was "selling like hotcakes," and companies could barely keep up with consumers' demands.

Three problems became apparent to the educated consumer. First, there is no such thing as spot-reducing; therefore, the claims could not be true. Second, five minutes of daily exercise burn hardly any calories and, therefore, have no effect on weight loss. Third, the intended abdominal (gut) muscles were not really involved during the exercise. The exercise engaged mostly the gluteal and lower back muscles. This piece of equipment could then be found at garage sales for about a tenth of its original cost!

Although people in the United States tend to be firm believers in the benefits of physical activity and positive lifestyle habits as a means to promote better health, most do not reap these benefits because they simply do not know how to put into practice a sound fitness and wellness program that will give them the results they want. Unfortunately, many uneducated wellness consumers are targets of deception by organizations making fraudulent claims for their products.

Deception is not limited to advertisements. Deceit is found all around us. One can find it in newspaper and magazine articles, trade books, radio, and television shows. To make a profit, popular magazines occasionally exaggerate health claims or leave out pertinent information to avoid offending advertisers. Some publishers print books on diets or self-treatment approaches that have no scientific foundation. Consumers should even be cautious about news reports of the latest medical breakthroughs. Reporters have been known to overlook important information or give certain findings greater credence than they deserve.

Precautions must also be taken when seeking health advice on the Internet. The Internet is full of both credible and dubious information. The following tips can help as you conduct a search on the Internet:

- Look for government, university, non-profit, or well-known medical school websites.
- Look for credentials of the person or organization sponsoring the site.
- Check when the site was last updated. Credible sites are updated often.
- Check the appearance of the information on the site. It should be presented in a professional manner. If every sentence ends with an exclamation point, you have good cause for suspicion.
- Be cautious if the site's sponsor is trying to sell a product. If so, be leery of opinions posted on the site. They could be biased, given that the company's main objective is to sell a product. Credible companies trying to sell a product on the Internet usually reference their sources of health information and provide additional links that support their product.
- Compare the content of a site to other credible sources. The content should compare favorably to that of other reputable sites or publications.
- Note the address and contact information for the company. A reliable company will list more than a post office box, an 800 number, and the company's e-mail address. When only the latter information is provided, consumers may never be able to locate the company for questions, concerns, or refunds.
- Be on the alert for companies that claim to be innovators while criticizing competitors or the government for being close-minded or trying to keep them from doing business.
- Watch for advertisers that use valid medical terminology in an irrelevant context or use vague pseudo-medical jargon to sell their product.
- Look for medical research presented in the information. Give more credence to reliable scientific evidence than opinions and testimonials.

Not all people who promote fraudulent products know they are doing so. Some may be convinced that the product is effective. If you have questions or concerns about a health product, you can search the Federal Trade Commission's website at http://www.consumer.ftc.gov under the topic "Health & Fitness" to get credible information on the latest market claims concerning healthy living, treatment and cures, weight loss, and fitness. As the nation's consumer protection agency, you can also file a complaint with the FTC about scams or dubious health claims at http://www.ftc.gov/complaint or call 1-877-382-4357.

Other consumer protection organizations offer to follow up on complaints about quackery and fraud. The existence of these organizations, however, should not give the consumer a false sense of security. The overwhelming number of complaints made each year to these organizations makes it impossible for them to follow up on each case individually.

The FDA's Center for Drug Evaluation Research, for example, has developed a priority system to determine which health fraud product it should regulate first. Products are rated on how great a risk they pose to the consumer. With this in mind, you can use the following list of organizations to make an educated decision before you spend your money. You can also report consumer fraud to these organizations:

- Better Business Bureau (BBB). The BBB can tell you whether other customers have lodged complaints about a product, a company, or a salesperson. You can find a listing for the local office in the business section of the phone book, or you can check its Web site at http://www.betterbusinessbureau.com/.
- Consumer Product Safety Commission (CPS). This independent federal regulatory agency targets products that threaten the safety of American families. Unsafe products can be researched and reported on its Web site at http://www.cpsc.gov/.
- U.S. Food and Drug Administration (FDA). The FDA regulates safety and labeling of health products and cosmetics. You can search for the office closest to you in the federal government listings (blue pages) of the phone book.
- Your state Attorney General. Attorneys General govern state consumer protection divisions to enforce local laws and investigate claims that protect consumers and businesses from deceptive acts and practices. Find a list of state Attorneys General at http://www.naag.org.
- Your local Consumer Protection Office. Find your local consumer protection office to report frauds and scams, or get help with a consumer complaint at http://www.consumeraction.gov.

GLOSSARY

Activities of daily living Everyday behaviors that people normally do to function in life (cross the street, carry groceries, lift objects, do laundry, and sweep floors).

Quackery/fraud The conscious promotion of unproven claims for profit.

Another way to get informed before you make your purchase is to seek the advice of a reputable professional. Ask someone who understands the product but does not stand to profit from the transaction. As examples, a physical educator or an exercise physiologist can advise you regarding exercise equipment, a registered dietitian can provide information on nutrition and weight control programs, and a physician can offer advice on nutritive supplements. Also, be alert to those who bill themselves as "experts." Look for qualifications, degrees, professional experience, certifications, and reputation.

Keep in mind that if it sounds too good to be true, it probably is. Fraudulent promotions often rely on testimonials or scare tactics and promise that their products will cure a long list of unrelated ailments. They use words such as quick-fix, time-tested, newfound, miraculous, special, secret, all natural, mail-order only, and money-back guarantee. Deceptive companies move often enough that customers have no way of contacting the company to ask for a reimbursement.

When claims are made, ask where the claims are published. Refereed scientific journals are the most reliable sources of information. When a researcher submits information for publication in a refereed journal, at least two qualified and reputable professionals in the field conduct blind reviews of the manuscript. A blind review means that the author does not know who will review the manuscript and the reviewers do not know who submitted the manuscript. Acceptance for publication is based on this input and relevant changes.

Q: What guidelines should I follow when looking for a reputable health/fitness facility?

A: As you follow a lifetime wellness program, you may want to consider joining a health/fitness facility. Or if you have mastered the contents of this book and your choice of fitness activity is one you can pursue on your own (walking, jogging, or cycling), you may not need to join a health club. Barring injuries, you may continue your exercise program outside the walls of a health club for the rest of your life. You also can conduct strength-training and stretching programs in your own home (see Chapter 3, Chapter 4, Appendix A, Appendix B, and Appendix C).

To stay up to date on fitness and wellness developments, you probably should buy a reputable and updated fitness/wellness book every four or five years. You also might subscribe to a credible health, fitness, nutrition, or wellness newsletter to stay current. You can also surf the Web—but be sure that the sites you are searching are from credible and reliable organizations.

If you are contemplating membership in a fitness facility, do all of the following:

- Make sure that the facility complies with the standards established by the American College of Sports Medicine (ACSM) for health and fitness facilities. These standards are given in Figure 9.5.
- Examine all exercise options in your community—health clubs/spas, YMCAs, gyms, colleges, schools, community centers, senior centers, and the like.
- Check to see if the facility's atmosphere is pleasurable and nonthreatening to you. Will you feel comfortable with the instructors and other people who go there? Is it clean and well kept up? If the answer is no, this may not be the right place for you.
- Analyze costs versus facilities, equipment, and programs. Take a look at your personal budget. Will you really use the facility? Will you exercise there regularly? Many people obtain memberships and have monthly membership dues withdrawn automatically from a local bank account, yet seldom attend the fitness center.
- Find out what types of facilities are available: walking/running track, basketball/tennis/racquetball courts, aerobic exercise room, strength-training room, pool, locker rooms, saunas, hot tubs, handicapped access, and so on.
- Check the aerobic and strength-training equipment available. Does the facility have treadmills, bicycle ergometers, elliptical trainers, cross-country skiing simulators, free weights, and strength-training machines? Make sure the facilities and equipment meet your activity interests.

Figure 9.5 American College of Sports Medicine standards for health and fitness facilities.

1. A facility must have an appropriate emergency plan.
2. A facility must offer each adult member a preactivity screening that is relevant to the activities that will be performed by the member.
3. Each person who has supervisory responsibility must be professionally competent.
4. A facility must post appropriate signs in those areas of a facility that present potential increased risk.
5. A facility that offers services or programs to youth must provide appropriate supervision.
6. A facility must conform to all relevant laws, regulations, and published standards.

SOURCE: From *ACSM's Health/Fitness Facility Standards and Guidelines* (Champaign, IL: Human Kinetics, 2006).

- Consider the location. Is the facility close, or do you have to travel several miles to get there? Distance often discourages participation.
- Check on times the facility is accessible. Is it open during your preferred exercise time (for example, early morning or late evening)?
- Work out at the facility several times before becoming a member. Are people standing in line to use the equipment, or is it readily available during your exercise time?
- Inquire about the instructors' knowledge and qualifications. Do the fitness instructors have college degrees or professional training certifications from organizations such as the ACSM, the American Council on Exercise (ACE), the National Strength and Conditioning Association (NSCA), or the National Academy of Sports Medicine (NASM)? These organizations have rigorous standards to ensure professional preparation and quality of instruction.
- Consider the approach to fitness (including all health-related components of fitness). Is it well rounded? Do the instructors spend time with members, or do members have to seek them out constantly for help and instruction?
- Ask about supplementary services. Does the facility provide or contract out for regular health and fitness assessments (cardiovascular endurance, body composition, blood pressure, or blood chemistry analysis)? Are wellness seminars (nutrition, weight control, and stress management) offered? Do these have hidden costs?

Q: What should one look for when selecting a personal trainer?

A: A **personal trainer** is an exercise specialist who works one on one with an individual and is typically paid by the hour or exercise session. A qualified personal trainer can help you start and maintain a safe exercise program, provide motivation and encouragement, design a time-effective exercise program, and provide objective health fitness information. Rates typically range between $20 and $50 an hour, or more for trainers that are highly specialized or in high demand.

Currently, anyone who prescribes exercise can call himself/herself a personal trainer without proof of education, experience, or certification. Although good trainers strive to maximize their own health and fitness, a good physique and previous athletic experience do not certify a person as a personal trainer.

Because of the high demand for personal trainers, more than 200 organizations now provide some type of certification to fitness specialists. This has led to great confusion by clients on how to evaluate the credentials of personal trainers. There is also a clear distinction between "certification" and a "certificate." Certification implies that the individual has met educational and professional standards of performance and competence. A certificate is typically awarded to individuals who attend a conference or workshop but are not required to meet any professional standards.

Presently, no licensing body is in place to oversee personal trainers. Thus, becoming a personal trainer is easy. At a minimum, personal trainers should have an undergraduate degree and certification from a reputable organization such as ACSM, ACE, NSCA, or NASM. Undergraduate (and graduate) degrees should be conferred in a fitness-related area such as exercise science, exercise physiology, kinesiology, sports medicine, or physical education. When looking for a personal trainer, always inquire about the trainer's education and certification credentials.

Before selecting a trainer, you need to establish your program goals. Below are sample questions you need to ask yourself and consider when interviewing potential trainers prior to selecting one.

- Can the potential personal trainer provide you with a resume?
- What type of professional education and certification does the potential trainer possess?
- How long has the person been a personal trainer and are references available upon request?
- Are you looking for a male or female trainer?
- What are the fees? Are multiple sessions cheaper than a single session? Can individuals be trained in groups? Are there cancellation fees if you are not able to attend a given session?
- How long will you need the services of the personal trainer: one session, multiple sessions, periodically, or indefinitely?
- What goals do you intend to achieve with the guidance of the personal trainer: weight loss, cardiorespiratory fitness, strength and/or flexibility fitness, improved health, or sport fitness conditioning?
- What type of personality are you looking for in the trainer—a motivator, a hard-challenging trainer, a gentle trainer, or professional counsel only?

GLOSSARY

Personal trainer An exercise specialist who works one on one with an individual and is typically paid by the hour or exercise session.

As a final word of caution when seeking fitness advice from a health/fitness trainer online: Be aware that certain services cannot be provided over the Internet. An online trainer is not able to directly administer fitness tests, motivate, observe exercise limitations, or respond effectively in an emergency situation (spotting, administering first aid or CPR), and thus is not able to design the most safe and effective exercise program for you.

Q: What factors should I consider before purchasing exercise equipment?

A: The first question you need to ask yourself is: Do I really need this piece of equipment? Most people buy on impulse because of television advertisements or because a salesperson convinced them it is a great piece of equipment that will do wonders for their health and fitness. With some creativity, you can implement an excellent and comprehensive exercise program with little, if any, equipment (see Chapter 3 and Chapter 4).

Many people buy expensive equipment only to find that they really do not enjoy that mode of activity. They do not remain regular users. Stationary bicycles (lower body only) and rowing ergometers were among the most popular pieces of equipment in the 1980s. Most of them now are seldom used and have become "fitness furniture" somewhere in the basement.

Exercise equipment does have its value for people who prefer to exercise indoors, especially during the winter months. It supports some people's motivation and

---

Behavior Modification Planning

Healthy Lifestyle Guidelines

1. Accumulate 30 to 60 minutes of moderate-intensity physical activity on most days of the week and avoid excessive sitting throughout each day.

2. Exercise aerobically in the proper cardiorespiratory training zone at least three times per week for a minimum of 20 minutes.

3. Accumulate at least 10,000 steps on a daily basis.

4. Strength train at least once a week (preferably twice per week) using a minimum of eight exercises that involve all major muscle groups of the body.

5. Perform flexibility exercises that involve all major joints of the body two to three times per week.

6. Eat a healthy diet that is rich in whole-wheat grains, fruits, and vegetables; incudes cold water fish two to three times per week; and is low in saturated and trans fats.

7. Eat a healthy breakfast every day.

8. Do not use tobacco in any form, avoid second-hand smoke, and avoid all other forms of substance abuse.

9. Maintain healthy body weight (achieve a range between the high-physical fitness and health/fitness standards for percent body fat).

10. Get 7 to 8 hours of sleep per night.

11. Practice safe sex every time you have sex and don't have sexual contact with anyone who doesn't practice safe sex.

12. Manage stress effectively.

13. Limit daily alcohol intake to two or less drinks per day if you are a man or one drink or less per day if you are a woman (or do not consume any alcohol at all).

14. Get 10 to 20 minutes of safe sun exposure on most days of the week.

15. Have at least one close friend or relative in whom you can confide and to whom you can express your feelings openly.

16. Be aware of your surroundings and take personal safety measures at all times.

17. Seek continued learning on a regular basis.

18. Subscribe to a reputable health/fitness/nutrition newsletter to stay up-to-date on healthy lifestyle guidelines.

19. Seek proper medical evaluations as necessary.

Try It

Now that you are about to complete this course, evaluate how many of the above healthy lifestyle guidelines have become part of your personal wellness program. Prepare a list of those that you still need to work on and write SMART goals and specific objectives that will help you achieve the desired behaviors. Remember that each one of the above guidelines will lead to a longer, healthier, and happier life.

adherence to exercise. The convenience of having equipment at home also allows for flexible scheduling. You can exercise before or after work or while you watch your favorite television show.

If you are going to purchase equipment, the best recommendation is to actually try it out several times before buying it. Ask yourself several questions: Did you enjoy the workout? Is the unit comfortable? Are you too short, tall, or heavy for it? Is it stable, sturdy, and strong? Do you have to assemble the machine? If so, how difficult is it to put together? How durable is it? Ask for references—people or clubs that have used the equipment extensively. Are they satisfied? Have they enjoyed using the equipment? Talk with professionals at colleges, sports medicine clinics, or health clubs.

Another consideration is to look at used units for signs of wear and tear. Quality is important. Cheaper brands may not be durable, so your investment would be wasted.

Finally, watch out for expensive gadgets. Monitors that provide exercise heart rate, work output, caloric expenditure, speed, grade, and distance may help motivate you, but they are expensive, need repairs, and do not enhance the actual fitness benefits of the workout. Look at maintenance costs and check for service personnel in your community.

Q: What is the greatest benefit of a lifetime wellness lifestyle?

A: There are many benefits derived from an active wellness lifestyle, including greater functional capacity, good health, less sickness, lower health care expenses and time under medical supervision, and a longer, more productive life. Without question, these benefits altogether translate into one great benefit: a higher quality of life, that is, the freedom to live life to its fullest without functional and health limitations. People go through life wishing that they could live without functional limitations. The power, nevertheless, is within each one of us to do so. You can accomplish such a lifestyle by taking action today and living a wellness way of life for the rest of your life.

9.7 *What's Next?*

The objective of this book is to provide you with the basic information necessary to implement your personal healthy lifestyle program. Your activities over the last few weeks or months may have helped you develop positive habits that you should try to carry on throughout life.

Now that you are about to finish this course, the real challenge will be a lifetime commitment to fitness and wellness. Adhering to the program in a structured setting is a lot easier. Fitness and wellness is a continuous process. As you proceed with the program, keep in mind that the greatest benefit is a higher quality of life.

In Activity 9.1 you have a chance to evaluate the fitness and Wellness lifestyle changes that you have implemented in recent weeks/months. Most people who adopt a wellness way of life recognize this new quality after only a few weeks into the program. For some people—especially individuals who have led a poor lifestyle for a long time—establishing positive habits and gaining feelings of well-being might take a few months. In the end, however, everyone who applies the principles of fitness and wellness will reap the desired benefits.

Critical Thinking

What impact has this course had on your personal fitness and healthy lifestyle program? • Have you implemented changes that are improving your quality of life?

Being diligent and taking control of yourself will provide you a better, happier, healthier, and more productive life. Be sure to maintain a program based on your needs and what you enjoy doing most. This will make the journey easier, and you'll have more fun along the way. Once you reach the top, you will know there is no looking back. Improving your longevity and quality of life now is in your hands. It will require persistence and commitment, but only you can take control of your lifestyle and thereby reap the benefits of wellness.

Activity 9.1   Fitness and Wellness Lifestyle Self Evaluation

Name _____   Date _____

Course _____   Section _____

I. Explain the exercise program that you implemented in this course. Express your feelings about the outcomes of this program and how well you accomplished your fitness goals.

_____

_____

_____

_____

_____

_____

_____

_____

_____

II. List nutritional or dietary changes that you were able to implement this term and the effects of these changes on your body composition and personal wellness.

_____

_____

_____

_____

_____

_____

_____

_____

_____

Activity 9.1 **Fitness and Wellness Lifestyle Self Evaluation** *(continued)*

III. List other lifestyle changes that you were able to make this term that may decrease your risk for disease. In a few sentences, explain how you feel about these changes and their impact on your overall well-being.

_____

_____

_____

_____

_____

_____

_____

_____

_____

IV. Please indicate:

Total number of daily steps at the beginning of the course: ☐

Current total number of daily steps: ☐

Total weekly minutes of physical activity at the beginning of the semester: ☐

Current total weekly minutes of physical activity: ☐

V. Briefly evaluate this course and its impact on your quality of life. Indicate what you feel will be needed for you to continue to adhere to an active and healthy lifestyle.

_____

_____

_____

_____

_____

_____

_____

_____

Assess Your Behavior

. . . .

1. Has your level of physical activity increased, compared with the beginning of the term?

2. Do you participate in a regular exercise program that includes cardiorespiratory endurance, muscular strength, and muscular flexibility training?

3. Is your diet healthier now, compared with a few weeks ago?

4. Are you able to take pride in the lifestyle changes that you have implemented over the last several weeks? Have you rewarded yourself for your accomplishments?

Assess Your Knowledge

. . . .

1. A regular aerobic exercise program
   a. makes a person immune to heart disease.
   b. significantly decreases the risk for cardiovascular disease.
   c. decreases HDL-cholesterol.
   d. increases triglycerides.
   e. All are correct choices.

2. Change
   a. is difficult for most people to accomplish.
   b. takes place when core values are addressed.
   c. happens when people are uncomfortable with how they feel.
   d. is most likely to happen when you associate with people who practice healthy habits.
   e. All of the above are correct.

3. The standard treatment for an acute injury is
   a. rest.
   b. cold application.
   c. compression.
   d. elevation.
   e. All choices apply.

4. Which of the following recommendations is false regarding exercise during pregnancy?
   a. Women who are accustomed to strenuous exercise may continue to do so in the early stages of pregnancy.
   b. After the first trimester, women should avoid exercises that require lying on the back.
   c. Exercise above 6,000 feet of altitude is not recommended.
   d. Women are encouraged to exercise above a "somewhat hard" exertion level.
   e. Women may accumulate 30 minutes of moderate-intensity physical activities on most days of the week.

5. From a functional point of view, typical sedentary people in the United States are about how many years older than their chronological age indicates?
   a. 2
   b. 8
   c. 15
   d. 25
   e. 50

6. A person suffering from heatstroke
   a. requires immediate medical attention.
   b. should be placed in a cool, humidity-controlled environment.
   c. should be sprayed with cool water and rubbed with cool towels.
   d. should not be given fluids if unconscious.
   e. All are correct choices.

7. Drinking about a cup of cool water every ___ minutes seems to be ideal to prevent dehydration during exercise in the heat.
   a. 5
   b. 15 to 20
   c. 30
   d. 30 to 45
   e. 60

8. Improvements in maximal oxygen uptake in older adults (compared with younger adults) as a result of cardiorespiratory endurance training are
   a. similar.
   b. higher.
   c. lower.
   d. difficult to determine.
   e. nonexistent.

9. Osteoporosis is
   a. a crippling disease.
   b. more prevalent in women.
   c. higher in people who were calcium-deficient at a young age.
   d. linked to heavy drinking and smoking.
   e. All are correct choices.

10. To protect yourself from consumer fraud when buying a new product,
    a. get as much information as you can from the salesperson.
    b. obtain details about the product from another salesperson.
    c. ask someone who understands the product but does not stand to profit from the transaction.
    d. obtain all the research information from the manufacturer.
    e. All choices are correct.

Correct answers can be found on page 307.

Appendices

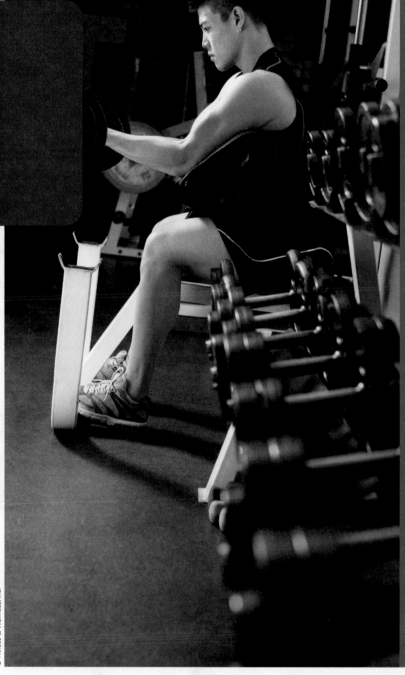

© Fitness & Wellness, Inc.

Strength-Training Exercises Without Weights

EXERCISE 1 Step-Up

ACTION: Step up and down using a box or chair approximately 12 to 15 inches high. Conduct one set using the same leg each time you go up and then conduct a second set using the other leg. You could also alternate legs on each step-up cycle. You may increase the resistance by holding a child or some other object in your arms (hold the child or object close to the body to avoid increased strain in the lower back).

MUSCLES DEVELOPED: Gluteal muscles, quadriceps, gastrocnemius, and soleus

EXERCISE 2 Rowing Torso

ACTION: Raise your arms laterally (abduction) to a horizontal position and bend your elbows to 90°. Have a partner apply enough pressure on your elbows to gradually force your arms forward (horizontal flexion) while you try to resist the pressure. Next, reverse the action, horizontally forcing the arms backward as your partner applies sufficient forward pressure to create resistance.

MUSCLES DEVELOPED: Posterior deltoid, rhombus, and trapezius

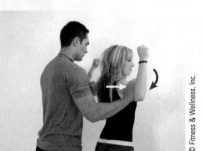

EXERCISE 3 Push-Up

ACTION: Maintaining your body as straight as possible, flex the elbows, lowering the body until you almost touch the floor, then raise yourself back up to the starting position. If you are unable to perform the push-up as indicated, you can decrease the resistance by supporting the lower body with the knees rather than the feet (see illustration c).

MUSCLES DEVELOPED: Triceps, deltoid, pectoralis major, erector spinae, and abdominals

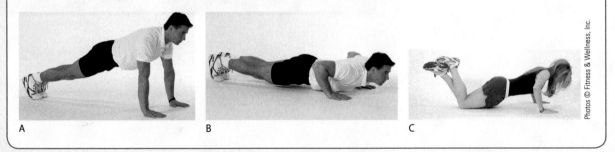

EXERCISE 4
Abdominal Crunch and Bent-Leg Curl-Up

ACTION: Start with your head and shoulders off the floor, arms crossed on your chest, and knees slightly bent (the greater the flexion of the knee, the more difficult the curl-up). Now curl up to about 30° (abdominal crunch—see illustration b) or curl all the way up (bent-leg curl-up), then return to the starting position without letting the head or shoulders touch the floor, or allowing the hips to come off the floor. If you allow the hips to rise off the floor and the head and shoulders to touch the floor, you will most likely "swing up" on the next sit-up, which minimizes the work of the abdominal muscles. If you cannot curl up with the arms on the chest, place the hands by the side of the hips or even help yourself up by holding on to your thighs (illustrations d and e). Do not perform the curl-up exercise with your legs completely extended, as this will cause strain on the lower back.

MUSCLES DEVELOPED: Abdominal muscles (crunch) and hip flexors (complete curl-up)

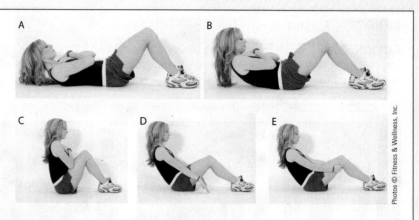

Photos © Fitness & Wellness, Inc.

NOTE: The bent-leg curl-up exercise should be used only by individuals of at least average fitness without a history of lower back problems. New participants and those with a history of lower back problems should use the abdominal crunch exercise in its place.

EXERCISE 5 Leg Curl

ACTION: Lie on the floor facedown. Cross the right ankle over the left heel. Apply resistance with your right foot, while you bring the left foot up to 90° at the knee joint. (Apply enough resistance so that the left foot can only be brought up slowly.) Repeat the exercise, crossing the left ankle over the right heel.

MUSCLES DEVELOPED: Hamstrings (and quadriceps)

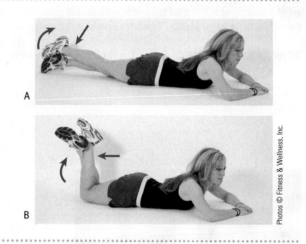

Photos © Fitness & Wellness, Inc.

EXERCISE 6 Modified Dip

ACTION: Place your hands on a box or gymnasium bleacher. The feet are supported and held in place by an exercise partner. Dip down at least a 90° angle at the elbow joint and then return to the starting position.

MUSCLES DEVELOPED: Triceps, deltoid, and pectoralis major

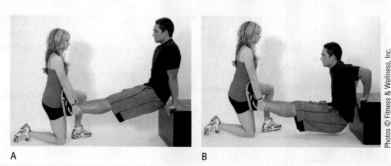

Photos © Fitness & Wellness, Inc.

EXERCISE 7   Pull-Up

ACTION: Suspend yourself from a bar with a pronated grip (thumbs in). Pull your body up until your chin is above the bar, then lower the body slowly to the starting position. If you are unable to perform the pull-up as described, have a partner hold your feet to push off and facilitate the movement upward—see illustrations c and d.

MUSCLES DEVELOPED: Biceps, brachioradialis, brachialis, trapezius, and latissimus dorsi

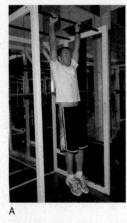
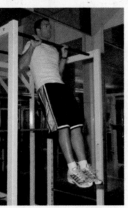
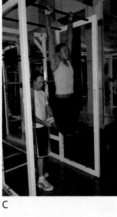
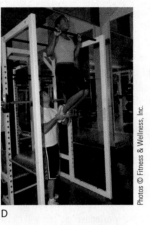

A   B   C   D

Photos © Fitness & Wellness, Inc.

EXERCISE 8   Arm Curl

ACTION: Using a palms-up grip, start with the arm completely extended (a), and with the aid of a sandbag or bucket filled (as needed) with sand or rocks, curl up as far as possible (b), then return to the initial position. Repeat the exercise with the other arm.

MUSCLES DEVELOPED: Biceps, brachioradialis, and brachialis

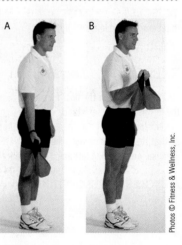

A   B

Photos © Fitness & Wellness, Inc.

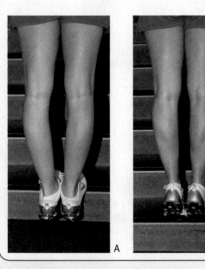

A   B

Photos © Fitness & Wellness, Inc.

EXERCISE 9   Heel Raise

ACTION: From a standing position with feet flat on the floor or at the edge of a step (a), raise and lower your body weight by moving at the ankle joint only (b). For added resistance, have someone else hold your shoulders down as you perform the exercise.

MUSCLES DEVELOPED: Gastrocnemius and soleus

EXERCISE 10 Leg Abduction and Adduction

ACTION: Both participants sit on the floor. The person on the left places the feet on the inside of the other participant's feet. Simultaneously, the person on the left presses the legs laterally (to the outside—abduction), while the one on the right presses the legs medially (adduction). Hold the contraction for 5 to 10 seconds. Repeat the exercise at all three angles, and then reverse the pressing sequence. The person on the left places the feet on the outside and presses inward, while the one on the right presses outward.

MUSCLES DEVELOPED: Hip abductors (rectus femoris, sartorius, gluteus medius and minimus) and adductors (pectineus, gracilis, adductor magnus, adductor longus, and adductor brevis)

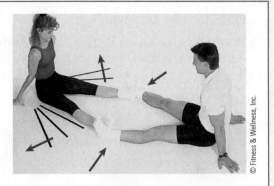

© Fitness & Wellness, Inc.

EXERCISE 11 Reverse Crunch

ACTION: Lie on your back with arms to the sides and knees and hips flexed at 90° (a). Now attempt to raise the pelvis off the floor by lifting vertically from the knees and lower legs (b). This is a challenging exercise that may be difficult for beginners to perform.

MUSCLES DEVELOPED: Abdominals

A   B

Photos © Fitness & Wellness, Inc.

EXERCISE 12 Pelvic Tilt

ACTION: Lie flat on the floor with the knees bent at about a 90° angle (a). Tilt the pelvis by tightening the abdominal muscles, flattening your back against the floor, and raising the lower gluteal area ever so slightly off the floor (b). Hold the final position for several seconds.

AREAS STRETCHED: Low back muscles and ligaments

AREAS STRENGTHENED: Abdominal and gluteal muscles

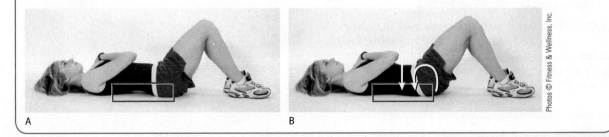

A   B

Photos © Fitness & Wellness, Inc.

EXERCISE 13   Lateral Plank

ACTION: Lie on your side with legs bent (a: easier version) or straight (b: harder version) and support the upper body with your arm. Straighten your body by raising the hip off the floor, and hold the position for several seconds. Repeat the exercise with the other side of the body.

MUSCLES DEVELOPED: Abdominals (obliques and transversus abdominus) and quadratus lumborum (lower back)

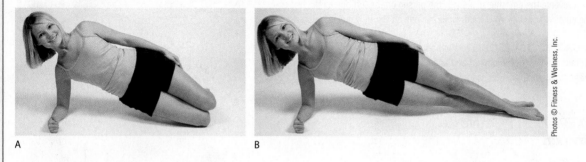

A   B

Photos © Fitness & Wellness, Inc.

EXERCISE 14   Prone Plank

ACTION: Starting in a prone position on a floor mat, balance yourself on the tips of your toes and elbows while attempting to maintain a straight body from heels to toes (do not arch your back—see illustration a). You can increase the difficulty of this exercise by placing your hands in front of you and straightening the arms (see illustration b).

MUSCLES DEVELOPED: Anterior and posterior muscle groups of the trunk and pelvis

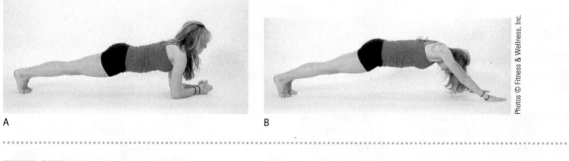

A   B

Photos © Fitness & Wellness, Inc.

EXERCISE 15   Supine Plank

ACTION: Lie face up on the floor with the knees bent at about 120°. Do a pelvic tilt (Exercise 12, page 275) and maintain the pelvic tilt while you raise the hips off the floor until the upper body and upper legs are in a straight line. Hold this position for up to 5 seconds.

AREAS STRENGTHENED: Gluteal and abdominal flexor muscles

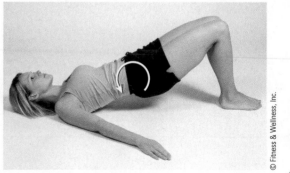

© Fitness & Wellness, Inc.

Strength-Training Exercises With Weights

EXERCISE 16   Arm Curl

ACTION: Using a supinated (palms-up) grip, start with the arms almost completely extended (a). Curl up as far as possible (b), then return to the starting position.

MUSCLES DEVELOPED: Biceps, brachioradialis, and brachialis

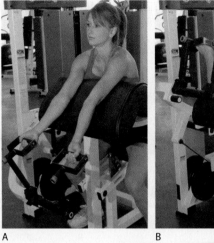
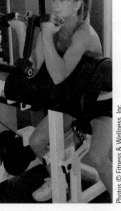

A   B

EXERCISE 17   Bench Press

ACTION: Lie down on the bench with the head by the weight stack and the bench press bar above the chest, and place the feet on the bench (a). Grasp the bar handles and press upward until the arms are completely extended (b), then return to the original position. Do not arch the back during this exercise.

MUSCLES DEVELOPED: Pectoralis major, triceps, and deltoid

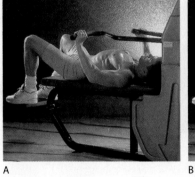
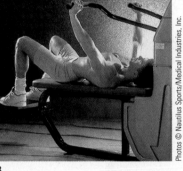

A   B

EXERCISE 18   Abdominal Crunch

ACTION: Sit in an upright position and grasp the handles over your shoulders and crunch forward. Slowly return to the original position.

MUSCLES DEVELOPED: Abdominals

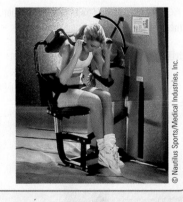

EXERCISE 19 Leg Press

ACTION: From a sitting position with the knees flexed at about 90° and both feet on the footrest (a), extend the legs fully (b), then return slowly to the starting position.

MUSCLES DEVELOPED: Quadriceps and gluteal muscles

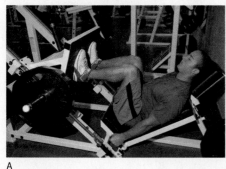 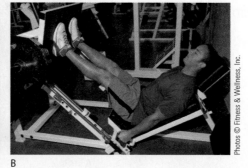

A   B

Photos © Fitness & Wellness, Inc.

EXERCISE 20
Leg Curl

ACTION: Lie with the face down on the bench, legs straight, and place the back of the feet under the padded bar (a). Curl up to at least 90° (b), and return to the original position.

MUSCLES DEVELOPED: Hamstrings

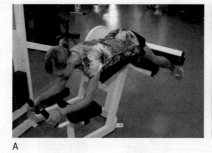

A   B

Photos © Fitness & Wellness, Inc.

EXERCISE 21 Lat Pull-Down

ACTION: Starting from a sitting position, hold the exercise bar with a wide grip (a). Pull the bar down in front of you until it reaches the base of the neck (b), then return to the starting position.

MUSCLES DEVELOPED: Latissimus dorsi, pectoralis major, and biceps

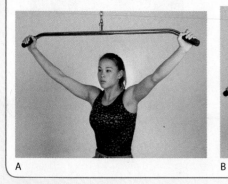 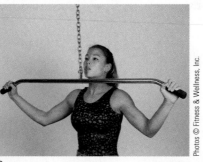

A   B

Photos © Fitness & Wellness, Inc.

EXERCISE 22   Heel Raise

ACTION: Start with your feet either flat on the floor or the front of the feet on an elevated block (a), then raise and lower yourself by moving at the ankle joint only (b). If additional resistance is needed, you can use a squat strength-training machine.

MUSCLES DEVELOPED: Gastrocnemius and soleus

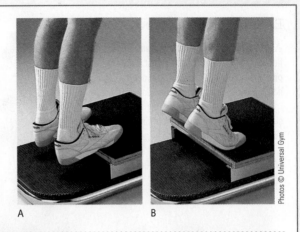

A   B

Photos © Universal Gym

EXERCISE 23   Triceps Extension

ACTION: Using a palms-down grip, grasp the bar slightly closer than shoulder width, and start with the elbows almost completely bent (a). Extend the arms fully (b), then return to starting position.

MUSCLES DEVELOPED: Triceps

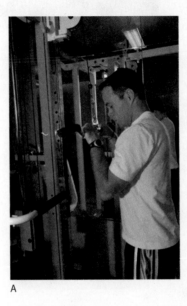
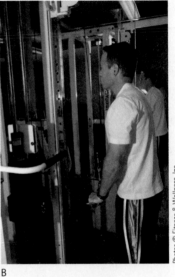

A   B

Photos © Fitness & Wellness, Inc.

EXERCISE 24   Rotary Torso

ACTION: Sit upright into the machine and place the elbows behind the padded bars. Rotate the torso as far as possible to one side and then return slowly to the starting position. Repeat the exercise to the opposite side.

MUSCLES DEVELOPED: Internal and external obliques (abdominal muscles)

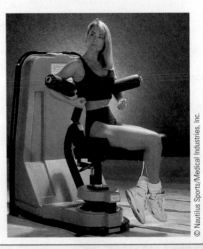

© Nautilus Sports/Medical Industries, Inc.

EXERCISE 25   **Seated Back**

ACTION: Sit in the machine with your trunk flexed and the upper back against the shoulder pad. Place the feet under the padded bar and hold on with your hands to the bars on the sides (a). Start the exercise by pressing backward, simultaneously extending the trunk and hip joints (b). Slowly return to the original position.

MUSCLES DEVELOPED: Erector spinae and gluteus maximus

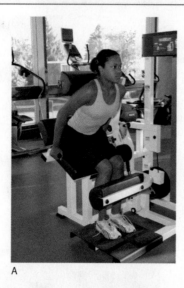
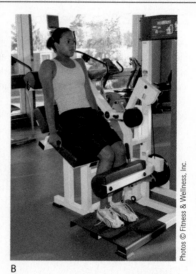

A   B

Photos © Fitness & Wellness, Inc.

EXERCISE 26   **Rowing Torso**

ACTION: Sit in the machine with your arms in front of you, elbows bent and resting against the padded bars (a). Press back as far as possible, drawing the shoulder blades together (b). Return to the original position.

MUSCLES DEVELOPED: Posterior deltoid, rhomboids, and trapezius

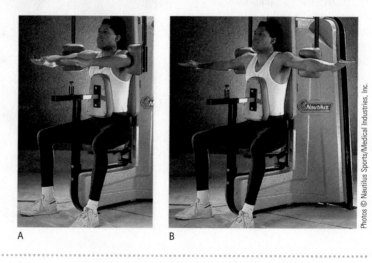

A   B

Photos © Nautilus Sports/Medical Industries, Inc.

EXERCISE 27   **Back Extension**

ACTION: Place your feet under the ankle rollers and the hips over the padded seat. Start with the trunk in a flexed position and the arms crossed over the chest (a). Slowly extend the trunk to a horizontal position (b), hold the extension for 2 to 5 seconds, then slowly flex (lower) the trunk to the original position.

MUSCLES DEVELOPED: Erector spinae, gluteus maximus, and quadratus lumborum (lower back)

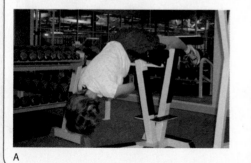
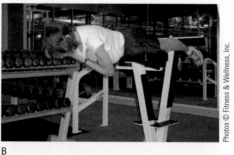

A   B

Photos © Fitness & Wellness, Inc.

EXERCISE 28 Lateral Head Tilt

ACTION: Slowly and gently tilt the head laterally. Repeat several times to each side.

AREAS STRETCHED: Neck flexors and extensors and ligaments of the cervical spine

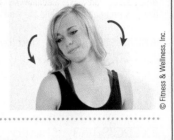

EXERCISE 29 Arm Circles

ACTION: Gently circle your arms all the way around. Conduct the exercise in both directions.

AREAS STRETCHED: Shoulder muscles and ligaments

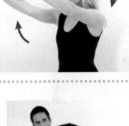

EXERCISE 30 Side Stretch

ACTION: Stand straight up, feet separated to shoulder width, and place your hands on your waist. Now move the upper body to one side and hold the final stretch for a few seconds. Repeat on the other side.

AREAS STRETCHED: Muscles and ligaments in the pelvic region

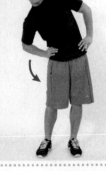

EXERCISE 31 Body Rotation

ACTION: Place your arms slightly away from your body and rotate the trunk as far as possible, holding the final position for several seconds. Conduct the exercise for both the right and left sides of the body. You can also perform this exercise by standing about 2 feet away from the wall (back toward the wall), and then rotating the trunk, placing the hands against the wall.

AREAS STRETCHED: Hip, abdominal, chest, back, neck, and shoulder muscles; hip and spinal ligaments

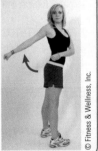

EXERCISE 32   Shoulder Stretch

ACTION: Place your hands on the shoulders of your partner, who will in turn push you down by your shoulders. Hold the final position for a few seconds.

AREAS STRETCHED: Chest (pectoral) muscles and shoulder ligaments

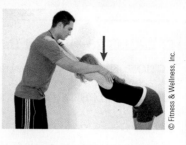

© Fitness & Wellness, Inc.

EXERCISE 33   Shoulder Hyperextension Stretch

ACTION: Have a partner grasp your arms from behind by the wrists and slowly push them upward. Hold the final position for a few seconds.

AREAS STRETCHED: Deltoid and pectoral muscles, and ligaments of the shoulder joint

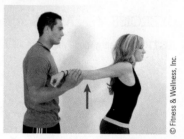

© Fitness & Wellness, Inc.

EXERCISE 34   Shoulder Rotation Stretch

ACTION: With the aid of surgical tubing or an aluminum or wood stick, place the tubing or stick behind your back and grasp the two ends using a reverse (thumbs-out) grip. Slowly bring the tubing or stick over your head, keeping the elbows straight. Repeat several times (bring the hands closer together for additional stretch).

AREAS STRETCHED: Deltoid, latissimus dorsi, and pectoral muscles; shoulder ligaments

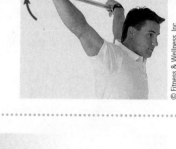

© Fitness & Wellness, Inc.

EXERCISE 35   Quad Stretch

ACTION: Lie on your side and move one foot back by flexing the knee. Grasp the front of the ankle and pull the ankle toward the gluteal region. Hold for several seconds. Repeat with the other leg.

AREAS STRETCHED: Quadriceps muscle, and knee and ankle ligaments

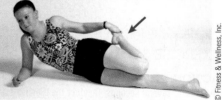

© Fitness & Wellness, Inc.

EXERCISE 36   Heel Cord Stretch

ACTION: Assume a push-up position, then bend one knee and stretch the opposite heel cord. Hold the stretched position for a few seconds. Alternate legs. You may also perform this exercise leaning against a wall or standing at the edge of a step, then stretch the heel downward.

AREAS STRETCHED: Heel cord (Achilles tendon), gastrocnemius, and soleus muscles

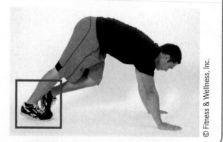

© Fitness & Wellness, Inc.

EXERCISE 37   Adductor Stretch

ACTION: Stand with your feet about twice shoulder width and place your hands slightly above the knee. Flex one knee and slowly go down as far as possible, holding the final position for a few seconds. Repeat with the other leg.

AREAS STRETCHED: Hip adductor muscles

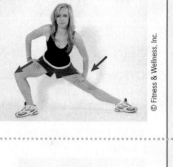

© Fitness & Wellness, Inc.

EXERCISE 38   Sitting Adductor Stretch

ACTION: Sit on the floor and bring your feet in close to you, allowing the soles of the feet to touch each other. Now place your forearms (or elbows) on the inner part of the thigh and push the legs downward, holding the final stretch for several seconds.

AREAS STRETCHED: Hip adductor muscles

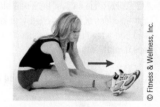

© Fitness & Wellness, Inc.

EXERCISE 39   Sit-And-Reach Stretch

ACTION: Sit on the floor with legs together and gradually reach forward as far as possible. Hold the final position for a few seconds. This exercise may also be performed with the legs separated, reaching to each side as well as to the middle.

AREAS STRETCHED: Hamstrings and lower back muscles, and lumbar spine ligaments

© Fitness & Wellness, Inc.

EXERCISE 40   Triceps Stretch

ACTION: Place the right hand behind your neck. Grasp the right arm above the elbow with the left hand. Gently pull the elbow backward. Repeat the exercise with the opposite arm.

AREAS STRETCHED: Back of upper arm (triceps muscle) and shoulder joint

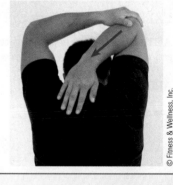

© Fitness & Wellness, Inc.

EXERCISE 41   Single-Knee-to-Chest Stretch

ACTION: Lie down flat on the floor. Bend one leg at approximately 100° and gradually pull the opposite leg toward your chest. Hold the final stretch for a few seconds. Switch legs and repeat the exercise.

AREAS STRETCHED: Lower back and hamstring muscles, and lumbar spine ligaments

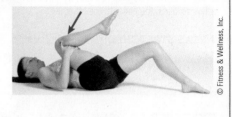

EXERCISE 42   Double-Knee-to-Chest Stretch

ACTION: Lie flat on the floor and then slowly curl up into a fetal position. Hold for a few seconds.

AREAS STRETCHED: Upper and lower back and hamstring muscles; spinal ligaments

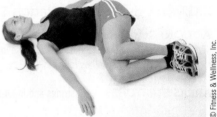
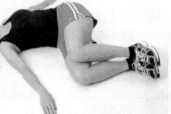

EXERCISE 43   Passive Spinal Twist

ACTION: Lie on your back and place your arms flat on the floor laterally out from the sides of the body. Lift your knees into a 90-degree angle. Keeping your head and torso flat and level, slowly lower both knees comfortably to one side. Repeat on the other side.

AREAS STRETCHED: Hip and lower back

EXERCISE 44   Upper and Lower Back Stretch

ACTION: Sit on the floor and bring your feet in close to you, allowing the soles of the feet to touch each other. Hold on to your feet and gently bring your head and upper chest toward your feet.

AREAS STRETCHED: Upper and lower back muscles and ligaments

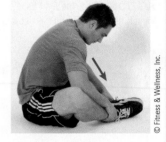

EXERCISE 45   Sit-and-Reach Stretch

See Exercise 39, page 283.

EXERCISE 46   Gluteal Stretch

ACTION: Sit on the floor, bend the right leg, and place your right ankle slightly above the left knee. Grasp the left thigh with both hands and gently pull the leg toward your chest. Repeat the exercise with the opposite leg.

AREAS STRETCHED: Buttock area (gluteal muscles)

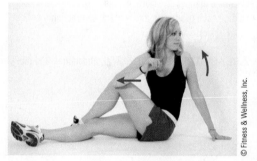

EXERCISE 47   Back Extension

ACTION: Lie facedown on the floor with the elbows by the chest, forearms on the floor, and the hands beneath the chin. Gently raise the trunk by extending the elbows until you reach an approximate 90° angle at the elbow joint. Be sure that the forearms remain in contact with the floor at all times. Hold the stretched position for a few seconds. DO NOT extend the back beyond this point. Hyperextension of the lower back may lead to or aggravate an already existing back problem.

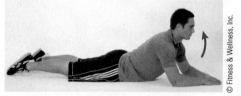

AREA STRETCHED: Abdominal region

ADDITIONAL BENEFIT: Restore lower back curvature

EXERCISE 48   Trunk Rotation and Lower Back Stretch

ACTION: Sit on the floor and bend the left leg, placing the left foot on the outside of the right knee. Place the right elbow on the left knee and push against it. At the same time, try to rotate the trunk to the left (counterclockwise). Hold the final position for a few seconds. Repeat the exercise with the other side.

AREAS STRETCHED: Lateral side of the hip and thigh; trunk and lower back

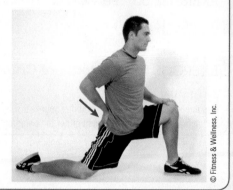

EXERCISE 49   Hip Flexors Stretch

ACTION: Kneel down on an exercise mat or a soft surface, or place a towel under your knees. Raise the left knee off the floor and place the left foot about 3 feet in front of you. Place your left hand over your left knee and the right hand over the back of the right hip. Keeping the lower back flat, slowly move forward and downward as you apply gentle pressure over the right hip. Repeat the exercise with the opposite leg forward.

AREAS STRETCHED: Flexor muscles in front of the hip joint

© Fitness & Wellness, Inc.

EXERCISE 50   Cat Stretch

ACTION: Kneel on the floor and place your hands in front of you (on the floor) about shoulder width apart. Relax your trunk and lower back (a). Now arch the spine and pull in your abdomen as far as you can and hold this position for a few seconds (b). Repeat the exercise four or five times.

AREAS STRETCHED: Low back muscles and ligaments

AREAS STRENGTHENED: Abdominal and gluteal muscles

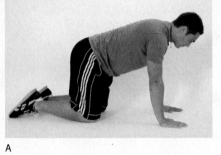
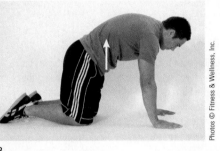

A   B

Photos © Fitness & Wellness, Inc.

EXERCISE 51   Pelvic Clock

ACTION: Lie face up on the floor with the knees bent at about 120°. Fully extend the hips as in the supine plank (Exercise 15, page 276). Now progressively rotate the hips in a clockwise manner (2 o'clock, 4 o'clock, 6 o'clock, 8 o'clock, 10 o'clock, and 12 o'clock), holding each position in an isometric contraction for about 1 second. Repeat the exercise counterclockwise.

AREAS STRETCHED: Gluteal, abdominal, and hip flexor muscles

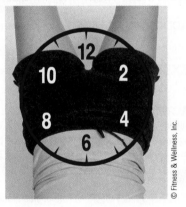

© Fitness & Wellness, Inc.

EXERCISE 52   Pelvic Tilt

See Exercise 12, page 275.

EXERCISE 53   Abdominal Crunch or Bent-Leg Curl-Up

See Exercise 4, page 273.
It is important that you do not stabilize your feet when performing either of these exercises because doing so decreases the work of the abdominal muscles. Also, remember not to "swing up" but, rather, to curl up as you perform these exercises.

Swan Stretch

Excessive strain on the spine; may harm intervertebral disks.

ALTERNATIVE: Flexibility Exercise 47, page 285

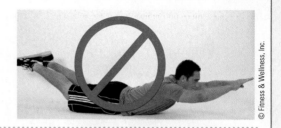

Cradle

Excessive strain on the spine, knees, and shoulders.

ALTERNATIVES: Flexibility Exercises 47, 35, and 33, pages 285 and 282

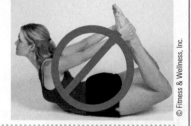

Windmill

Excessive strain on the spine and knees.

ALTERNATIVES: Flexibility Exercises 39 and 48, pages 283 and 285

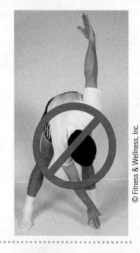

Hurdler Stretch

Excessive strain on the bent knee.

ALTERNATIVES: Flexibility Exercises 35 and 39, pages 282 and 283

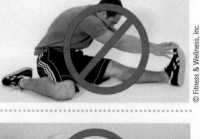

The Hero

Excessive strain on the knees.

ALTERNATIVES: Flexibility Exercises 35 and 49, pages 282 and 285

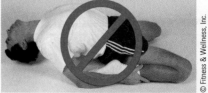

© Fitness & Wellness, Inc.

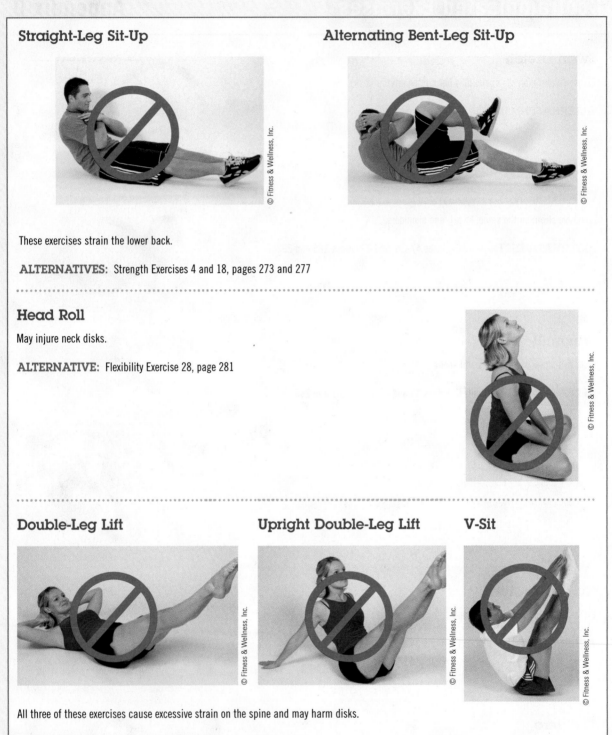

Straight-Leg Sit-Up

Alternating Bent-Leg Sit-Up

© Fitness & Wellness, Inc.

These exercises strain the lower back.

ALTERNATIVES: Strength Exercises 4 and 18, pages 273 and 277

Head Roll

May injure neck disks.

ALTERNATIVE: Flexibility Exercise 28, page 281

© Fitness & Wellness, Inc.

Double-Leg Lift

Upright Double-Leg Lift

V-Sit

© Fitness & Wellness, Inc.

All three of these exercises cause excessive strain on the spine and may harm disks.

ALTERNATIVES: Strength Exercises 4 and 18, pages 273 and 277

Sit-Up With Hands Behind The Head

Excessive strain on the neck.

ALTERNATIVES: Strength Exercises 4 and 18, pages 273 and 277

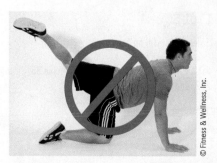

Donkey Kick

Excessive strain on the back, shoulders, and neck.

ALTERNATIVES: Flexibility Exercises 47, 49, and 28, pages 285 and 281

Knees To Chest

Excessive strain on the knees.

ALTERNATIVES: Flexibility Exercises 41 and 42, page 284

STANDING TOE TOUCH

Excessive strain on the knee and lower back.

ALTERNATIVE: Flexibility Exercise 39, page 283

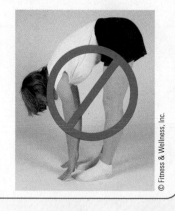

Yoga Plow

Excessive strain on the spine, neck, and shoulders.

ALTERNATIVES: Flexibility Exercises 39, 41, 42, 44, and 46, pages 283, 284, and 285

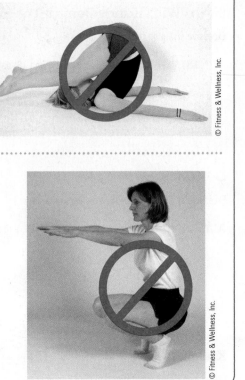

© Fitness & Wellness, Inc.

Full Squat

Excessive strain on the knees.

ALTERNATIVES: Flexibility Exercise 35, Strength Exercises 1 and 19, pages 282, 272, and 278

© Fitness & Wellness, Inc.

Food Description	Qty	Measure	Energy (cal)	Protein (g)	Carb (g)	Dietary Fiber (g)	Fat(g)	SatFat(g)	TransFat (g)	Cholesterol (mg)
Almonds, dry roasted, no salt added	¼	cup(s)	206	8	7	4	18	1.40	—	0
Apples, raw medium, w/peel	1	item(s)	72	<1	19	3	<1	0.04	—	0
Applesauce, sweetened, canned	½	cup(s)	97	<1	25	2	<1	0.04	—	0
Apricot, fresh w/o pits	4	item(s)	67	2	16	3	1	0.04	—	0
Apricot, halves w/skin, canned in heavy syrup	½	cup(s)	107	1	28	2	<1	0.01	—	0
Asparagus, boiled, drained	½	cup(s)	20	2	4	2	0.19	0.06	—	0
Avocado, California, whole, w/o skin or pit	1	item(s)	284	3	15	12	26	3.59	—	0
Bacon, cured, broiled, pan fried, or roasted	2	slice(s)	68	5	<1	0	5	1.73	0	14
Bagel chips, plain	3	item(s)	130	3	19	1	5	0.50	—	0
Bagel, plain, enriched, toasted	1	item(s)	195	7	38	2	1	0.16	0	0
Banana, fresh whole, w/o peel	1	item(s)	105	1	27	3	<1	0.13	—	0
Beans, black, boiled	½	cup(s)	114	8	20	7	<1	0.12	—	0
Beans, Fordhook lima, frozen, boiled, drained	½	cup(s)	88	5	16	5	<1	0.07	—	0
Beans, mung, sprouted, boiled, drained	½	cup(s)	13	1	3	<1	<1	0.02	—	0
Beans, red kidney, canned	½	cup(s)	109	7	20	8	<1	0.06	—	0
Beans, refried, canned	½	cup(s)	119	7	20	7	2	0.60	—	10
Beans, yellow snap, string or wax, boiled, drained	½	cup(s)	22	1	5	2	<1	0.04	—	0
Beef, chuck, arm pot roast, lean & fat, ¼" fat, braised	3	ounce(s)	282	23	0	0	20	7.97	—	84
Beef, corned, canned	3	ounce(s)	213	23	0	0	13	5.25	—	73
Beef, ground, lean, broiled, well	3	ounce(s)	238	24	0	0	15	5.89	—	86
Beef, ground, regular, broiled, medium	3	ounce(s)	246	20	0	0	18	6.91	—	77
Beef, liver, pan fried	3	ounce(s)	149	23	4	0	4	1.27	0.17	324
Beef, rib steak, small end, lean, ¼" fat, broiled	3	ounce(s)	188	24	0	0	10	3.84	—	68
Beef, rib, whole, lean and fat, ¼" fat, roasted	3	ounce(s)	320	19	0	0	27	10.71	—	72
Beef, short loin, T-bone steak, lean, ¼" fat, broiled	3	ounce(s)	174	23	0	0	9	3.05	—	50
Beer	12	fluid ounce(s)	118	1	6	<1	<1	0.00	—	0
Beer, light	12	fluid ounce(s)	99	1	5	0	0	0.00	0	0
Beets, sliced, canned, drained	½	cup(s)	26	1	6	1	<1	0.02	—	0
Biscuits	1	item(s)	121	3	16	1	5	1.40	0	<1
Blueberries, raw	½	cup(s)	41	1	10	2	<1	0.02	—	0
Bologna, beef	1	slice(s)	90	3	1	0	8	3.50	—	20
Bologna, turkey	1	slice(s)	50	3	1	0	4	1.00	—	20
Brazil nuts, unblanched, dried	¼	cup(s)	230	5	4	3	23	5.30	—	0
Bread, cracked wheat	1	slice(s)	65	2	12	1	1	0.23	—	0
Bread, French	1	slice(s)	69	2	13	1	1	0.16	—	0
Bread, mixed grain	1	slice(s)	65	3	12	2	1	0.21	—	0
Bread, pita	1	item(s)	165	5	33	1	1	0.10	—	0
Bread, pumpernickel	1	slice(s)	80	3	15	2	1	0.14	—	0
Bread, rye	1	slice(s)	83	3	15	2	1	0.20	—	0
Bread, white	1	slice(s)	67	2	13	1	1	0.18	—	0
Bread, whole wheat	1	slice(s)	128	4	24	3	2	0.37	—	0
Broccoli, chopped, boiled, drained	½	cup(s)	27	2	6	3	<1	0.06	—	0
Brownie, prepared from mix	1	item(s)	112	1	12	1	7	1.76	—	18
Brussels sprouts, boiled, drained	½	cup(s)	28	2	6	2	<1	0.08	—	0
Bulgur, cooked	½	cup(s)	76	3	17	4	<1	0.04	—	0
Buns, hamburger, plain	1	item(s)	120	4	21	1	2	0.47	—	0
Butter	1	tablespoon(s)	108	<1	<1	0	12	6.13	—	32
Buttermilk, low fat	1	cup(s)	98	8	12	0	2	1.34	—	10
Cabbage, boiled, drained, no salt added	1	cup(s)	33	2	7	3	1	0.08	—	0
Cabbage, raw, shredded	1	cup(s)	17	1	4	2	<1	0.01	—	0
Cake, angel food, from mix	1	slice(s)	129	3	29	<1	<1	0.02	—	0
Cake, butter pound, ready to eat, commercially prepared	1	slice(s)	291	4	37	<1	15	8.67	—	166
Cake, carrot, cream cheese frosting, from mix	1	slice(s)	484	5	52	1	29	5.43	—	60
Cake, chocolate, chocolate icing, commercially prepared	1	slice(s)	235	3	35	2	10	3.05	—	27
Cake, devil's food cupcake, chocolate frosting	1	item(s)	120	2	20	1	4	1.80	—	19

Food Description	Qty	Measure	Energy (cal)	Protein (g)	Carb (g)	Dietary Fiber (g)	Fat(g)	SatFat(g)	TransFat (g)	Cholesterol (mg)
Cake, white, coconut frosting, from mix	1	slice(s)	399	5	71	1	12	4.36	—	1
Candy, Almond Joy bar	1	item(s)	240	2	29	2	13	9.00	0	3
Candy, Life Savers	1	item(s)	8	0	2	0	<1	0.00	0	0
Candy, M&M's peanut chocolate candy, small bag	1	item(s)	250	5	30	2	13	5.00	—	5
Candy, M&M's plain chocolate candy, small bag	1	item(s)	240	2	34	1	10	6.00	—	5
Candy, milk chocolate bar	1	item(s)	483	8	53	2	28	16.69	—	22
Candy, Milky Way bar	1	item(s)	270	2	41	1	10	5.00	—	5
Candy, Reese's peanut butter cups	2	piece(s)	250	5	25	1	14	5.00	0	3
Candy, Special Dark chocolate bar	1	item(s)	220	2	24	3	13	8.00	0	3
Candy, Starburst fruit chews, original fruits	1	package	240	0	48	0	5	1.00	—	0
Candy, York peppermint patty	1	item(s)	170	1	34	1	3	2.00	0	0
Cantaloupe	½	cup(s)	27	1	7	1	<1	0.04	—	0
Carrots, raw	½	cup(s)	25	1	6	2	<1	0.02	0	0
Carrots, sliced, boiled, drained	½	cup(s)	27.29	0.59	6.41	2.33	0.14	0.02	—	0
Cashews, dry roasted	¼	cup(s)	197	5	11	1	16	3.14	—	0
Catsup/ketchup	1	tablespoon(s)	14	<1	4	<1	<1	0.01	—	0
Cauliflower, boiled, drained	½	cup(s)	14	1	3	2	<1	0.04	—	0
Celery, stalk	2	item(s)	11	1	2	1	<1	0.03	—	0
Cereal, All-Bran	1	cup(s)	160	8	46	20	2	0.00	0	0
Cereal, All-Bran Buds	1	cup(s)	212	6	73	42	3	—	0	0
Cereal, Bran Flakes, Post	1	cup(s)	133	4	32	7	1	0.00	—	0
Cereal, Cap'n Crunch	1	cup(s)	144	2	30	1	2	0.53	—	0
Cereal, Cheerios	1	cup(s)	110	3	22	3	2	0.00	—	0
Cereal, Complete wheat bran flakes	1	cup(s)	120	4	31	7	1	—	0	0
Cereal, Corn Flakes	1	cup(s)	100	2	24	1	0	0.00	0	0
Cereal, Corn Pops	1	cup(s)	120	1	28	0	0	0.00	0	0
Cereal, Cracklin' Oat Bran	1	cup(s)	266	5	47	7	9	2.70	0	0
Cereal, Cream of Wheat, instant, prepared	½	cup(s)	61	2	13	<1	<1	0.01	0	0
Cereal, Frosted Flakes	1	cup(s)	160	1	37	1	0	0.00	0	0
Cereal, Frosted Mini-Wheats	5	item(s)	180	5	41	5	1	0.00	0	0
Cereal, granola, prepared	½	cup(s)	299	9	32	5	15	2.76	—	0
Cereal, Kashi puffed	1	cup(s)	70	3	13	2	1	0.00	—	0
Cereal, Life	1	cup(s)	160	4	33	3	2	0.35	—	0
Cereal, Multi-Bran Chex	1	cup(s)	200	4	49	7	2	0.00	0	0
Cereal, Nutri-Grain golden wheat	1	cup(s)	133	4	31	5	1	0.00	—	0
Cereal, oatmeal, cooked w/water	½	cup(s)	74	3	13	2	1	0.19	—	0
Cereal, Product 19	1	cup(s)	100	2	25	1	0	0.00	0	0
Cereal, Raisin Bran	1	cup(s)	190	4	47	8	1	0.00	—	0
Cereal, Rice Chex	1	cup(s)	96	2	22	<1	0	0.00	0	0
Cereal, Rice Krispies	1	cup(s)	96	2	23	0	0	0.00	0	0
Cereal, Shredded Wheat	1	cup(s)	88	3	20	3	1	0.04	—	0
Cereal, Smacks	1	cup(s)	133	3	32	1	1	0.00	—	0
Cereal, Special K	1	cup(s)	110	7	22	1	0	0.00	0	0
Cereal, Total whole grain	1	cup(s)	146	3	31	4	1	0.00	—	0
Cereal, Wheaties	1	cup(s)	110	3	24	3	1	0.00	—	0
Cheese, American, processed	1	ounce(s)	106	6	<1	0	9	5.58	—	27
Cheese, blue, crumbled	1	ounce(s)	100	6	1	0	8	5.29	—	21
Cheese, cheddar, shredded	¼	cup(s)	114	7	<1	0	9	5.96	—	30
Cheese, feta	1	ounce(s)	74	4	1	0	6	4.18	—	25
Cheese, Monterey jack	1	ounce(s)	104	7	<1	0	8	5.34	—	25
Cheese, mozzarella, part skim milk	1	ounce(s)	71	7	1	0	4	2.83	—	18
Cheese, Parmesan, grated	1	tablespoon(s)	22	2	<1	0	1	0.87	—	4
Cheese, ricotta, part skim milk	¼	cup(s)	85	7	3	0	5	3.03	—	19
Cheese, Swiss	1	ounce(s)	106	8	2	0	8	4.98	—	26
Cherries, sweet, raw	½	cup(s)	46	1	12	2	<1	0.03	—	0
Chicken, broiler breast, meat & skin, flour coated, fried	3	ounce(s)	189	27	1	<0.1	8	2.08	—	76
Chicken, broiler drumstick, meat & skin, flour coated, fried	3	ounce(s)	208	23	1	<0.1	12	3.11	—	77
Chicken, light meat, roasted	3	ounce(s)	130	23	0	0	3	0.92	—	64
Chicken, roasted (meat only)	3	ounce(s)	142	21	0	0	6	1.54	—	64
Chickpeas or bengal gram, garbanzo beans, boiled	½	cup(s)	134	7	22	6	2	0.22	—	0
Chocolate milk, low fat	1	cup(s)	158	8	26	1	3	1.54	—	8
Cilantro	1	teaspoon(s)	<1	<0.1	<0.1	<0.1	<0.1	0.00	—	0

Food Description	Qty	Measure	Energy (cal)	Protein (g)	Carb (g)	Dietary Fiber (g)	Fat(g)	SatFat(g)	TransFat (g)	Cholesterol (mg)
Cocoa, hot, prepared w/milk	1	cup(s)	193	9	27	3	6	3.58	0.18	20
Coconut, dried, not sweetened	¼	cup(s)	393	4	14	10	38	34.06	—	0
Cod, Atlantic cod or scrod, baked or broiled	3	ounce(s)	46	10	0	0	<1	0.07	—	24
Coffee, brewed	8	fluid ounce(s)	9	<1	0	0	0	0.00	0	0
Collard greens, boiled, drained	½	cup(s)	25	2	5	3	<1	0.04	—	0
Cookies, animal crackers	12	piece(s)	134	2	22	<1	4	1.03	—	0
Cookies, chocolate chip	1	item(s)	140	2	16	1	8	2.09	0	13
Cookies, chocolate sandwich, extra crème filling	1	item(s)	65	<1	9	<1	3	0.50	1.10	0
Cookies, Fig Newtons	1	item(s)	55	1	10	1	1	0.50	0.50	0
Cookies, oatmeal	1	item(s)	234	6	45	3	4	0.70	0	<.1
Cookies, peanut butter	1	item(s)	163	4	17	1	9	1.65	0	13
Cookies, sugar	1	item(s)	61	1	7	<1	3	0.63	0	18
Corn, yellow sweet, frozen, boiled, drained	½	cup(s)	66	2	16	2	1	0.08	—	0
Cornbread	1	piece(s)	141	5	18	1	5	2.09	0	21
Cornmeal, yellow whole grain	½	cup(s)	221	5	47	4	2	0.31	—	0
Cottage cheese, low fat, 1% fat	½	cup(s)	81	14	3	0	1	0.73	—	5
Cottage cheese, low fat, 2% fat	½	cup(s)	102	16	4	0	2	1.38	—	9
Crab, blue, canned	2	ounce(s)	56	12	0	0	1	0.14	—	50
Crackers, cheese (mini)	30	item(s)	151	3	17	1	8	2.81	—	4
Crackers, honey graham	4	item(s)	118	2	22	1	3	0.43	—	0
Crackers, matzo, plain	1	item(s)	112	3	24	1	<1	0.06	—	0
Crackers, Ritz	5	item(s)	80	1	10	1	4	0.50	—	0
Crackers, rye crispbread	1	item(s)	37	1	8	2	<1	0.01	—	0
Crackers, saltine	5	item(s)	65	1	11	<1	2	0.44	0.54	0
Crackers, wheat	10	item(s)	142	3	19	1	6	1.55	—	0
Cranberry juice cocktail	½	cup(s)	72	0	18	<1	<1	0.01	—	0
Cream cheese	2	tablespoon(s)	101	2	1	0	10	6.37	—	32
Cream, heavy whipping, liquid	1	tablespoon(s)	52	<1	<1	0	6	3.45	—	21
Cream, light whipping, liquid	1	tablespoon(s)	44	,1	,1	0	5	2.90	—	17
Croissant, butter	1	item(s)	231	5	26	1	12	6.59	—	38
Cucumber	¼	item(s)	11	<1	3	<1	<.1	0.03	—	0
Danish pastry, nut	1	item(s)	280	5	30	1	16	3.78	—	30
Dates, domestic, whole	¼	cup(s)	126	1	33	4	<1	0.01	—	0
Distilled alcohol, 90 proof	1	fluid ounce(s)	73	0	0	0	0	0.00	0	0
Doughnut, cake	1	item(s)	198	2	23	1	11	1.70	—	17
Doughnut, glazed	1	item(s)	242	4	27	1	14	3.49	—	4
Egg substitute, Egg Beaters	¼	cup(s)	30	6	1	0	0	0.00	0	0
Eggs, fried	1	item(s)	92	6	<1	0	7	1.98	—	210
Eggs, hard boiled	1	item(s)	78	6	1	0	5	1.63	—	212
Eggs, poached	1	item(s)	74	6	<1	0	5	1.54	—	211
Eggs, raw, white	1	item(s)	17	4	<1	0	<0.1	0.00	—	0
Eggs, raw, whole	1	item(s)	74	6	<1	0	5	1.55	—	212
Eggs, raw, yolk	1	item(s)	53	3	1	0	4	1.59	—	205
Eggs, scrambled, prepared w/milk & butter	2	item(s)	203	14	3	0	15	4.49	—	429
Figs, raw, medium	2	item(s)	74	1	19	3	<1	0.06	—	0
Fish fillets, batter coated or breaded, fried	3	ounce(s)	197.19	12.46	14.42	0.42	10.44	2.39	—	28.89
Flounder, baked	3	ounce(s)	114	15	<1	<0.1	6	1.15	0	44
Flour, all purpose, white, bleached, enriched	½	cup(s)	228	6	48	2	1	0.10	—	0
Flour, whole wheat	½	cup(s)	203	8	44	7	1	0.19	—	0
Frankfurter, beef & pork	1	item(s)	174	7	1	1	16	6.14	—	29
Frankfurter, beef	1	item(s)	149	5	2	0	13	5.26	—	24
Frankfurter, turkey	1	item(s)	102	6	1	0	8	2.65	—	48
Frozen yogurt, chocolate, soft serve	½	cup(s)	115	3	18	2	4	2.61	—	4
Frozen yogurt, vanilla, soft serve	½	cup(s)	117	3	17	0	4	2.46	—	1
Fruit cocktail, canned in heavy syrup	½	cup(s)	91	<1	23	1	<0.1	0.01	—	0
Fruit cocktail, canned in juice	½	cup(s)	55	1	14	1	<0.1	0.00	—	0
Granola bar, plain, hard	1	item(s)	115	2	16	1	5	0.58	—	0
Grape juice, sweetened, added vitamin C, from frozen concentrate	½	cup(s)	64	<1	16	<1	<1	0.04	—	0
Grapefruit juice, pink, sweetened, canned	½	cup(s)	58	1	14	<1	<1	0.02	—	0
Grapefruit juice, white	½	cup(s)	48	1	11	<1	<1	0.02	—	0
Grapefruit, raw, pink or red	½	cup(s)	48	1	12	2	<1	0.02	—	0
Grapes, European, red or green, adherent skin	½	cup(s)	55	1	14	1	<1	0.04	—	0
Haddock, baked or broiled	3	ounce(s)	50	11	0	0	<1	0.07	—	33

Food Description	Qty	Measure	Energy (cal)	Protein (g)	Carb (g)	Dietary Fiber (g)	Fat(g)	SatFat(g)	TransFat (g)	Cholesterol (mg)
Halibut, Atlantic & Pacific, cooked, dry heat	3	ounce(s)	119	23	0	0	2	0.35	—	35
Ham, cured, boneless, 11% fat, roasted	3	ounce(s)	151	19	0	0	8	2.65	—	50
Ham, deli sliced, cooked	1	slice(s)	30	5	1	0	1	0.50	—	15
Honey	1	tablespoon(s)	64	<0.1	17	<0.1	0	0.00	0	0
Honeydew melon	½	cup(s)	32	<1	8	1	<1	0.03	—	0
Ice cream, chocolate	½	cup(s)	143	3	19	1	7	4.49	—	22
Ice cream, chocolate, soft serve	½	cup(s)	177	3	24	1	8	5.17	—	22
Ice cream, light vanilla	½	cup(s)	109	4	18	<1	3	1.71	—	17
Jams, jellies, preserves, all flavors	1	tablespoon(s)	56	<0.1	14	<1	<0.1	0.00	—	0
Jams, jellies, preserves, all flavors, low sugar	1	tablespoon(s)	25	<0.1	6	<1	<0.1	0.00	—	0
Kale, frozen, chopped, boiled, drained	½	cup(s)	20	2	3	1	<1	0.04	—	0
Kiwifruit	1	item(s)	53	1	11	3	1	0.02	—	0
Lamb, chop, loin, domestic, lean & fat, ¼" fat, broiled	3	ounce(s)	269	21	0	0	20	8.36	—	85
Lamb, leg, domestic, lean & fat, ¼" fat, cooked	3	ounce(s)	250	21	0	0	18	7.51	—	82
Lemon juice	1	tablespoon(s)	4	<0.1	1	<0.1	0	0.00	—	0
Lemonade, from frozen concentrate	8	fluid ounce(s)	131	<1	34	<1	<1	0.02	—	0
Lentils, boiled	½	cup(s)	115	9	20	8	<1	0.05	—	0
Lentils, sprouted	1	cup(s)	82	7	17	0	<1	0.04	—	0
Lettuce, butterhead, Boston, or bibb	1	cup(s)	7	1	1	1	<1	0.02	—	0
Lettuce, romaine, shredded	1	cup(s)	10	1	2	1	<1	0.02	—	0
Lobster, northern, cooked, moist heat	3	ounce(s)	83	17	1	0	1	0.09	—	61
Macadamias, dry roasted, no salt added	¼	cup(s)	241	3	4	3	25	4.00	—	0
Mayonnaise w/soybean oil	1	tablespoon(s)	99	<1	1	0	11	1.64	0.04	5
Mayonnaise, low calorie	1	tablespoon(s)	37	<0.1	3	0	3	0.53	—	4
Milk, fat free, nonfat, or skim	1	cup(s)	83	8	12	0	<1	0.29	—	5
Milk, fat free, nonfat, or skim, w/nonfat milk solids	1	cup(s)	91	9	12	0	1	0.40	—	5
Milk, low fat, 1%	1	cup(s)	102	8	12	0	2	1.54	—	12
Milk, low fat, 1%, w/nonfat milk solids	1	cup(s)	105	9	12	0	2	1.48	—	10
Milk, reduced fat, 2%	1	cup(s)	122	8	11	0	5	2.35	—	20
Milk, reduced fat, 2%, w/nonfat milk solids	1	cup(s)	125	9	12	0	5	2.93	—	20
Milk, whole, 3.3%	1	cup(s)	146	8	11	0	8	4.55	—	24
Milk, whole, evaporated, canned	2	tablespoon(s)	42	2	3	0	2	1.45	—	9
Milkshakes, chocolate	1	cup(s)	270	7	48	1	6	3.81	—	25
Muffin, English, plain, enriched	1	item(s)	134	4	26	2	1	0.15	—	0
Muffin, English, wheat	1	item(s)	127	5	26	3	1	0.16	—	0
Muffins, blueberry	1	item(s)	160	3	23	1	6	0.87	0	20
Mushrooms, raw	½	cup(s)	8	1	1	<1	<1	0.02	—	0
Mustard greens, frozen, boiled, drained	½	cup(s)	14	2	2	2	<1	0.01	—	0
Oil, canola	1	tablespoon(s)	120	0	0	0	14	0.97	—	0
Oil, corn	1	Tablespoon(s)	120	0	0	0	14	1.73	0.04	0
Oil, olive	1	tablespoon(s)	119	0	0	0	14	1.82	—	0
Oil, peanut	1	tablespoon(s)	119	0	0	0	14	2.28	—	0
Oil, safflower	1	tablespoon(s)	120	0	0	0	14	0.84	—	0
Oil, soybean w/cottonseed oil	1	tablespoon(s)	120	0	0	0	14	2.45	—	0
Okra, sliced, boiled, drained	½	cup(s)	18	1	4	2	<1	0.04	—	0
Onions, chopped, boiled, drained	½	cup(s)	47	1	11	1	<1	0.03	—	0
Orange juice, unsweetened, from frozen concentrate	½	cup(s)	56	1	13	<1	<0.1	0.01	—	0
Orange, raw	1	item(s)	62	1	15	3	<1	0.02	—	0
Oysters, eastern, farmed, raw	3	ounce(s)	50	4	5	0	1	0.38	—	21
Oysters, eastern, wild, cooked, moist heat	3	ounce(s)	116	12	7	0	4	1.31	—	89
Pancakes, blueberry, from recipe	3	item(s)	253	7	33	1	10	2.26	—	64
Pancakes, from mix w/egg & milk	3	item(s)	249	9	33	2	9	2.33	—	81
Papaya, raw	½	cup(s)	27	<1	7	1	<0.1	0.03	—	0
Pasta, egg noodles, enriched, cooked	½	cup(s)	106	4	20	1	1	0.25	0.02	26
Pasta, macaroni, enriched, cooked	½	cup(s)	99	3	20	1	<1	0.07	—	0
Pasta, spaghetti, al dente, cooked	½	cup(s)	95	4	20	1	1	0.05	—	0
Pasta, spaghetti, whole wheat, cooked	½	cup(s)	87	4	19	3	<1	0.07	—	0
Pasta, tricolor vegetable macaroni, enriched, cooked	½	cup(s)	86	3	18	3	<0.1	0.01	—	0
Peach, halves, canned in heavy syrup	½	cup(s)	97	1	26	2	<1	0.01	—	0
Peach, halves, canned in water	½	cup(s)	29	1	7	2	<0.1	0.01	—	0

Food Description	Qty	Measure	Energy (cal)	Protein (g)	Carb (g)	Dietary Fiber (g)	Fat(g)	SatFat(g)	TransFat (g)	Cholesterol (mg)
Peach, raw, medium	1	item(s)	38	1	9	1	<1	0.02	—	0
Peanut butter, smooth	1	Tablespoon(s)	96	4	3	1	8	1.60	—	0
Peanuts, oil roasted, salted	¼	cup(s)	216	10	5	3	19	3.12	—	0
Pear, halves, canned in heavy syrup	½	cup(s)	98	<1	25	2	<1	0.01	—	0
Pear, raw	1	item(s)	96	1	26	5	<1	0.01	—	0
Peas, green, canned, drained	½	cup(s)	59	4	11	3	<1	0.05	—	0
Peas, green, frozen, boiled, drained	½	cup(s)	62	4	11	4	<1	0.04	—	0
Pecans, dry roasted, no salt added	¼	cup(s)	403	5	8	5	42	3.56	—	0
Pepperoni, beef & pork	1	slice(s)	55	2	<1	0	5	1.77	—	9
Peppers, green bell or sweet, raw	½	cup(s)	15	1	3	1	<1	0.04	—	0
Pickle relish, sweet	1	tablespoon(s)	20	<0.1	5	<1	<0.1	0.01	—	0
Pickle, dill	1	ounce(s)	5	<1	1	<1	<0.1	0.01	—	0
Pie crust, frozen, ready to bake, enriched, baked	1	slice(s)	82	1	8	<1	5	1.69	—	0
Pie crust, prepared w/water, baked	1	slice(s)	100	1	10	<1	6	1.54	—	0
Pie, apple, from home recipe	1	slice(s)	411	4	58	2	19	4.73	—	0
Pie, pecan, from home recipe	1	slice(s)	503	6	64	0	27	4.87	—	106
Pie, pumpkin, from home recipe	1	slice(s)	316	7	41	0	14	4.92	—	65
Pineapple, canned in extra heavy syrup	½	cup(s)	108	<1	28	1	<1	0.01	—	0
Pineapple, canned in juice	½	cup(s)	75	1	20	1	<0.1	0.01	—	0
Pineapple, raw, diced	½	cup(s)	37	<1	10	1	<0.1	0.01	—	0
Pinto beans, boiled, drained, no salt added	½	cup(s)	25	2	5	0	<1	0.04	—	0
Pomegranate	1	item(s)	105	1	26	1	<1	0.06	—	0
Popcorn, air popped	1	cup(s)	31	1	6	1	<1	0.05	—	0
Popcorn, popped in oil	1	cup(s)	165	3	19	3	9	1.61	—	0
Pork, ribs, loin, country style, lean and fat, roasted	3	ounce(s)	279	20	0	0	22	7.83	—	78
Potato chips, salted	20	item(s)	152	2	15	1	10	3.11	—	0
Potatoes, au gratin mix, prepared w/water, whole milk, and butter	½	cup(s)	106	3	15	1	5	2.94	—	17
Potatoes, baked, flesh and skin	1	item(s)	220	5	51	4	<1	0.05	—	0
Potatoes, baked, flesh only	½	cup(s)	57	1	13	1	<0.1	0.02	—	0
Potatoes, hashed brown	½	cup(s)	207	2	27	2	10	1.11	—	0
Potatoes, mashed, from dehydrated granules w/ milk, water, and margarine	½	cup(s)	122	2	17	1	5	1.27	—	2
Pretzels, plain, hard, twists	5	item(s)	114	3	24	1	1	0.23	—	0
Prune juice, canned	1	cup(s)	182	2	45	3	<0.1	0.01	—	0
Prunes, dried	2	item(s)	40	<1	11	1	<0.1	0.01	—	0
Pudding, chocolate	½	cup(s)	154	5	23	1	5	2.78	0	35
Pudding, tapioca, ready to eat	1	item(s)	169	3	28	<1	5	0.85	—	1
Pudding, vanilla	½	cup(s)	116	5	17	<0.1	3	1.31	0	35
Quinoa, dry	½	cup(s)	318	11	59	5	5	0.50	—	0
Raisins, seeded, packed	¼	cup(s)	122	1	32	3	<1	0.07	—	0
Raspberries, raw	½	cup(s)	32	1	7	4	<1	0.01	—	0
Raspberries, red, sweetened, frozen	½	cup(s)	129	1	33	6	<1	0.01	—	0
Rice, brown, long grain, cooked	½	cup(s)	108	3	22	2	1	0.18	—	0
Rice, white, long grain, boiled	½	cup(s)	103	2	22	<1	<1	0.06	—	0
Rice, wild brown, cooked	½	cup(s)	82.81	3.27	17.49	1.47	0.27	0.04	—	0
Roll, hard	1	item(s)	167	6	30	1	2	0.35	—	0
Salad dressing, blue cheese	2	tablespoon(s)	154	1	2	0	16	3.03	—	5
Salad dressing, French	2	tablespoon(s)	143	<1	5	0	14	1.76	—	0
Salad dressing, French, low fat	2	tablespoon(s)	76	<1	10	<1	4	0.36	—	0
Salad dressing, Italian	2	tablespoon(s)	86	<1	3	0	8	1.32	—	0
Salad dressing, Italian, diet	2	tablespoon(s)	23	<1	1	0	2	0.14	—	2
Salad dressing, ranch	2	tablespoon(s)	146	<1	2	<0.1	16	2.32	—	1
Salad dressing, Thousand Island	2	tablespoon(s)	115	<1	5	<1	11	1.59	—	8
Salad dressing, Thousand Island, low calorie	2	tablespoon(s)	62	<1	7	<1	4	0.23	—	<1
Salami, pork, dry or hard	1	slice(s)	52	3	<1	0	4	1.52	—	10
Salmon, broiled or baked w/butter	3	ounce(s)	155	23	0	0	6	1.16	—	40
Salmon, smoked chinook (lox)	2	ounce(s)	66	10	0	0	2	0.52	—	13
Salsa	2	tablespoon(s)	4	<1	1	<1	<0.1	0.00	—	0
Sardines, Atlantic, with bones, canned in oil	2	item(s)	50	6	0	0	3	0.36	—	34
Sauerkraut, canned	½	cup(s)	22	1	5	3	<1	0.04	—	0
Sausage, Italian, pork, cooked	1	item(s)	220	14	1	0	17	6.14	—	53
Sausage, smoked, pork link	1	piece(s)	295	17	2	—	24	8.58	—	52

Food Description	Qty	Measure	Energy (cal)	Protein (g)	Carb (g)	Dietary Fiber (g)	Fat(g)	SatFat(g)	TransFat (g)	Cholesterol (mg)
Scallops, mixed species, breaded, fried	3	item(s)	100	8	5	0	5	1.24	—	28
Seaweed, spirulina, dried	½	cup(s)	22	4	2	<1	1	0.20	—	0
Shrimp, mixed species, breaded, fried	3	ounce(s)	205.69	18.18	9.74	0.34	10.43	1.77	—	150.44
Shrimp, mixed species, cooked, moist heat	3	ounce(s)	84	18	0	0	1	0.25	—	166
Soda, Coca-Cola Classic cola	12	fluid ounce(s)	146	0	41	0	0	0.00	0	0
Soda, Coke diet cola	12	fluid ounce(s)	2	0	<1	0	0	0.00	0	0
Soda, cola	12	fluid ounce(s)	179	<1	46	0	0	0.00	—	0
Soda, ginger ale	12	fluid ounce(s)	124	0	32	0	0	0.00	0	0
Soda, lemon lime	12	fluid ounce(s)	147	0	38	0	0	0.00	—	0
Soda, root beer	12	fluid ounce(s)	152	0	39	0	0	0.00	0	0
Sour cream	2	tablespoon(s)	51	1	1	0	5	3.13	—	11
Sour cream, fat free	2	tablespoon(s)	24	1	5	0	0	0.00	0	3
Soy sauce	1	tablespoon(s)	10	1	2	0	<0.1	0.00	—	0
Spinach, canned, drained	½	cup(s)	25	3	4	3	1	0.09	—	0
Spinach, chopped, boiled, drained	½	cup(s)	21	3	3	2	<1	0.04	—	0
Spinach, raw, chopped	1	cup(s)	7	1	1	1	<1	0.02	—	0
Squash, acorn, baked	½	cup(s)	57	1	15	5	<1	0.03	—	0
Squash, summer, all varieties, sliced, boiled, drained	½	cup(s)	18	1	4	1	<1	0.06	—	0
Squash, winter, all varieties, baked, mashed	½	cup(s)	38	1	9	3	<1	0.13	—	0
Squid, mixed species, fried	3	ounce(s)	149	15	7	0	6	1.60	—	221
Strawberries, raw	½	cup(s)	23	<1	6	1	<1	0.01	—	0
Strawberries, sweetened, frozen, thawed	½	cup(s)	99	1	27	2	<1	0.01	—	0
Sugar, brown, packed	1	teaspoon(s)	17	0	4	0	0	0.00	0	0
Sugar, white, granulated	1	teaspoon(s)	15	0	4	0	0	0.00		
Sweet potatoes, baked, peeled	½	cup(s)	90	2	21	3	<1	0.03	—	0
Syrup, maple	¼	cup(s)	209	0	54	0	<1	0.03	—	0
Taco shell, hard	1	item(s)	62	1	8	1	3	0.43	—	0
Tangerine, raw	1	item(s)	37	1	9	2	<1	0.02	—	0
Tea, decaffeinated, prepared	8	fluid ounce(s)	2	0	1	0	0	0.00	0	0
Tea, herbal, prepared	8	fluid ounce(s)	2	0	<1	0	0	0.00	0	0
Tea, prepared	8	fluid ounce(s)	2	0	1	0	0	0.00	0	0
Teriyaki sauce	1	Tablespoon(s)	15	1	3	<0.1	0	0.00	0	0
Tofu, firm	3	ounce(s)	80	8	2	1	4	0.50	—	0
Tomato juice, canned	½	cup(s)	21	1	5	<1	<0.1	0.01	—	0
Tomato sauce	½	cup(s)	46	2	8	2	1	0.18	0	0
Tomatoes, fresh, ripe, red	1	item(s)	22.13	1.08	4.82	1.47	0.24	0.05	—	0
Tomatoes, stewed, canned, red	½	cup(s)	33	1	8	1	<1	0.03	—	0
Tortilla chips, plain	6	item(s)	142	2	18	2	7	1.43	—	0
Tortillas, corn, soft	1	item(s)	58	1	12	1	1	0.09	—	0
Tortillas, flour	1	item(s)	104	3	18	1	2	0.56	—	0
Tuna, light, canned in oil, drained	2	ounce(s)	113	17	0	0	5	0.87	—	10
Tuna, light, canned in water, drained	2	ounce(s)	66	14	0	0	<1	0.13	—	17
Turkey, breast, processed, oven roasted, fat free	1	slice(s)	25	4	1	0	0	0.00	0	10
Turkey, breast, processed, traditional carved	2	slice(s)	40	9	0	0	1	0.00	—	20
Turkey, roasted, dark meat, meat only	3	ounce(s)	159	24	0	0	6	2.06	—	72
Turkey, roasted, light meat, meat only	3	ounce(s)	133	25	0	0	3	0.88	—	59
Turnip greens, chopped, boiled, drained	½	cup(s)	14	1	3	3	<1	0.04	—	0
Turnips, cubed, boiled, drained	½	cup(s)	17	1	4	2	<0.1	0.01	—	0
Vegetables, mixed, canned, drained	½	cup(s)	40	2	8	2	<1	0.04	—	0
Vinegar, balsamic	1	tablespoon(s)	10	0	2	0	0	0.00	0	0
Waffle, plain, frozen, toasted	2	item(s)	174	4	27	2	5	0.95	—	16
Walnuts, dried black, chopped	¼	cup(s)	193	8	3	2	18	1.05	—	0
Watermelon	½	cup(s)	23	<1	6	<1	<1	0.01	—	0
Wheat germ, crude	2	tablespoon(s)	52	3	7	2	1	0.24	—	0
Wine cooler	10	fluid ounce(s)	150	<1	18	<0.1	<0.1	0.01	—	0
Wine, red, California	5	fluid ounce(s)	125	<1	4	0	0	0.00	0	0
Wine, sparkling, domestic	5	fluid ounce(s)	105	<1	4	0	0	0.00	0	0
Wine, white	5	fluid ounce(s)	100	<1	1	0	0	0.00	0	0
Yogurt, custard style, fruit flavors	6	ounce(s)	190	7	32	0	4	2.00	—	15
Yogurt, fruit, low fat	1	cup(s)	243	10	46	0	3	1.82	—	12
Yogurt, fruit, nonfat, sweetened w/low-calorie sweetener	1	cup(s)	122	11	19	1	<1	0.21	—	3

Food Description	Qty	Measure	Energy (cal)	Protein (g)	Carb (g)	Dietary Fiber (g)	Fat(g)	SatFat(g)	TransFat (g)	Cholesterol (mg)
Yogurt, plain, low fat	1	cup(s)	154	13	17	0	4	2.45	—	15
VEGETARIAN FOODS										
Prepared										
Macaroni and cheese (lacto)	8	ounce(s)	181	8	17	<1	9	4.37	0	22
Steamed rice and vegetables (vegan)	8	ounce(s)	265	5	40	3	10	1.84	0	0
Vegan spinach enchiladas (vegan)	1	piece(s)	93	5	15	2	2	0.34	—	0
Vegetable chow mein (vegan)	8	ounce(s)	166	6	22	2	6	0.65	0	0
Vegetable lasagna (lacto)	8	ounce(s)	177	12	25	2	4	1.92	0	10
Vegetarian chili (vegan)	8	ounce(s)	116	6	21	7	2	0.24	0	<1
Vegetarian vegetable soup (vegan)	8	ounce(s)	92	3	14	2	4	0.77	0	0
Boca burger										
All American flamed grilled patty	1	item(s)	110	14	6	4	4	1.00	0	3
Boca meatless ground burger	½	cup(s)	70	11	7	4	1	0.00	—	0
Breakfast links	2	item(s)	100	10	6	5	4	0.00	0	0
Breakfast patties	1	item(s)	80	8	5	3	4	0.00	0	0
Vegan original patty	1	item(s)	90	13	4	0	1	0.00	0	0
Gardenburger										
Black bean burger	1	item(s)	80	8	11	4	2	0.00	0	0
Chik'n grill	1	item(s)	100	13	5	3	3	0.00	0	0
Meatless breakfast sausage	1	item(s)	50	5	2	2	4	0.00	0	0
Meatless meatballs	6	item(s)	110	12	8	4	5	1.00	0	0
Original	3	ounce(s)	132	7	19	4	4	1.80	0	24
Morningstar Farms										
America's Original Veggie Dog links	1	item(s)	80	11	6	1	1	0.00	0	0
Better n Eggs egg substitute	¼	cup(s)	20	5	0	0	0	0.00	0	0
Breakfast links	2	item(s)	80	9	3	2	3	0.50	0	0
Breakfast strips	2	item(s)	60	2	2	1	5	0.50	0	0
Garden veggie patties	1	item(s)	100	10	9	4	3	0.50	0	0
Spicy black bean veggie burger	1	item(s)	150	11	16	5	5	0.50	0	0
MIXED FOODS, SOUPS, SANDWICHES										
Mixed Dishes										
Bean burrito	1	item(s)	327	17	33	6	15	8.30	0	38
Beef and vegetable fajita	1	item(s)	397	23	35	3	18	5.50	—	45
Chicken and vegetables w/broccoli, onion, bamboo shoots in soy based sauce	1	cup(s)	287	22	6	1	19	5.13	—	84
Chicken cacciatore	1	cup(s)	266	28	5	1	14	3.98	0	103
Chicken Waldorf salad	½	cup(s)	178	14	6	1	11	1.76	0	42
Fettuccine alfredo	1	cup(s)	247	11	42	1	3	1.61	0	9
Hummus	½	cup(s)	218	6	25	5	11	1.38	—	0
Lasagna w/ground beef	1	cup(s)	288	18	22	2	15	7.47	0	68
Macaroni and cheese	1	cup(s)	393	15	40	1	19	8.18	—	30
Meat loaf	1	slice(s)	244	17	7	<1	16	6.15	0	85
Potato salad	½	cup(s)	179	3	14	2	10	1.79	—	85
Spaghetti and meatballs w/tomato sauce, prepared	1	cup(s)	330	19	39	3	12	3.90	—	89
Spicy thai noodles (pad thai)	8	ounce(s)	222	9	36	3	6	0.83	0	37
Sushi w/vegetables in seaweed	6	piece(s)	182	3	41	1	<1	0.10	—	0
Tuna salad	½	cup(s)	192	16	10	0	9	1.58	0	13
Soups										
Chicken noodle, condensed, prepared w/water	1	cup(s)	75	4	9	1	2	0.65	—	7
Cream of chicken, condensed, prepared w/milk	1	cup(s)	191	7	15	<1	11	4.64	—	27
Cream of mushroom, condensed, prepared w/milk	1	cup(s)	203	6	15	<1	14	5.13	—	20
Manhattan clam chowder, condensed, prepared w/water	1	cup(s)	78	2	12	1	2	0.38	—	2
Minestrone, condensed, prepared w/water	1	cup(s)	82	4	11	1	3	0.55	—	2
New England clam chowder, condensed, prepared w/milk	1	cup(s)	164	9	17	1	7	2.95	—	22
Split pea	1	cup(s)	85	4	19	2	<1	0.07	0	0
Tomato, condensed, prepared w/milk	1	cup(s)	161	6	22	3	6	2.90	—	17
Tomato, condensed, prepared w/water	1	cup(s)	85	2	17	<1	2	0.37	—	0
Vegetable beef, condensed, prepared w/water	1	cup(s)	78	6	10	<1	2	0.85	—	5
Vegetarian vegetable, condensed, prepared w/water	1	cup(s)	72	2	12	—	2	0.29	—	0

Food Description	Qty	Measure	Energy (cal)	Protein (g)	Carb (g)	Dietary Fiber (g)	Fat(g)	SatFat(g)	TransFat (g)	Cholesterol (mg)
Sandwiches										
Bacon, lettuce, and tomato w/mayonnaise	1	item(s)	349	11	34	2	19	4.54	—	20
Cheeseburger, large, plain	1	item(s)	609	30	47	0	33	14.84	—	96
Cheeseburger, large, w/bacon, vegetables, and condiments	1	item(s)	608	32	37	2	37	16.24	—	111
Club w/bacon, chicken, tomato, lettuce, and mayonnaise	1	item(s)	555	31	48	3	26	5.94	—	72
Cold cut submarine w/cheese and vegetables	1	item(s)	456	22	51	2	19	6.81	—	36
Egg salad	1	item(s)	278	10	29	1	13	2.96	—	217
Hamburger, double patty, large, w/condiments and vegetables	1	item(s)	540	34	40	0	27	10.52	—	122
Hamburger, large, plain	1	item(s)	426	23	32	2	23	8.38	—	71
Hot dog w/bun, plain	1	item(s)	242	10	18	2	15	5.11	—	44
Pastrami	1	item(s)	331	14	27	2	18	6.18	—	51
Peanut butter and jelly	1	item(s)	330	11	42	3	15	3.00	—	1
FAST FOOD										
Arby's										
Au jus sauce	1	serving(s)	5	<1	1	<0.1	<0.1	0.02	—	0
Beef 'n cheddar sandwich	1	item(s)	480	23	43	2	24	8.00	—	90
Curly fries, medium	1	serving(s)	400	5	50	4	20	5.00	—	0
Market Fresh grilled chicken Caesar salad w/o dressing	1	serving(s)	230	33	8	3	8	3.50	—	80
Roast beef deluxe sandwich, light	1	item(s)	296	18	33	6	10	3.00	—	42
Roast beef sandwich, giant	1	item(s)	480	32	41	3	23	10.00	—	110
Roast beef sandwich, regular	1	item(s)	350	21	34	2	16	6.00	—	85
Roast chicken deluxe sandwich, light	1	item(s)	260	23	33	3	5	1.00	—	40
Burger King										
BK Broiler chicken sandwich	1	item(s)	550	30	52	3	25	5.00	—	105
Croissanwich w/sausage, egg, and cheese	1	item(s)	520	19	24	1	39	14.00	1.93	210
Fish Filet sandwich	1	item(s)	520	18	44	2	30	8.00	1.12	55
French fries, medium, salted	1	item(s)	360	4	46	4	18	5.00	4.50	0
Onion rings, medium	1	serving(s)	320	4	40	3	16	4.00	3.50	0
Whopper	1	item(s)	710	31	52	4	43	13.00	1	85
Whopper w/cheese	1	item(s)	800	36	53	4	50	18.00	2	110
Chick-Fil-A										
Chargrilled chicken garden salad	1	item(s)	180	22	9	3	6	3.00	0	70
Chargrilled deluxe chicken sandwich	1	item(s)	290	27	31	2	7	1.50	0	70
Chicken biscuit w/cheese	1	item(s)	450	19	43	2	23	7.00	2.85	45
Chicken salad sandwich	1	item(s)	350	20	32	5	15	3.00	0	65
Chick-n-Strips	4	item(s)	290	29	14	1	13	2.50	0	65
Coleslaw	1	item(s)	210	1	14	2	17	2.50	0	20
Dairy Queen										
Banana split	1	item(s)	510	8	96	3	12	8.00	0	30
Chocolate chip cookie dough blizzard, small	1	item(s)	720	12	105	0	28	14.00	2.50	50
Chocolate malt, small	1	item(s)	650	15	111	0	16	10.00	0.50	55
Vanilla soft serve	½	cup(s)	140	3	22	0	5	3.00	0	15
Domino's										
Classic hand tossed pizza										
America's favorite feast, 12"	2	slice(s)	508	22	57	4	22	9.20	—	49
Pepperoni feast, extra pepperoni & cheese, 12"	2	slice(s)	534	24	56	3	25	10.92	—	57
Vegi feast, 12"	2	slice(s)	439	19	57	4	16	7.09	—	34
Thin crust pizza										
Extravaganzza, 12"	¼	item(s)	425	20	34	3	24	9.41	—	53
Pepperoni, extra pepperoni & cheese, 12"	¼	item(s)	420	20	32	2	24	10.46	—	54
Vegi, 12"	¼	item(s)	338	16	34	3	17	7.08	—	34
Ultimate deep dish pizza										
America's favorite, 12"	2	slice(s)	617	26	59	4	33	12.88	—	58
Pepperoni, extra pepperoni & cheese, 12"	2	slice(s)	629	26	57	4	34	13.57	—	61
Vegi, 12"	2	slice(s)	547	22	59	4	26	10.19	—	41
In-n-Out Burger										
Cheeseburger w/mustard and ketchup	1	item(s)	400	22	41	3	18	9.00	—	55
Chocolate shake	1	item(s)	690	9	83	0	36	24.00	—	95
Double-Double cheeseburger w/mustard and ketchup	1	item(s)	590	37	42	3	32	17.00	—	115

Food Description	Qty	Measure	Energy (cal)	Protein (g)	Carb (g)	Dietary Fiber (g)	Fat(g)	SatFat(g)	TransFat (g)	Cholesterol (mg)
FAST FOOD (continued)										
In-n-Out Burger (continued)										
French fries	1	item(s)	400	7	54	2	18	5.00	—	0
Hamburger w/mustard and ketchup	1	item(s)	310	16	41	3	10	4.00	—	35
Jack in the Box										
Chicken club salad	1	item(s)	310	28	15	5	16	6.00	0	65
Hamburger	1	item(s)	250	12	30	2	9	3.50	0.88	30
Jack's Spicy Chicken sandwich	1	item(s)	580	24	53	3	31	6.00	2.81	60
Jumbo Jack hamburger w/cheese	1	item(s)	690	26	60	3	38	16.00	1.55	75
Sourdough Jack	1	item(s)	700	30	36	3	49	16.00	2.98	80
Jamba Juice										
Banana berry smoothie	24	fluid ounce(s)	470	5	112	5	2	0.50	—	5
Chocolate mood smoothie	24	fluid ounce(s)	690	16	142	2	8	4.50	—	25
Jamba powerboost smoothie	24	fluid ounce(s)	440	6	103	7	2	0.00	—	0
Orange juice, freshly squeezed	16	fluid ounce(s)	220	3	52	1	1	0.00	—	0
Protein berry pizzaz smoothie	24	fluid ounce(s)	440	20	92	6	2	0.00	—	0
Kentucky Fried Chicken (KFC)										
Extra Crispy chicken, breast	1	item(s)	470	34	19	0	28	8.00	4.50	135
Hot and spicy chicken, whole wing	1	item(s)	180	11	9	0	11	3.00	0	60
Original Recipe chicken, drumstick	1	item(s)	140	14	4	0	8	2.00	1	75
Long John Silver's										
Baked cod	1	serving(s)	120	22	1	0	5	1.00		90
Batter dipped fish sandwich	1	item(s)	440	17	48	3	20	5.00	—	35
Clam chowder	1	item(s)	220	9	23	0	10	4.00	—	25
Crunchy shrimp basket	21	item(s)	340	12	32	2	19	5.00	—	105
McDonald's										
Big Mac hamburger	1	item(s)	590	24	47	3	34	11.00	1.48	85
Cheeseburger	1	item(s)	330	15	36	2	14	6.00	1.02	45
Chicken McNuggets	4	item(s)	210	10	12	1	13	2.50	1.13	35
Egg McMuffin	1	item(s)	300	18	29	2	12	4.50	0.42	235
Filet-o-Fish sandwich	1	item(s)	470	15	45	1	26	5.00	1.11	50
French fries, small	1	serving(s)	210	3	26	2	10	1.50	2.30	0
Fruit 'n yogurt parfait	1	item(s)	380	10	76	2	5	2.00	0.18	15
Hash browns	1	item(s)	130	1	14	1	8	1.50	2	0
Honey sauce	1	item(s)	45	0	12	0	0	0.00	—	0
McSalad Shaker garden salad	1	item(s)	100	7	4	2	6	3.00	—	75
McSalad Shaker grilled chicken caesar salad	1	item(s)	100	17	3	2	3	1.50	—	40
Newman's Own creamy Caesar salad dressing	1	item(s)	190	2	4	0	18	3.50	0.29	20
Plain hotcakes w/syrup & margarine	3	item(s)	600	9	104	0	17	3.00	4	20
Quarter Pounder hamburger	1	item(s)	430	23	37	2	21	8.00	1.01	70
Quarter Pounder hamburger w/cheese	1	item(s)	530	28	38	2	30	13.00	1.51	95
Sausage McMuffin w/egg	1	item(s)	450	20	29	2	28	10.00	0.59	255
Vanilla milkshake	8	fluid ounce(s)	254	9	40	0	7	4.28	—	27
Pizza Hut										
Pepperoni Lovers stuffed crust pizza	1	slice(s)	480	23	44	3	24	11.00	1.05	65
Pepperoni Lovers thin 'n crispy pizza	1	slice(s)	270	13	22	2	14	7.00	0.51	40
Personal Pan supreme pizza	1	slice(s)	170	8	19	1	7	3.00	0.95	15
Veggie Lovers stuffed crust pizza	1	slice(s)	370	17	45	3	14	7.00	0.53	35
Veggie Lovers thin 'n crispy pizza	1	slice(s)	190	8	23	2	7	3.00	0.54	15
Starbucks										
Cappuccino, tall	12	fluid ounce(s)	120	7	10	0	6	4.00	—	25
Cinnamon spice mocha, tall nonfat w/o whipped cream	12	fluid ounce(s)	170	11	32	0	0	0.50	0	5
Frappuccino, tall chocolate	12	fluid ounce(s)	290	13	52	1	5	1.00	—	3
Latte, tall w/nonfat milk	12	fluid ounce(s)	123	12	17	0	1	0.40	0	6
Latte, tall w/whole milk	12	fluid ounce(s)	212	11	17	0	11	6.90	—	46
Macchiato, tall caramel w/whole milk	12	fluid ounce(s)	190	6	27	0	7	4.00	—	25
Tazo chai black tea, tall nonfat	12	fluid ounce(s)	170	6	37	0	0	0.00	0	5
Subway										
Chocolate chip cookie	1	item(s)	209	3	29	1	10	3.50	1.07	12
Classic Italian B.M.T. sandwich, 6", white bread	1	item(s)	453	21	40	3	24	8.00	0	56
Meatball sandwich, 6", white bread	1	item(s)	501	23	46	4	25	10.00	0.75	56
Roast beef sandwich, 6", white bread	1	item(s)	264	18	39	3	5	1.00	0	20

Food Description	Qty	Measure	Energy (cal)	Protein (g)	Carb (g)	Dietary Fiber (g)	Fat(g)	SatFat(g)	TransFat (g)	Cholesterol (mg)
FAST FOOD (continued)										
Subway (continued)										
Roasted chicken breast sandwich, 6", white bread	1	item(s)	311	25	40	3	6	1.50	0	48
Tuna sandwich, 6", white bread	1	item(s)	419	18	39	3	21	5.00	—	42
Turkey breast sandwich, 6", white bread	1	item(s)	254	16	39	3	4	1.00	0	15
Taco Bell										
7-layer burrito	1	item(s)	530	18	67	10	22	8.00	3	25
Beef burrito supreme	1	item(s)	440	18	51	7	18	8.00	2	40
Grilled chicken burrito	1	item(s)	390	19	49	3	13	4.00	—	40
Taco	1	item(s)	170	8	13	3	10	4.00	0.50	25
Veggie fajita wrap supreme	1	item(s)	470	11	55	3	22	7.00	—	30
CONVENIENCE MEALS										
Budget Gourmet										
Cheese manicotti w/meat sauce	1	item(s)	420	18	38	4	22	11.00	—	85
Chicken w/fettuccine	1	item(s)	380	20	33	3	19	10.00	—	85
Light beef stroganoff	1	item(s)	290	20	32	3	7	4.00	—	35
Light sirloin of beef in herb sauce	1	item(s)	260	19	30	5	7	4.00	—	30
Light vegetable lasagna	1	item(s)	290	15	36	5	9	1.79	—	15
Healthy Choice										
Chicken enchilada suprema meal	1	item(s)	360	13	59	8	7	3.00	—	30
Lemon pepper fish meal	1	item(s)	280	11	49	5	5	2.00	—	30
Traditional salisbury steak meal	1	item(s)	360	23	45	5	9	3.50	—	45
Traditional turkey breasts meal	1	item(s)	330	21	50	4	5	2.00	—	35
Zucchini lasagna	1	item(s)	280	13	47	5	4	2.50	—	10
Stouffer's										
Cheese enchiladas with Mexican rice	1	serving(s)	370	12	48	5	14	5.00	—	25
Chicken pot pie	1	item(s)	740	23	56	4	47	18.00	—	65
Homestyle beef pot roast and potatoes	1	item(s)	270	16	25	3	12	4.50	—	35
Homestyle roast turkey breast w/stuffing and mashed potatoes	1	item(s)	300	16	34	2	11	3.00	—	35
Lean Cuisine Everyday Favorites chicken chow mein w/rice	1	item(s)	210	12	33	2	3	1.00	0	30
Lean Cuisine Everyday Favorites lasagna w/meat sauce	1	item(s)	300	19	41	3	8	4.00	0	30
Weight Watchers										
Smart Ones chicken enchiladas suiza entree	1	serving(s)	270	15	33	2	9	3.50	—	50
Smart Ones garden lasagna entrée	1	item(s)	270	14	36	5	7	3.50	—	30
Smart Ones pepperoni pizza	1	item(s)	390	23	46	4	12	4.00	—	45
Smart Ones spicy penne pasta and ricotta	1	item(s)	280	11	45	4	6	2.00	—	5
Smart Ones spicy Szechuan style vegetables and chicken	1	item(s)	220	11	39	3	2	0.50	—	10

Notes

Chapter 1

Notes

1. World Health Organization "Chronic Diseases and Health Promotion," available at http://www.who.int/chp/en/, accessed March 20, 2015.
2. U.S. Department of Health and Human Services, Centers for Disease Control and Prevention, National Center for Health Statistics, *National Vital Statistics Reports, Deaths: Preliminary Data for 2011*, 61:6 (October 10, 2012).
3. Institute for Health Metrics and Evaluation, "U.S. County Profiles, 2013," http://www.healthdata.org/us-county-profiles, accessed March 11, 2015.
4. OECD (2013), Health at a Glance 2013: OECD Indicators, OECD Publishing, http://www.oecd-ilibrary.org/social-issues-migration-health/health-at-a-glance-2013-en, downloaded February 28, 2014.
5. Heart Disease and Stroke Statistics—2014 Update: A Report from the American Heart Association," http://circ.ahajournals.org/content/129/3/e28.extract, downloaded February 28, 2014.
6. Alere Wellbeing, "The Economic Impacts of Obesity," April 2012, http://www.alerewellbeing.com/_assets/cms_uploads/WP_Economic%20Impact%20of%20Obesity_4.12.pdf, accessed March 20, 2015.
7. American College of Sports Medicine, *ACSM's Guidelines for Exercise Testing and Prescription* (Philadelphia: Wolters Kluwer/Lippincott Williams & Wilkins, 2010).
8. JA Lavine, "Non-exercise activity thermogenesis (NEAT)," *Best Practice & Research Clinical Endocrinology & Metabolism* 2002 Dec; 16(4):679–702. James A. Levin, "The 'NEAT Defect' in Human Obesity: The Role of Nonexercise Activity Thermogenesis," Mayo Clinic Endocrinology Update 2 no. 1: 1–2.
9. W. L. Haskell, et al., "Physical Activity and Public Health: Updated Recommendation for Adults from the American College of Sports Medicine and the American Heart Association," *Medicine & Science in Sports & Exercise* 39 (2007): 1423–1434.
10. U.S. Department of Health and Human Services, *Physical Activity and Health: A Report of the Surgeon General* (Atlanta, GA: Centers for Disease Control and Prevention, National Center for Chronic Disease Prevention and Health Promotion, 1996).
11. U.S. Department of Health and Human Services, *2008 Physical Activity Guidelines for Americans*, http://health.gov/-paguidelines, downloaded October 15, 2008.
12. U.S. Department of Health and Human Services, *2008 Physical Activity Guidelines for Americans* (Washington, DC: DHHS, 2008); U.S. Department of Health and Human Services and U.S. Department of Agriculture, *Dietary Guidelines for Americans 2010* (Washington, DC: DHHS, 2010).
13. National Academy of Sciences, Institute of Medicine, *Dietary Reference Intakes for Energy, Carbohydrates, Fiber, Fat, Fatty Acids, Cholesterol, Protein and Amino Acids (Macronutrients)* (Washington, DC: National Academy Press, 2005).
14. U.S. Department of Health and Human Services and Department of Agriculture, *Dietary Guidelines for Americans*, 2005 (Washington, DC: DHHS, 2005).
15. R. S. Paffenbarger, Jr., R. T. Hyde, A. L. Wing, and C. H. Steinmetz, "A History of Athleticism and Cardiovascular Health," *Journal of the American Medical Association*, 252 (1984): 491–495.
16. S. N. Blair, H. W. Kohl III, R. S. Paffenbarger, Jr., D. G. Clark, K. H. Cooper, and L. W. Gibbons, "Physical Fitness and All-Cause Mortality: A Prospective Study of Healthy Men and Women," *Journal of the American Medical Association*, 262 (1989): 2395–2401.
17. S. N. Blair, H. W. Kohl III, C. E. Barlow, R. S. Paffenbarger, Jr., L. W. Gibbons, and C. A. Macera, "Changes in Physical Fitness and All-Cause Mortality: A Prospective Study of Healthy and Unhealthy Men," *Journal of the American Medical Association*, 273 (1995): 1193–1198.
18. Huseyin Naci, John P. A. Ioannidis, "Comparative Effectiveness of Exercise and Drug Interventions on Mortality Outcomes: Metaepidemiological Study," *BMJ* (2013), 347:f5577; Jane E. Brody, "Sweaty Answer for Chronic Ills," *New York Times*, Jan. 27, 2015, D5.
19. I. Lee, C. Hsieh, and R. S. Paffenbarger, Jr., "Exercise Intensity and Longevity in Men: The Harvard Alumni Health Study," *Journal of the American Medical Association*, 273 (1995): 1179–1184; D. P. Swain, "Moderate- or Vigorous-Intensity Exercise: What Should We Prescribe?" *ACSM's Health & Fitness Journal* 10, no. 5 (2007): 7–11.
20. P. T. Williams, "Physical Fitness and Activity as Separate Heart Disease Risk Factors: A Meta-analysis," *Medicine & Science in Sports & Exercise* 33 (2001): 754–761; D. P. Swain and B. A. Franklin, "Comparative Cardioprotective Benefits of Vigorous vs. Moderate Intensity Aerobic Exercise," *American Journal of Cardiology* 97 (2006): 141–147.
21. American College of Sports Medicine, "Exercise Is Medicine," http://www.exerciseismedicine.org/, downloaded January 10, 2012.
22. American Heart Association, *Heart Disease & Stroke Statistics—20154 Update*, http://circ.ahajournals.org/content/131/4/e29.extracthttp://circ.ahajournals.org/content/129/3/e28.extract, downloaded March 11, 2015.
23. J. O. Prochaska, J. C. Norcross, and C. C. DiClemente, *Changing for Good* (New York: William Morrow and Co., 1994).

Chapter 2

Notes

1. R. B. O'Hara, et al., "Increased Volume Resistance Training: Effects upon Predicted Aerobic Fitness in a Select Group of Air Force Men," *ACSM's Health and Fitness Journal* 8, no. 4 (2004): 16–25.

2. W. L. Haskell, et al., "Physical Activity and Public Health: Updated Recommendation for Adults from the American College of Sports Medicine and the American Heart Association," *Medicine & Science in Sports & Exercise* 39 (2007): 1423–1434.

3. American College of Sports Medicine, *ACSM's Guidelines for Exercise Testing and Prescription* (Philadelphia: Wolters Kluwer/Lippincott Williams & Wilkins, 2010).

4. S. J. Fitzgerald, et al., "Muscular Fitness and All-cause Mortality: Prospective Observations," *Journal of Physical Activity and Health* 1 (2004): 7–18.

5. W. J. Evans, "Exercise Nutrition and Aging," *Journal of Nutrition,* 122 (1992), 786–801.

6. R. Kjorstad, *Validity of Two Field Tests of Abdominal Strength and Muscular Endurance,* Unpublished master's thesis, Boise State University, 1997.

7. G. L. Hall, R. K. Hetzler, D. Perrin, and A. Weltman, "Relationship of Timed Sit-Up Tests to Isokinetic Abdominal Strength," *Research Quarterly for Exercise and Sport,* 63 (1992), 80–84.

8. American College of Obstetricians and Gynecologists, *Guidelines for Exercise During Pregnancy,* 2003.

9. "Stretch Yourself Younger," *Consumer Reports on Health* 11 (August 1999), 6–7.

10. K. M. Flegal, M. D. Carrol, R. J. Kuczmarski, and C. L. Johnson, "Overweight and Obesity in the United States: Prevalence and Trends, 1960–1994," *International Journal of Obesity and Related Metabolic Disorders* 22 (1998): 39–47.

11. C. Bouchard, G. A. Bray, and V. S. Hubbard, "Basic and Clinical Aspects of Regional Fat Distribution," *American Journal of Clinical Nutrition* 52 (1990): 946–950; G. Hu, et al., "Joint Effects of Physical Activity, Body Mass Index, Waist Circumference, and Waist-to-Hip Ratio on the Risk of Heart Failure," *Circulation* 121 (2010): 237–244; D. Canoy, et al., "Body Fat Distribution and Risk of Coronary Heart Disease in Men and Women in the European Prospective Investigation Into Cancer and Nutrition in Norfolk Cohort," *Circulation* 116 (2007): 2933–2943; J. P. Després, I. Lemieux, and D. Prudhomme, "Treatment of Obesity: Need to Focus on High Risk Abdominally Obese Patients," *British Medical Journal* 322 (2001): 716–720.

12. T. Pischon, et al., "General and Abdominal Adiposity and Risk of Death in Europe," *New England Journal of Medicine* 359 (2008): 2105–2120.

13. M. Ashwell, "Charts Based on Body Mass Index and Waist-to-Height Ratio to Assess the Health Risks of Obesity," *The Open Obesity Journal* 3 (2011): 78–84.

14. M. Ashwell, P. Gunn, and S. Gibson, "Waist-to-Height Ratio is a Better Screening Tool than Waist Circumference and BMI for Adult Cardiometabolic Risk Factors: Systematic Review and Meta-Analysis," *Obesity Review* 13 (2012): 275–86.

15. Ashwell M, et al., "Waist-to-Height Ratio Is More Accurate than Body Mass Index to Quantify Reduced Life Expectancy," *Euro Congress Obesity* 2013; Abstract T3T4:P.013.

Chapter 3

Notes

1. W. W. K. Hoeger, L. Bond, L. Ransdell, J. M. Shimon, and S. Merugu, "One-Mile Step Count at Walking and Running Speeds," *ACSM's Health & Fitness Journal* 12, no. 1 (2008): 14–19.

2. American College of Sports Medicine, "Position Stand: Quantity and Quality of Exercise for Developing and Maintaining Cardiorespiratory, Musculoskeletal, and Neuromotor Fitness in Apparently Healthy Adults: Guidance for Prescribing Exercise," *Medicine and Science in Sports and Exercise* 43 (2011): 1334–1359.

3. American College of Sports Medicine, *ACSM's Guidelines for Exercise Testing and Prescription* (Philadelphia: Wolters Kluwer/Lippincott Williams & Wilkins, 2014).

4. See note 3, ACSM.

5. W. L. Haskell et al., "Physical Activity and Public Health: Updated Recommendation for Adults from the American College of Sports Medicine and the American Heart Association," *Medicine & Science in Sports & Exercise* 39 (2007): 1423–1434.

6. S. E. Gormley et al., "Effect of Intensity of Aerobic Training on VO_{2max}," *Medicine & Science in Sports & Exercise* 40 (2008): 1336–1343.

7. R. L. Gellish et al., "Longitudinal Modelling of the Relationship Between Age and Maximal Heart Rate," *Medicine & Science in Sports & Exercise* 39 (2007): 822–829.

8. U.S. Department of Health and Human Services, *Physical Activity and Health: A Report of the Surgeon General* (Atlanta, GA: Centers for Disease Control and Prevention, National Center for Chronic Disease Prevention and Health Promotion, 1996).

9. D. P. Swain, "Moderate- or Vigorous-Intensity Exercise: What Should We Prescribe?" *ACSM's Health & Fitness Journal* 10, no. 5 (2006): 7–11.

10. D. P. Swain and B. A. Franklin, "Comparative Cardio-protective Benefits of Vigorous vs. Moderate Intensity Aerobic Exercise," *American Journal of Cardiology* 97, no. 1 (2006): 141–147.

11. See note 5, Haskell et al.

12. R. F. DeBusk, U. Stenestrand, M. Sheehan, and W. L. Haskell, "Training Effects of Long Versus Short Bouts of Exercise in Healthy Subjects," *American Journal of Cardiology* 65 (1990): 1010–1013.

13. National Academy of Sciences, Institute of Medicine, *Dietary Reference Intakes for Energy, Carbohydrates, Fiber, Fat, Protein and Amino Acids (Macronutrients)* (Washington, DC: National Academy Press, 2002).

14. U.S. Department of Health and Human Services, Department of Agriculture, *Dietary Guidelines for Americans 2005* (Washington, DC: DHHS, 2005).

15. W. Dunstan et al., "Television Viewing Time and Mortality: The Australian Diabetes, Obesity, and Lifestyle Study (AusDiab)," *Circulation* 121 (2010): 384–391.

16. P. T. Katzmarzyk et al., "Sitting Time and Mortality from All Causes, Cardiovascular Disease, and Cancer," *Medicine & Science in Sports & Exercise* 41 (2009): 998–1005.

17. See note 3, ACSM.

18. American College of Sports Medicine, "Position Stand: Progression Models in Resistance Training for Healthy Adults," *Medicine & Science in Sports & Exercise* 41 (2009): 687–708.

19. W. W. K. Hoeger, D. R. Hopkins, S. L. Barette, and D. F. Hale, "Relationship Between Repetitions and Selected Percentages of One Repetition Maximum: A Comparison Between Untrained and Trained Males and Females," *Journal of Applied Sport Science Research* 4, no. 2 (1990): 47–51.

20. See note 3, ACSM.

21. W. J. Kraemer and M. S. Fragala, "Personalize It: Program Design in Resistance Training," *ACSM's Health & Fitness Journal* 10, no. 4 (2006): 7–17.

22. K. J. Hartman, A. J. Bruenger, and J. T. Lemmer, "Timing Protein Intake Increases Energy Expenditure 24 h After Resistance Training," *Medicine & Science in Sports & Exercise* 42 (2010): 998–1003

23. P. Cribb and A. Hayes, "Effect of Supplement Timing on Skeletal Muscle Hypertrophy," *Medicine & Science in Sports & Exercise* 38 (2006): 1918–1925.

24. J. L. Areta, et al., "Timing and Distribution of Protein Ingestion During Prolonged Recovery from Resistance Exercise Alters Myofibrillar Protein Synthesis," *Journal of Physiology* (2013): 1-13, DOI: 10.1113/jphysiol.2012.244897; D. R. Moore, et al., "Daytime Pattern of Post-exercise Protein Intake Affects Whole-Body Protein Turnover in Resistance-Trained Males," *Nutrition & Metabolism* 9, no. 1 (2012): 91, DOI:10.1186/1743-7075-9-91.

25. See note 3, ACSM.

26. K. B. Fields, C. M. Burnworth, and M. Delaney, "Should Athletes Stretch Before Exercise?" *Gatorade Sports Science Institute: Sports Science Exchange* 30, no. 1 (2007): 1–5.

27. L. Simic, N. Sarabon, and G. Markovic, "Does Pre-exercise Static Stretching Inhibit Maximal Muscular Performance? A Meta-analytical Review," *Scandinavian Journal of Medicine & Science in Sports,* 23, no. 2 (2013): 131–148.

28. "Stretching: 35 Exercises to Improve Flexibility and Reduce Pain," *Harvard Health Publications Special Health Report* (2014).

29. D. B. J. Andersson, L. J. Fine, and B. A. Silverstein, "Musculoskeletal Disorders," *Occupational Health: Recognizing and Preventing Work-Related Disease,* edited by B. S. Levy and D. H. Wegman (Boston: Little, Brown, 1995).

30. M. R. Bracko, "Can We Prevent Back Injuries?" *ACSM's Health & Fitness Journal* 8, no. 4 (2004): 5–11.

31. H. B. Albert et al., *European Spine Journal* 22 (2013): 690–696.

32. H. B. Albert et al., "Antibiotic Treatment in Patients with Chronic Low Back Pain and Vertebral Bone Edema (Modic Type 1 Changes): A Double-blind Randomized Clinical Controlled Trial of Efficacy," *European Spine Journal* 22 (2013): 697–707.

33. B. W. Nelson et al., "Can Spinal Surgery Be Prevented by Aggressive Strengthening Exercise? A Prospective Study of Cervical and Lumbar Patients," *Archives of Physical Medicine and Rehabilitation* 80 (1999): 20–25.

34. B.A. Roy, Greg Vanichkachorn, "Low Back Pain," *ACSM's Health & Fitness Journal* 17, no. 2, (2013): 5.

35. J. A. Hides, G. A. Jull, and C. A. Richardson, "Long-Term Effects of Specific Stabilizing Exercises for First-Episode Low Back Pain," *Spine* 26 (2001): E243–248.

36. "Position Yourself to Stay Well," *Consumer Reports on Health* 18 (February 2006): 8–9.

37. A. Brownstein, "Chronic Back Pain Can Be Beaten," *Bottom Line/Health* 13 (October 1999): 3–4.

Chapter 4

Notes

1. J. L. Christi et al., "Cardiovascular Regulation During Head-out Water Immersion Exercise," *Journal of Applied Physiology* 69 (1990): 657–664; L. M. Sheldahl, F. E. Tristani, P. S. Clifford, C. V. Hughes, K. A. Sobocinski, and R. D. Morris, "Effect of Head-out Water Immersion on Cardio-respiratory Response to Dynamic Exercise," *Journal of American College of Cardiology* 10 (1987): 1254–1258; J. Svedenhang and J. Seger, "Running on Land and in Water: Comparative Exercise Physiology," *Medicine & Science in Sports & Exercise* 24 (1992): 1155–1160.

2. W. W. K. Hoeger, D. Hopkins, and D. Barber, "Physiologic Responses to Maximal Treadmill Running and Water Aerobic Exercise," *National Aquatics Journal* 11 (1995): 4–7.

3. W. W. K. Hoeger, T. A. Spitzer-Gibson, N. Kaluhiokalani, R. K. M. Cardejon, and J. Kokkonen, "A Comparison of Physiological Responses to Self-Paced Water Aerobics and Self-Paced Treadmill Running," *International Council for Health, Physical Education, Recreation, Sport, and Dance Journal* 30, no. 4 (2004): 27–30.

4. W. W. K. Hoeger, T. S. Gibson, J. Moore, and D. R. Hopkins, "A Comparison of Selected Training Responses to Low-Impact Aerobics and Water Aerobics," *National Aquatics Journal* 9 (1993): 13–16.

5. E. J. Marcinick, J. Potts, G. Schlabach, S. Will, P. Dawson, and B. F. Hurley, "Effects of Strength Training on Lactate Threshold and Endurance Performance," *Medicine & Science in Sports & Exercise* 23 (1991): 739–743.

6. B. Klika and C. Jordan, "High-Intensity Circuit Training Using Body Weight: Maximum Results with Minimal Investment," *ACSM's Health & Fitness Journal* 17 no. 3 (2013): 8–13.

7. American College of Sports Medicine, *ACSM's Guidelines for Exercise Testing and Prescription* (Philadelphia: Wolters Kluwer/Lippincott Williams & Wilkins, 2014).

Chapter 5

Notes

1. A. Pan, et al., "Red Meat Consumption and Mortality: Results from 2 Prospective Cohort Studies," *Archives of Internal Medicine* 172 (2012): 555–563.

2. National Academy of Sciences, Institute of Medicine. *Dietary Reference Intakes for Energy, Carbohydrates, Fiber, Fat, Protein and Amino Acids (Macronutrients)* (Washington, DC: National Academy Press, 2002).

3. G. Bjelakovic et al., "Mortality in Randomized Trials of Antioxidant Supplements for Primary and Secondary Prevention," *Journal of the American Medical Association* 297 (2007): 842–857.

4. M. L. Neuhouser et al., "Multivitamin Use and Risk of Cancer and Cardiovascular Disease in the Women's Health Initiative Cohorts," *Archives of Internal Medicine* 169 (2009): 294–304.

5. "Ride the D Train: Research Finds Even More Reasons to Get Vitamin D," *Environmental Nutrition* 28, no. 9 (2005): 1, 4.

6. "Vitamin D May Help You Dodge Cancer; How to Be Sure You Get Enough," *Environmental Nutrition* 30, no. 6 (2007): 1, 4.

7. "Understanding Vitamin D Cholecalciferol," Vitamin D Council, http://www.vitamindcouncil.org/, downloaded July 30, 2009.

8. American Dietetic Association, "Position of the American Dietetic Association: Nutrient Supplementation," *Journal of the American Dietetic Association* 109 (2009): 2073–2085.

9. "Eating Fish: Rewards Outweigh Risks," *Tufts University Health & Nutrition Letter* (January 2007).

10. D. Mozaffarian and E. B. Rimm, "Fish Intake, Contaminants, and Human Health," *Journal of the American Medical Association* 296 (2006): 1885–1899.

11. American Psychiatric Association, *Diagnostic and Statistical Manual of Mental Disorders* (Washington, DC: APA, 1994).

12. See note 11. American Psychiatric Association.

13. Van den Brandt, P. A., "The Impact of a Mediterranean Diet and Healthy Lifestyle on Premature Mortality in Men and Women," *American Journal of Clinical Nutrition* 94 (2011): 913–920.

14. R. Estrutch, "Primary Prevention of Cardiovascular Disease with a Mediterranean Diet," *New England Journal of Medicine* 368 (2013): 1279–1290.

Chapter 6

Notes

1. A. H. Mokdad, J. S. Marks, D. F. Stroup, and J. L. Gerberding, "Actual Causes of Death in the United States, 2000," *Journal of the American Medical Association* 291 (2004): 1238–1241.

2. R. Sturm and K. B. Wells, "Does Obesity Contribute as Much to Morbidity as Poverty or Smoking?" *Public Health* 115 (2001): 229–235.

3. E. E. Calle et al., "Overweight, Obesity, and Mortality from Cancer in a Prospectively Studied Cohort of U.S. Adults," *New England Journal of Medicine* 348 (2003): 1625–1638.

4. A. Peeters et al., "Obesity in Adulthood and Its Consequences for Life Expectancy: A Life-Table Analysis," *Annals of Internal Medicine* 138 (2003): 2432.

5. K. R. Fontaine et al., "Years of Life Lost Due to Obesity," *Journal of the American Medical Association* 289 (2003): 187–193.

6. American College of Sports Medicine, "Position Stand: Appropriate Physical Activity Intervention Strategies for Weight Loss and Prevention of Weight Regain for Adults," *Medicine & Science in Sports & Exercise* 41 (2009): 459–471.

7. S. Thomsen, "A Steady Diet of Images," *BYU Magazine* 57, no. 3 (2003): 20–21.

8. C. D. Gardner et al., "Comparison of the Atkins, Zone, Ornish, and LEARN Diets for Change in Weight and Related Risk Factors Among Overweight Premenopausal Women," *Journal of the American Medical Association* 297 (2007): 969–977; G. D. Foster et al., "A Randomized Trial of a Low-Carbohydrate Diet for Obesity," *New England Journal of Medicine* 348 (2003): 2082–2090.

9. R. L. Leibel, M. Rosenbaum, and J. Hirsh, "Changes in Energy Expenditure Resulting from Altered Body Weight," *New England Journal of Medicine* 332 (1995): 621–628.

10. A. Eliasson et al., "Sleep Is a Critical Factor in the Maintenance of Healthy Weight," chapter doi: 10.1164/ajrccm-conference.2009.179.1_MeetingAbstracts .A211310.1164/ajrccm-conference.2009.179.1_Meeting Abstracts.A2113 (2009).

11. S. Pattel et al., "Sleep Your Way to Weight Loss?" ScienceDaily, 29 May 2006.

12. K. Knutson, "Impact of Sleep and Sleep Loss on Glucose Homeostasis and Appetite Regulation," *Sleep Medicine Clinic* 2 (2007): 187–197.

13. S. Taheri et al., "Short Sleep Duration Is Associated with Reduced Leptin, Elevated Ghrelin, and Increased Body Mass Index," *PLoS Medicine* 1 (2004): e62. doi:10.1371/ -journal.pmed.0010062.

14. National Academy of Sciences, Institute of Medicine, *Dietary Reference Intakes for Energy, Carbohydrates, Fiber, Fat, Protein and Amino Acids (Macronutrients)* (Washington, DC: National Academy Press, 2002).

15. E. T. Poehlman et al., "Effects of Endurance and Resistance Training on Total Daily Energy Expenditure in Young Women: A Controlled Randomized Trial," *Journal of Clinical Endocrinology and Metabolism* 87 (2002): 1004–1009; L. M. Van Etten et al., "Effect of an 18-wk Weight-Training Program on Energy Expenditure and Physical Activity," *Journal of -Applied Physiology* 82 (1997): 298–304; W. W. Campbell, M. C. Crim, V. R. Young, and W. J. Evans, "Increased Energy Requirements and Changes in Body Composition with Resistance Training in Older Adults," *American Journal of Clinical Nutrition* 60 (1994): 167–175; Z. Wang et al., "Resting Energy Expenditure: Systematic Organization and Critique of Prediction Methods," *Obesity Research* 9 (2001): 331–336.

16. J. R. Karp and W. L. Wescott, "The Resting Metabolic Rate Debate," *Fitness Management* 23, no. 1 (2007): 44–47.

17. American College of Sports Medicine, *ACSM's Guidelines for Exercise Testing and Prescription* (Baltimore: Williams & Wilkins, 2006).

18. Schmitz, K. H., et al., "Strength Training and Adiposity in Premenopausal Women: Strong, Healthy, and Empowered Study," *The American Journal of Clinical Nutrition* 86 no. 3 (2007): 566–572.

19. Rania A. Mekary, R. A., et al., "Weight Training, Aerobic Physical Activities, and Long-term Waist Circumference Change in Men," *Obesity*, 2014; doi: 10.1002/oby.20949.

20. A. M. Knab, et al., "A 45-Minute Vigorous Exercise Bout Increases Metabolic Rate for 14 Hours," *Medicine and Science in Sports and Exercise* 43 (2011): 1643–1648.

21. A. Tremblay, J. A. Simoneau, and C. Bouchard, "Impact of Exercise Intensity on Body Fatness and Skeletal Muscle Metabolism," *Metabolism* 43 (1994): 814–818.

22. T. S. Church et al., "Changes in Weight, Waist Circumference and Compensatory Responses with Different Doses of Exercise Among Sedentary, Overweight Postmenopausal Women," *PLoS ONE* 4, no. 2 (2009): e4515. doi:10.1371/-journal.pone.0004515.

23. I. Lee et al., "Physical Activity and Weight Gain Prevention," *Journal of the American Medical Association* 303 (2010): 1173–1179.

24. T. A. Hagobian and B. Braun, "Physical Activity and Hormonal Regulation of Appetite: Sex Differences and Weight Control," *Exercise and Sport Sciences Reviews* 38 (2010): 25–30.

25. W. W. K. Hoeger, C. Harris, E. M. Long, and D. R. Hopkins, "Four-Week Supplementation with a Natural Dietary Compound Produces Favorable Changes in Body Composition," *Advances in Therapy* 15, no. 5 (1998): 305–313; W. W. K. Hoeger, et al., "Dietary Supplementation with Chromium Picolinate/L-Carnitine Complex in Combination with Diet and Exercise Enhances Body Composition," *Journal of the American Nutraceutical Association* 2, no. 2 (1999): 40–45.

26. D. Mozaffarian, et al., "Changes in Diet and Lifestyle and Long-Term Weight Gain in Women and Men," *New England Journal of Medicine* 364 (2011): 2392–2404.

27. N. A. Christakis and J. H. Fowler, "The Spread of Obesity in a Large Social Network over 32 Years," *New England Journal of Medicine* 357 (2007): 370–379.

Chapter 7

Notes

1. H. E. Selye, *Stress Without Distress* (New York: Signet, 1974).
2. R. Rosenman, "Do You Have Type 'A' Behavior?" *Health and Fitness* (supplement): 1987; H. Friedman, *The Self-Healing Personality* (New York: Henry Holt & Co., 1991).
3. R. Williams, *The Trusting Heart: Great News About Type A Behavior* (New York: Times Books, Division of Random House, 1989).
4. D. A. Girdano, D. E. Dusek, and G. S. Everly. *Controlling Stress and Tension* (San Francisco: Benjamin Cummings, 2012).
5. S. Bodian, "Meditate Your Way to Much Better Health," *Bottom Line Health* 18 (June 2004): 11–13.
6. D. Mueller, "Yoga Therapy," *ACSM's Health & Fitness Journal* 6, no. 1 (2002): 18–24.
7. A. Lazaridou, P. Philbrook, A.A. Rzika, "Yoga and Mindfulness as Therapeutic Interventions for Stroke Rehabilitation: A Systematic Review," *Evidence-Based Complementary and Alternative Medicine* (May 2013).
8. M. Samuels, "Use Your Mind to Heal Your Body," *Bottom Line/Health* 19 (February 2005): 13–14.

Chapter 8

Notes

1. L. Dossey, "Can Spirituality Improve Your Health?" *Bottom Line/Health* 15 (July 2001): 11–13.
2. Centers for Disease Control and Prevention, Death and Mortality 2013, NCHS FastStats Web site. http://www.cdc.gov/nchs/fastats/deaths.htm, accessed March 11, 2015.
3. See note 2, Centers for Disease Control and Prevention.
4. American Heart Association, *Heart Disease and Stroke Statistics: 2013 Update* (Dallas, TX: American Heart Association, 2013).
5. S. N. Blair, H. W. Kohl III, R. S. Paffenbarger Jr., D. G. Clark, K. H. Cooper, and L. W. Gibbons, "Physical Fitness and All-Cause Mortality: A Prospective Study of Healthy Men and Women," *Journal of the American Medical Association* 262 (1989): 2395–2401.
6. S. C. Moore, et al., "Leisure Time Physical Activity of Moderate to Vigorous Intensity and Mortality: A Large Pooled Cohort Analysis," *PLOS Medicine* 9, no. 11 (2012): e1335. doi:10.1371/journal.pmed.001001335.
7. L. S. Pescatello, et al., "Exercise and Hypertension Position Stand," *Medicine and Science in Sports and Exercise* 36 (2004): 533–553.
8. C. A. Slentz et al., "Inactivity, Exercise, and Visceral Fat. STRRIDE: A Randomized, Controlled Study of Exercise Intensity and Amount," *Journal of Applied Physiology* 99 (2005): 1613–1618.
9. "Lipid Research Clinics Program: The Lipid Research Clinic Coronary Primary Prevention Trial Results," *Journal of the American Medical Association* 251 (1984): 351–364.
10. See note 4, American Heart Association.
11. American Heart Association, *Heart and Stroke Facts* (Dallas, TX: AHA, 1999).
12. R. Singa, et al., "Meat Intake and Mortality: A Prospective Study of Over Half a Million People," *Archives of Internal Medicine* 169 (2009): 562–571
13. A. E. Buyken, et al., "Modifications in Dietary Fat Are Associated with Changes in Serum Lipids of Older Adults Independently of Lipid Medication," *Journal of Nutrition* 140 (2010): 88–94.
14. P. W. Siri-Tarino, Q. Sun, F. B. Hu, and R. M. Krauss, "Saturated Fat, Carbohydrate, and Cardiovascular Disease," *The American Journal of Clinical Nutrition* 91 (2010): 502–509.
15. D. Mozaffarian, R. Micha, and S. Wallace, "Effects on Coronary Heart Disease of Increasing Polyunsaturated Fat in Place of Saturated Fat: A Systematic Review of Meta-Analysis of Randomized Controlled Trials," *PLoS Medicine* 7 (2010): 7:e1000252.
16. G. M. Reaven, T. K. Strom, and B. Fox, *Syndrome X: Overcoming the Silent Killer That Can Give You a Heart Attack* (New York: Simon & Schuster, 2000).
17. M. Guarneri, "What Most People Don't Know about Heart Disease," *Bottom Line/Health* 21 (July 2007): 11–12.
18. See note 4, American Heart Association.
19. American Cancer Society, *2015 Cancer Facts and Figures* (New York: ACS, 2015).
20. J. E. Enstrom, "Health Practices and Cancer Mortality Among Active California Mormons," *Journal of the National Cancer Institute* 81 (1989): 1807–1814.
21. A. S. Ford, et al., "Healthy Living is the Best Revenge: Findings from the European Prospective Investigation into Cancer and Nutrition—Potsdam Study," *Archives of Internal Medicine* 169 (2009): 1355–1362.
22. N. Ahmad et al., "Green Tea Constituent Epigallocatechin-3-Gallate and Induction of Apoptosis and Cell Cycle

Arrest in Human Carcinoma Cells," *Journal of the National Cancer Institute* 89 (1997): 1881–1886.

23. N. E. Allen et al., "Moderate Alcohol Intake and Cancer Incidence in Women," *Journal of the National Cancer Institute* 101 (2009): 296–305.

24. C. A. Thomson and P. A. Thomson, "Healthy Lifestyle and Cancer Prevention," *ACSM's Health & Fitness Journal* 12, no. 3 (2008): 18–26

25. S. W. Farrell et al., "Cardiorespiratory Fitness, Different Measures of Adiposity, and Cancer Mortality in Men," *Obesity* 15 (2007): 3140–3149.

26. L. Byberg et al., "Total Mortality After Changes in Leisure Time Physical Activity in 50 Year Old Men: 35 Year Follow-up of Population Based Cohort," *British Medical Journal* (2009): 338. doi:10.1136.

27. E. L. Giovannucci, "A Prospective Study of Physical Activity and Incident and Fatal Prostate Cancer," *Archives of Internal Medicine* 165 (2005): 1005–1010.

28. L. Ratnasinghe et al., *Exercise and Breast Cancer Risk: A Multinational Study*, (Beltsville, MD: Genomic Nanosystems, BioServe Biotechnologies, Ltd., 2009).

29. C. W. Matthews et al., "Physical Activity and Risk of Endometrial Cancer: A Report from the Shanghai Endometrial Cancer Study," *Cancer Epidemiology Biomarkers & Prevention* 14 (2005): 779–785.

30. M. D. Holmes et al., "Physical Activity and Survival After Breast Cancer Diagnosis," *Journal of the American Medical Association* 293 (2005): 2479–2486.

31. J. R. Ruiz, "Muscular Strength and Adiposity as Predictors of Adulthood Cancer Mortality in Men," *Cancer Epidemiology, Biomarkers & Prevention* 18 (2009): 1468–1476.

32. D. Servan-Schreiber, "The Anticancer Life Plan," *Bottom Line Health* 23, no. 5 (May 2009).

33. R. Horowitz, et al., "Herpes Simplex Virus Infection in a University Health Population: Clinical Manifestations, Epidemiology, and Implications," *The Journal of American College Health*, 59, no. 2 (2011): 69–74.

Chapter 9

Notes

1. R. S. Paffenbarger Jr., R. T. Hyde, A. L. Wing, and C. H. Steinmetz, "A Natural History of Athleticism and Cardiovascular Health," *Journal of the American Medical Association* 252 (1984): 491–495.

2. S. N. Blair, H. W. Kohl III, R. S. Paffenbarger Jr., D. G. Clark, K. H. Cooper, and L. W. Gibbons, "Physical Fitness and All-Cause Mortality: A Prospective Study of Healthy Men and Women," *Journal of the American Medical Association* 262 (1989): 2395–2401.

3. R. Hambrecht et al., "Various Intensities of Leisure Time Physical Activity in Patients with Coronary Artery Disease: Effects on Cardiorespiratory Fitness and Progression of Coronary Atherosclerotic Lesions," *Journal of the American College of Cardiology* 22 (1993): 468–477.

4. M. K. Torstveit et al., "The Female Athlete Triad: Are Elite Athletes at Increased Risk?" *Medicine & Science in Sports & Exercise* 37 (2005): 184–193.

5. American College of Obstetricians and Gynecologists, "Exercise During Pregnancy and the Postpartum Period," ACOG Committee Opinion No. 267, *International Journal of Gynecology and Obstetrics* 77 (2002): 79–81.

6. F. W. Kash, J. L. Boyer, S. P. Van Camp, L. S. Verity, and J. P. Wallace, "The Effect of Physical Activity on Aerobic Power in Older Men (A Longitudinal Study)," *The Physician and Sports Medicine* 18, no. 4 (1990): 73–83.

7. American College of Sports Medicine, "Exercise and Physical Activity for Older Adults," *Medicine & Science in Sports & Exercise* 41 (2009): 1510–1530.

Answer Key

Chapter 1
1. a   2. e   3. d   4. c   5. c   6. b
7. b   8. d   9. a   10. e

Chapter 2
1. e   2. a   3. e   4. e   5. c   6. b
7. b   8. a   9. d   10. c

Chapter 3
1. d   2. c   3. c   4. d   5. a   6. c
7. b   8. c   9. e   10. e

Chapter 4
1. d   2. a   3. c   4. d   5. c   6. a
7. e   8. d   9. a   10. b

Chapter 5
1. b   2. e   3. c   4. d   5. d   6. a
7. a   8. c   9. a   10. e

Chapter 6
1. c   2. d   3. e   4. a   5. b   6. c
7. a   8. c   9. d   10. e

Chapter 7
1. a   2. c   3. c   4. e   5. b   6. e
7. e   8. a   9. e   10. c

Chapter 8
1. e   2. a   3. b   4. e   5. b   6. e
7. e   8. b   9. d   10. c

Chapter 9
1. b   2. e   3. e   4. d   5. d   6. e
7. b   8. a   9. e   10. c

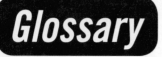
Glossary

Acquired immunodeficiency syndrome (AIDS) End stage of HIV infection, manifested by any of a number of diseases that arise when the body's immune system is compromised by HIV.

Action stage Stage of change in which people are actively changing a negative behavior or adopting a new, healthy behavior.

Actions Steps required to reach a goal.

Active static stretch Stretching exercise wherein the position is held by the strength of the muscle being stretched.

Activities of daily living Everyday behaviors that people normally do to function in life (cross the street, carry groceries, lift objects, do laundry, and sweep floors).

Activity tracker An electronic device that contains an accelerometer (a unit that measures gravity, changes in movement, and counts footsteps). These devices can also determine distance, calories burned, speeds, and time spent being physically active.

Adequate Intakes (AI) The recommended amount of a nutrient intake when sufficient evidence is not available to calculate the EAR and subsequent RDA.

Advanced glycation end products (AGEs) Derivatives of glucose-protein and glucose-lipid interactions that are linked to aging and chronic diseases.

Aerobic exercise Activity that requires oxygen to produce the necessary energy to carry out the activity.

Aerobics A series of exercise routines that include a combination of stepping, walking, jogging, skipping, kicking, and arm swinging movements performed to music.

Alcoholism Disease in which an individual loses control over drinking alcoholic beverages.

Altruism True concern for and action on behalf of others (opposite of egoism); a sincere desire to serve others above one's personal needs.

Amenorrhea Absence (primary amenorrhea) or cessation (secondary amenorrhea) of normal menstrual function.

Amino acids The basic building blocks of protein.

Android obesity Obesity pattern seen in individuals who tend to store fat in the trunk or abdominal area.

Angiogenesis Capillary (blood vessel) formation into a tumor.

Anorexia nervosa An eating disorder characterized by self-imposed starvation to lose weight and then maintain very low body weight.

Antibodies Substances produced by the white blood cells in response to an invading agent.

Antioxidants Compounds that prevent oxygen from combining with other substances it might damage.

Arrhythmias Irregular heart rhythms.

Atherosclerosis Fatty/cholesterol deposits in the walls of the arteries leading to formation of plaque.

Ballistic stretching Stretching exercises performed with jerky, rapid, and bouncy movements.

Basal metabolic rate (BMR) Lowest level of caloric intake necessary to sustain life.

Behavior modification The process used to permanently change negative behaviors in favor of positive behaviors that will lead to better health and well-being.

Benign Noncancerous.

Binge-eating disorder An eating disorder characterized by uncontrollable episodes of eating excessive amounts of food within a relatively short time.

Blood lipids (fat) Cholesterol and triglycerides.

Blood pressure A measure of the force exerted against the walls of the vessels by the blood flowing through them.

Body composition The fat and nonfat components of the human body.

Body mass index (BMI) An index that incorporates height and weight to estimate critical fat values at which risk for disease increases.

Bulimia nervosa An eating disorder characterized by a pattern of binge eating and purging.

Calorie The amount of heat necessary to raise the temperature of 1 gram of water 1°C; used to measure the energy value of food and the cost of physical activity.

Cancer Group of diseases characterized by uncontrolled growth and spread of abnormal cells into malignant tumors.

Carbohydrates Compounds composed of carbon, hydrogen, and oxygen that the body uses as its major source of energy.

Carcinogens Substances that contribute to the formation of cancers.

Carcinoma in situ Encapsulated malignant tumor that is found at an early stage and has not spread.

Cardiomyopathy A disease affecting the heart muscle.

Cardiorespiratory endurance Ability of the lungs, heart, and blood vessels to deliver adequate amounts of oxygen to the cells to meet the demands of prolonged physical activity.

Cardiorespiratory training zone The range of intensity at which a person should exercise to develop the cardiorespiratory system.

Cardiovascular diseases The array of conditions that affect the heart and blood vessels.

Carotenoids Pigment substances (more than 600) in plants, about 50 of which are precursors to vitamin A; the most potent carotenoid is beta-carotene.

Cholesterol A waxy substance, technically a steroid alcohol, found only in animal fats and oil; used in making cell membranes, as a building block for some hormones, in the fatty sheath around nerve fibers, and in other necessary substances.

Chronic diseases Illnesses that develop and last over a long time.

Chronic lower respiratory disease (CLRD) A group of diseases that limits airflow, such as chronic obstructive pulmonary disease, emphysema, and chronic bronchitis (all diseases of the respiratory system).

Chronological age Calendar age.

Chylomicrons Molecules that transport triglycerides in the blood.

Cirrhosis A disease characterized by scarring of the liver.

Clinical study A research study in which the investigator intervenes (makes certain changes or uses certain interventions or programs) to prevent or treat a disease.

Concentric Shortening of a muscle during muscle contraction.

Concentric muscle contraction A dynamic contraction in which the muscle shortens as it develops tension.

Contemplation stage Stage of change in which people are considering changing behavior in the next six months.

Contraindicated exercises Exercises that are not recommended because they pose potentially high risk for injury.

Controlled ballistic stretching Exercises done with slow, short, gentle, and sustained movements.

Cool-down A period at the end of an exercise session when exercise is tapered off.

Coronary heart disease (CHD) Condition in which the arteries that supply the heart muscle with oxygen and nutrients are narrowed by fatty deposits such as cholesterol and triglycerides.

C-reactive protein (CRP) A protein whose level in the blood increases with inflammation (which may be hidden deep in the body); elevation of this protein is an indicator of potential cardiovascular events.

Cruciferous vegetables Plants that produce cross-shaped leaves (cauliflower, broccoli, cabbage, Brussels sprouts, and kohlrabi); these seem to have a protective effect against cancer.

Daily Values (DVs) Reference values for nutrients and food components used in food labels.

Deoxyribonucleic acid (DNA) Genetic substance of which genes are made; molecule that bears a cell's genetic code.

Diabetes mellitus A condition in which blood glucose is unable to enter the cells because the pancreas either stops producing insulin or does not produce enough to meet the body's needs.

Diastolic blood pressure Pressure exerted by the blood against the walls of the arteries during the relaxation phase (diastole) of the heart.

Dietary Reference Intakes (DRIs) Four types of nutrient standards that are used to establish adequate amounts and maximum safe nutrient intakes in the diet: Estimated Average Requirements (EAR), Recommended Dietary Allowances (RDA), Adequate Intakes (AI), and Tolerable Upper Intake Levels (UL).

Distress Negative or harmful stress under which health and performance begin to deteriorate.

Duration of exercise Time exercising per session.

Dynamic exercise Strength training with muscle contraction that produces movement.

Dynamic stretching Stretching exercises that require speed of movement, momentum, and active muscular effort to help increase the range of motion about a joint or group of joints.

Dysmenorrhea Painful menstruation.

Eating Disorder Not Otherwise Specified (EDNOS) A medical condition used to diagnose individuals who don't fall into the most commonly known eating disorder categories but who have troubled relationships with food or distorted body images.

Eccentric Lengthening of a muscle during muscle contraction.

Eccentric muscle contraction A dynamic contraction in which the muscle lengthens as it develops tension.

Electrocardiogram (ECG or EKG) A recording of the electrical activity of the heart.

Emotional eating The consumption of large quantities of food to suppress negative emotions.

Energy-balancing equation A body weight formula stating that when caloric intake equals caloric output, weight remains unchanged.

Epidemiological Of the study of epidemic diseases.

Essential fat Body fat needed for normal physiological functions.

Essential nutrients Carbohydrates, fats, protein, vitamins, minerals, and water—the nutrients the human body requires for survival.

Estimated Average Requirements (EAR) The amount of a nutrient that meets the dietary needs of half the people.

Estimated energy requirement (EER) The average dietary energy (caloric) intake that is predicted to maintain energy balance in a healthy adult of defined age, gender, weight, height, and level of physical activity, consistent with good health.

Estrogen Female sex hormone; essential for bone formation and conservation of bone density.

Eustress Positive stress.

Exercise A type of physical activity that requires planned, structured, and repetitive bodily movement done to improve or maintain one or more components of physical fitness.

Fats (lipids) A class of nutrients that the body uses as a source of energy.

Female athlete triad Three interrelated disorders—disordered eating, amenorrhea, and bone mineral disorders—seen in some highly trained female athletes.

Ferritin Iron stored in the body.

Fiber Plant material that human digestive enzymes cannot digest.

Fight or flight A series of physical responses activated automatically in response to environmental stressors.

Fitness boot camp A military-style vigorous-intensity group exercise training program that combines calisthenics, running, interval training, strength training, plyometrics, and competitive games.

Fixed-resistance Exercise with strength-training equipment that provides a constant amount of resistance through the range of motion.

Flexibility The achievable range of motion at a joint or group of joints without causing injury.

Free radicals Oxygen compounds produced in normal metabolism.

Free weights Barbells and dumbbells.

Frequency of exercise How often a person engages in an exercise session.

Functional fitness The physical capacity of the individual to meet ordinary and unexpected demands of daily life safely and effectively.

Functional independence Ability to carry out activities of daily living without assistance from other individuals.

General adaptation syndrome (GAS) A theoretical model that explains the body's adaptation to sustained stress; it includes three stages: alarm reaction, resistance, and exhaustion/recovery.

Goal The ultimate aim toward which effort is directed.

Gynoid obesity Obesity pattern seen in people who store fat primarily around the hips and thighs.

Hatha yoga A yoga style that incorporates a series of static-stretching postures performed in specific sequences.

Health fitness standard The lowest fitness requirements for maintaining good health, decreasing the risk for chronic diseases, and lowering the incidence of muscular/skeletal injuries.

Health-related fitness A physical state encompassing cardiorespiratory endurance, muscular strength and endurance, muscular flexibility, and body composition.

Heart rate reserve (HRR) The difference between the maximal heart rate (MHR) and resting heart rate (RHR).

Hemoglobin Protein-iron compound in red blood cells that transports oxygen in the blood.

High-density lipoprotein (HDL) Cholesterol-transporting molecules in the blood (good cholesterol).

High-impact aerobics (HIA) Exercises incorporating movements in which both feet are off the ground at the same time momentarily.

High-intensity circuit training (HICT) An exercise modality that combines high-intensity aerobic and bodyweight-strength training exercises with limited rest between exercises.

High-intensity interval training (HIIT) A training program consisting of high- to very high-intensity intervals (80 percent to 90 percent of maximal capacity) that are interspersed with low- to moderate-intensity recovery intervals.

Homeostasis A natural state of equilibrium. The body attempts to maintain this equilibrium by constantly reacting to external forces that attempt to disrupt this fine balance.

Homocysteine Intermediate amino acid in the interconversion of two other amino acids: methionine and cysteine.

Human immunodeficiency virus (HIV) Virus that leads to acquired immunodeficiency syndrome (AIDS).

Hypertension Chronically elevated blood pressure.

Hypokinetic diseases Diseases related to a lack of physical activity.

Hypothermia A breakdown in the body's ability to generate heat, resulting in body temperature below 95°F.

Imagery Mental visualization of relaxing images and scenes to induce body relaxation in times of stress or as an aid in the treatment of certain medical conditions such as cancer, hypertension, asthma, chronic pain, and obesity.

Insulin-dependent diabetes mellitus (IDDM or type 1) A form of diabetes in which the pancreas produces little or no insulin.

Intensity (for flexibility exercises) Degree of stretch when doing flexibility exercises.

Intensity of exercise How hard a person has to exercise to improve cardiorespiratory endurance.

Interval training A repeated series of exercise work bouts (intervals) interspersed with low-intensity or rest intervals.

Isokinetic exercise Strength training method in which the speed of the muscle contraction is kept constant because the equipment (machine) provides an accommodating resistance to match the user's force through the full range of motion.

Isometric exercise Strength training with muscle contraction that produces little or no movement.

Isotonic exercise See Dynamic exercise.

Lean body mass Nonfat component of the body.

Life expectancy Number of years a person is expected to live based on the person's birth year.

Locus of control The extent to which a person believes he or she can influence the external environment.

Low-density lipoprotein (LDL) Cholesterol-transporting molecules in the blood (bad cholesterol).

Low-impact aerobics (LIA) Exercises in which at least one foot is in contact with the ground or floor at all times.

Lymphocytes Immune system cells responsible for waging war against disease or infection.

Macronutrients The nutrients the body needs in proportionately large amounts: carbohydrates, fats, proteins, and water are examples.

Maintenance stage Stage of change in which people maintain behavioral change for up to five years.

Malignant Cancerous.

Maximal oxygen uptake (VO$_{2max}$) Maximum amount of oxygen the human body is able to utilize per minute of physical activity.

Meditation A mental exercise in which the objective is to gain control over one's attention, clearing the mind and blocking out stressors.

Megadoses For most vitamins, 10 times the RDA or more; for vitamins A and D, 5 and 2 times the RDA, respectively.

Melanoma The most virulent, rapidly spreading form of skin cancer.

Metabolic fitness Denotes improvements in the metabolic profile through a moderate-intensity exercise program despite little or no improvement in cardiorespiratory fitness.

Metabolic profile Result of the assessment of diabetes and cardiovascular disease risk through plasma insulin, glucose, lipid, and lipoprotein levels.

Metabolic syndrome An array of metabolic abnormalities that contribute to the development of atherosclerosis triggered by resistance to insulin; these conditions include low HDL-cholesterol, high triglycerides, high blood pressure, and an increased blood-clotting mechanism.

Metastasis Movement of bacteria or body cells from one part of the body to another.

MET Short for metabolic equivalent; represents the rate of energy expenditure while sitting quietly at rest. This energy expenditure is approximately 3.5 milliliters of oxygen per kilogram of body weight per minute (mL/kg/min) or 1.2 calories per minute for a 70-kilogram person. A 3-MET activity requires three times the energy expenditure of sitting quietly at rest.

Micronutrients The nutrients the body needs in small quantities— vitamins and minerals—that serve specific roles in transformation of energy and body tissue synthesis.

Mindfulness A mental state of heightened awareness of the present moment.

Minerals Inorganic elements needed by the body.

Mode of exercise Form of exercise (e.g., aerobic).

Moderate-impact aerobics (MIA) Aerobics that include plyometric training.

Moderate-intensity aerobic physical activity Defined as the equivalent of a brisk walk that noticeably increases the heart rate.

Moderate physical activity Any activity that requires an energy expenditure of 150 calories per day, or 1,000 calories per week.

Motivation The desire and will to do something.

Muscular endurance Ability of a muscle to exert submaximal force repeatedly over a period of time.

Muscular fitness A term used to define good levels of both muscular strength and muscular endurance.

Muscular hypertrophy An increase in muscle mass or size.

Muscular strength Ability to exert maximum force against resistance.

Myocardial infarction Heart attack; damage or death of an area of the heart muscle as a result of an obstructed artery to that area.

Myofibrillar hypertrophy Muscle hypertrophy as a result of increased protein synthesis in the myosin and actin myofibrils.

Negative resistance The lowering or eccentric phase of a repetition during the performance of a strength-training exercise.

Nitrosamines Potentially cancer-causing compounds formed when nitrites and nitrates—which are used to prevent the growth of harmful bacteria in processed meats—combine with other chemicals in the stomach.

Non-exercise activity thermogenesis (NEAT) Energy expended doing everyday activities not related to exercise.

Non-insulin-dependent diabetes mellitus (NIDDM or type 2) A form of diabetes in which the pancreas either does not produce sufficient insulin or produces adequate amounts but the cells become insulin-resistant, keeping glucose from entering the cell.

Nonresponders Individuals who exhibit small or no improvements in fitness as compared with others who undergo the same training program.

Nutrients Substances found in food that provide energy, regulate metabolism, and help with growth and repair of body tissues.

Nutrition The science that studies the relationship of foods to optimal health and performance.

Obesity A chronic disease characterized by an excessively high amount of body fat (about 20 percent above recommended weight or a BMI at 30 or above).

Oligomenorrhea Irregular menstrual cycles.

One repetition maximum (1 RM) The maximal amount of resistance a person is able to lift in a single effort.

Opportunistic infections Diseases that arise in the absence of a healthy immune system that would fight them off in healthy people.

Osteoporosis Softening, deterioration, or loss of bone.

Overload principle Training concept holding that the demands placed on a body system must be increased systematically and progressively over time to cause physiologic adaptation.

Overweight Excess body weight when compared to a given standard such as height or recommended percent body fat.

Passive static stretch Stretching exercise performed with the aid of an external force applied by either another individual or an external apparatus.

Pedometer An activity tracker that counts footsteps. Some pedometers also record distance, calories burned, speeds, and time spent being physically active.

Percent body fat (fat mass) Fat component of the body.

Periodization A training approach that divides the season into cycles using a systematic variation in intensity and volume of training to enhance fitness and performance.

Personal trainer An exercise specialist who works one on one with an individual and is typically paid by the hour or exercise session.

Physical activity Bodily movement produced by skeletal muscles that requires energy expenditure and produces progressive health benefits.

Physical fitness The general capacity to adapt and respond favorably to physical effort.

Physical fitness standard Required criteria to achieve a high level of physical fitness; ability to do moderate-to-vigorous physical activity without undue fatigue.

Physiological age Age based on the individual's functional and physical capacity.

Phytonutrients Compounds found in fruits and vegetables that block formation of cancerous tumors and disrupt the process of cancer.

PLAC blood test A blood test that measures the level of Lipoprotein-associated Phospholipase A_2, an enzyme produced inside the plaque when the arteries are inflamed and indicates risk for plaque rupture.

Plyometric training A form of exercise that requires forceful jumps or springing off the ground immediately after landing from a previous jump.

Positive resistance The lifting, pushing, or concentric phase of a repetition during the performance of a strength-training exercise.

Precontemplation stage Stage of change in which people are unwilling to change their behavior.

Preparation stage Stage of change in which people are getting ready to make a change within the coming month.

Principle of individuality Training concept that states that genetics plays a major role in individual responses to exercise training and that these differences must be considered when designing exercise programs for different people.

Progressive muscle relaxation A relaxation technique that involves contracting, then relaxing muscle groups in the body in succession.

Progressive resistance training A gradual increase of resistance over a period of time.

Proprioceptive neuromuscular facilitation (PNF) Mode of stretching that uses reflexes and neuromuscular principles to relax the muscles being stretched.

Proteins A class of nutrients that the body uses to build and repair body tissues.

Quackery/fraud The conscious promotion of unproven claims for profit.

Recommended body weight The weight at which there appears to be no harm to human health.

Recommended Dietary Allowances (RDA) The daily amount of a nutrient (statistically determined from the EARs) considered adequate to meet the known nutrient needs of almost 98 percent of all healthy people in the United States.

Registered dietitian (RD) A person with a college degree in dietetics who meets all certification and continuing education requirements of the American Dietetic Association or Dietitians of Canada.

Relapse Slipping or falling back into unhealthy behavior(s) or failing to maintain healthy behaviors.

Repetitions The number of times a movement is performed.

Resistance Amount of weight lifted.

Responders Individuals who exhibit improvements in fitness as a result of exercise training.

Resting metabolism The energy requirement to maintain the body's vital processes in the resting state.

Ribonucleic acid (RNA) Genetic material involved in the formation of cell proteins.

Risk factors Characteristics that predict the chances for developing a certain disease.

Risk factors Lifestyle and genetic variables that may lead to disease.

RM zone A range of repetitions that are to be performed maximally during one set. For example, an 8 to 12 RM zone implies that the individual will perform anywhere from 8 to 12 repetitions, but cannot perform any more following the completion of the final repetition (e.g., 9 RM and could not perform a 10th repetition).

Sarcopenia Age-related loss of lean body mass, strength, and function.

Sarcoplasmic hypertrophy Muscle hypertrophy as a result of an increase in sarcoplasm.

Sedentary Death Syndrome (SeDS) Deaths that are attributed to a lack of regular physical activity.

Set The number of repetitions performed for a given exercise.

Setpoint Body weight and body fat percentage unique to each person that are regulated by genetic and environmental factors.

Sexually transmitted infections (STIs) Communicable infections spread through sexual contact.

Skill-related fitness Components of fitness important for successful motor performance in athletic events and in lifetime sports and activities.

SMART An acronym for Specific, Measurable, Acceptable, Realistic, and Time-specific goals.

Specificity of training A principle holding that, for a muscle to increase in strength or endurance, the training program must be specific to obtain the desired effects.

Spirituality A sense of meaning and direction in life, a relationship to a higher being; encompasses freedom, prayer, faith, love, closeness to others, peace, joy, fulfillment, and altruism.

Static stretching (slow-sustained stretching) Exercises in which the muscles are lengthened gradually through a joint's complete range of motion.

Step aerobics (SA) A form of exercise that combines stepping up onto and down from a bench with arm movements.

Storage fat Body fat stored in adipose tissue.

Stress The mental, emotional, and physiological response of the body to any situation that is new, threatening, frightening, or exciting.

Stress electrocardiogram (stress ECG) An exercise test during which the workload is gradually increased (until the subject reaches maximal fatigue), with blood pressure and 12-lead electrocardiographic monitoring throughout the test.

Stressor Stress-causing agent.

Stretching Moving the joints beyond the accustomed range of motion.

Substrates Foods that are used as energy sources (carbohydrates, fat, protein).

Sun protection factor (SPF) Degree of protection offered by ingredients in sunscreen lotion; at least SPF 15 is recommended.

Supplements Tablets, pills, capsules, liquids, or powders that contain vitamins, minerals, amino acids, herbs, or fiber that are taken to increase the intake of these substances.

Synergistic action The result of mixing two or more drugs, the effects of which can be much greater than the sum of two or more drugs acting by themselves.

Synergy A reaction in which the result is greater than the sum of its two parts.

Systolic blood pressure Pressure exerted by the blood against the walls of the arteries during the forceful contraction (systole) of the heart.

Technostress Stress resulting from the inability to adapt or cope with digital technologies in a healthy way.

Termination/adoption stage Stage of change in which people have eliminated an undesirable behavior or maintained a positive behavior for more than five years.

Tolerable Upper Intake Levels (UL) The highest level of nutrient intake that appears to be safe for most healthy people without an increased risk of adverse effects.

Tolerable weight A realistic body weight that is close to the health fitness percent body fat standard.

Triglycerides Fats formed by glycerol and three fatty acids.

Type A Behavior pattern characteristic of a hard-driving, overambitious, aggressive, at times hostile, and overly competitive person.

Type B Behavior pattern characteristic of a calm, casual, relaxed, and easygoing individual.

Variable-resistance Exercise that utilizes special equipment with mechanical devices that provide differing amounts of resistance through the range of motion.

Vegetarians Individuals whose diet is of vegetable or plant origin.

Vigorous exercise An exercise intensity that is either above 6 METs, 60 percent of maximal oxygen uptake, or one that provides a "substantial" challenge to the individual.

Vigorous-intensity aerobic physical activity Defined as an activity similar to jogging that causes rapid breathing and a substantial increase in heart rate.

Vitamins Organic substances essential for normal bodily metabolism, growth, and development.

Waist circumference (WC) A waist girth measurement to assess potential risk for disease based on intra- abdominal fat content.

Waist-to-height ratio (WHtR) A ratio to determine health risks associated with obesity.

Warm-up A period preceding exercise when exercise begins slowly.

Wellness The constant and deliberate effort to stay healthy and achieve the highest potential for well-being.

Yoga A school of thought in the Hindu religion that seeks to help the individual attain a higher level of spirituality and peace of mind.

Index

Note: Page numbers in bold are exercises.